Sepsis and Systemic Inflammatory Syndromes

Editors

MANU SHANKAR-HARI
LIEUWE D.J. BOS

CRITICAL CARE CLINICS

www.criticalcare.theclinics.com

Consulting Editor
GREGORY S. MARTIN

October 2026 • Volume 42 • Number 4

ELSEVIER

1818 Market Street • Suite 3323 • Philadelphia, Pennsylvania, 19103-2899

http://www.theclinics.com

CRITICAL CARE CLINICS Volume 42, Number 4
October 2026 ISSN 0749-0704, ISBN-13: 978-0-443-43280-4

Editor: Joanna Gascoine
Developmental Editor: Anirban Mukherjee

Publishing Office: *Critical Care Clinics* (ISSN 0749-0704) is published bimonthly by Elsevier Inc., 1818 Market Street, Philadelphia, PA 19103, United States. Periodicals postage paid at New York, NY and additional mailing offices. **USA POSTMASTER:** Send address changes to *Critical Care Clinics*, Elsevier Customer Service Department, 3251 Riverport Lane, Maryland Heights, MO 63043, USA. Months of issue are January, April, July, and October. Customer Service Office: 6277 Sea Harbor Drive, Orlando, FL 32887-4800. Periodicals postage paid at New York, NY and additional mailing offices. Subscription prices are $297.00 per year for US individuals, $100.00 per year for US students and residents, $330.00 per year for Canadian individuals, $377.00 per year for international individuals, $100.00 per year for Canadian students/residents, and $150.00 per year for foreign students/residents. For institutional access pricing please contact Customer Service via the contact information below. To receive student/resident rate, orders must be accompanied by name of affiliated institution, date of term, and the signature of program/residency coordinator on institution letterhead. Orders will be billed at individual rate until proof of status is received. Foreign air speed delivery is included in all *Clinics* subscription prices. All prices are subject to change without notice. Orders, claims, and journal inquiries: Please visit our Support Hub page https://service.elsevier.com for assistance.

Reprints. For copies of 100 or more of articles in this publication, please contact the Commercial Reprints Department, Elsevier Inc., 360 Park Avenue South, New York, NY 10010-1710. Tel.: 212-633-3874; Fax: 212-633-3820; E-mail: reprints@elsevier.com.

Critical Care Clinics is also published in Spanish by Editorial Inter-Medica, Junin 917, 1[er] A, 1113, Buenos Aires, Argentina.

Critical Care Clinics is covered in *MEDLINE/PubMed (Index Medicus), EMBASE/Excerpta Medica, Current Concepts/Clinical Medicine, ISI/BIOMED, and Chemical Abstracts*.

Contributors

CONSULTING EDITOR

GREGORY S. MARTIN, MD, MSc
Professor, Division of Pulmonary, Allergy, Critical Care and Sleep Medicine, Research Director, Emory Critical Care Center, Director, Emory/Georgia Tech Predictive Health Institute, Co-Director, Atlanta Center for Microsystems Engineered Point-of-Care Technologies, President, Society of Critical Care Medicine, Atlanta, Georgia, USA

EDITORS

MANU SHANKAR-HARI, MSc, FFICM, MD, PhD, FRSE
Professor, School of Immunology & Microbial Sciences, King's College London, London, UK

LIEUWE D.J. BOS, MD, PhD
Associate Professor, Department of Intensive Care, Amsterdam UMC, Amsterdam, The Netherlands

AUTHORS

DUARTE ABECASIS, MBBS
MD Student, Faculdade de Medicina da Universidade de Lisboa, Lisboa, Portugal

ELEONORA BALZANI, MD
Clinical Associate, Centre for Medical Sciences-CISMed, University of Trento, Trento, Italy

SIVASUBRAMANIUM V. BHAVANI, MD
Assistant Professor, Department of Medicine, Emory University, Atlanta, Georgia, USA

TRISTAN COUWENBERGH, MD
PhD Candidate, Medical Doctor, Department of Internal Medicine, Radboud University Medical Center (Radboudumc), Nijmegen, Gelderland, the Netherlands

GUILLAUME DUMAS, MD, PhD
Assistant Professor, Department of Critical Care Medicine, Universite Grenobles-Alpes, Grenobles, France

ANA C. GALES, MD, PhD
Professor, Division of Infectious Diseases, Department of Internal Medicine, Universidade Federal de São Paulo, Antimicrobial Resistance Institute of São Paulo, São Paulo, São Paulo, Brazil

MARGARET HERRIDGE, MD, MSc
Professor, Interdepartmental Division of Critical Care Medicine, University of Toronto, Toronto, Ontario, Canada

NICOLE P. JUFFERMANS, MD, PhD
Professor of Translational Intensive Care, Department of Intensive Care, The Emergency, Perioperative and Intensive Care Laboratory (EPIC Lab), Erasmus Medial Center, Rotterdam, the Netherlands

ANDRE C. KALIL, MD, MPH
Professor, Division of Infectious Diseases, Department of Internal Medicine, University of Nebraska Medical Center, Omaha, Nebraska, USA

WILSON F. KÄYSER-ABDO, MD, PhD
Assistant Professor, Intensivist, Department of Intensive Care Medicine, Radboud University Medical Center, Nijmegen, The Netherlands

LIES LANGOUCHE, MSc, PhD
Professor, Clinical Division and Laboratory of Intensive Care Medicine, Department of Cellular and Molecular Medicine, KU Leuven, Leuven, Belgium

ALEKSANDRA LELIGDOWICZ, MD, PhD
Assistant Professor, Department of Critical Care Medicine, University of Western Ontario, London, Ontario, Canada

LUCY McGEOCH, MBChB, FRCP(UK)
Consultant Rheumatologist, Centre for Rheumatic Diseases, Glasgow Royal Infirmary, Glasgow, United Kingdom

IAIN McINNES, PhD, FRCP(Gla), FRCP(Edin), FRSE, FMedSci
Arthritis UK Professor of Rheumatology, Vice Principal and Head, Muirhead Chair of Medicine, College of Medical, Veterinary and Life Sciences, University of Glasgow, Glasgow, United Kingdom

ROSS McMULLAN, MB BCh, BAO
Clinical Research Fellow, School of Medicine, Dentistry and Biomedical Sciences, Wellcome-Wolfson Institute for Experimental Medicine, Queen's University of Belfast, Belfast, United Kingdom

PAULO MERGULHAO, MD
Professor, Intensive Care Department, Hospital Lusíadas Porto, Grupo de Infeção e Desenvolvimento em Sepsis, Faculdade de Medicina da Universidade do Porto, Porto, Portugal

LUIS F. MOITA, MD, PhD
Associate Professor, Center for Disease Mechanisms Research, Medicine ULisboa for Health Clinical Research and Innovation (MUHCRI), Faculdade de Medicina da Universidade de Lisboa, Lisboa, Portugal

ELIZABETH S. MUNROE, MD, MSc
Assistant Professor, Department of Pulmonary and Critical Care Medicine, Intermountain Medical Center, Murray, Utah, USA

LAVEENA MUNSHI, MD, MSc
Associate Professor, Department of Critical Care Medicine, University of Toronto, Toronto, Ontario, Canada

MIHAI G. NETEA, MD, PhD
Professor, Department of Internal Medicine, Radboud Center for Infectious Diseases, Radboud University Medical Center, Nijmegen, the Netherlands; Department of

Immunology and Metabolism, Life and Medical Sciences Institute (LIMES), University of Bonn, Bonn, Germany

NATHAN D. NIELSEN, MD, MSc
Professor, Division of Pulmonary, Critical Care and Sleep Medicine, Section of Transfusion Medicine and Therapeutic Pathology, University of New Mexico School of Medicine, Albuquerque, New Mexico, USA

ITHAN D. PELTAN, MD, MSc
Associate Professor, Medical Director for Acute Care/Pulmonary and Critical Care Medicine Research, Department of Pulmonary and Critical Care Medicine, Intermountain Medical Center, Murray, Utah, USA

PETER PICKKERS, MD, PhD
Professor, Department of Intensive Care Medicine, Radboud University Medical Center, Nijmegen, The Netherlands

HALLIE C. PRESCOTT, MD, MSc
Professor, Division of Pulmonary and Critical Care Medicine, Department of Internal Medicine, University of Michigan, Ann Arbor, Michigan, USA

VALENTIM RODRIGUES, MBBS
MD Student, Faculdade de Medicina da Universidade de Lisboa, Lisboa, Portugal

MAYRA ROMIJNDERS, MSc
PhD Candidate, Department of Intensive Care Medicine, Radboud University Medical Center, Nijmegen, The Netherlands

CLARK D. RUSSELL, MBChB, PhD
NES/CSO Clinical Lecturer in Infectious Diseases, Centre for Inflammation Research, Institute for Regeneration and Repair, University of Edinburgh, Edinburgh, United Kingdom

ERMINIO SANTANGELO, MD
Fellow, Interdepartmental Division of Critical Care Medicine, University of Toronto, Toronto, Ontario, Canada

DAPHNE SCHOUTEN, MD, PhD Candidate
PhD candidate, Centre for Infection and Molecular Medicine, Amsterdam UMC, University of Amsterdam, Amsterdam, the Netherlands

PRATIK SINHA, MB ChB, PhD, FFICM, FRCEM
Associate Professor, Department of Anesthesia, Washington University in St. Louis, St Louis, Missouri, USA

BRAM SNOEK, MSc
PhD Candidate, Department of Intensive Care Medicine, Radboud University Medical Center, Nijmegen, The Netherlands

JASON THOMAS, MB BCH, BAO, MCH
Clinical Research Fellow, College of Medical, Veterinary and Life Sciences, University of Glasgow, Glasgow, United Kingdom

WOUTER A. VAN DER HEIJDEN, MD, PhD
Senior Scientist and Physician, Department of Intensive Care, Radboud Center for Infectious Diseases, Radboud University Medical Center, Nijmegen, The Netherlands

LUC VAN OSS, MSc
PhD Candidate, Department of Intensive Care Medicine, Radboud University Medical Center, Nijmegen, The Netherlands

LONNEKE VAN VUGHT, MD, PhD
Assistant Professor, Department of General Practice and Nursing Science, Julius Center for Health Sciences and Primary Care, University Medical Center Utrecht, Utrecht University, Utrecht, Netherlands

ANNETTE C. WESTGEEST, MD, PhD
Fellow in Infectious Diseases, Leiden University Center of Infectious Diseases, Leiden University Medical Center, Leiden, The Netherlands

W. JOOST WIERSINGA, MD, PhD
Professor, Division of Infectious Diseases, Department of Medicine, Center for Infection and Molecular Medicine, Amsterdam Institute for Infection and Immunity, Amsterdam UMC, University of Amsterdam, Amsterdam, The Netherlands

HANNAH WOZNIAK, MD
Clinical Associate, Intensive Care Unit, Department of Acute Medicine, Geneva University Hospitals, Faculty of Medicine, University of Geneva, Geneva, Switzerland

ANN ZALUCKY, MD, MSc
Assistant Professor, Department of Critical Care Medicine, University of Calgary, Calgary, Alberta, Canada

ALEXANDRE P. ZAVASCKI, MD, PhD
Professor, Department of Internal Medicine, Universidade Federal do Rio Grande do Sul, Infectious Diseases Service, Hospital de Clinicas de Porto Alegre, Infectious Diseases and Infection Control Service, Hospital Moinhos de Vento, Porto Alegre, Brazil

Contents

CRITICAL CARE CLINICS

FORTHCOMING ISSUES

January 2027
The ICU Workforce
Ankita Agarwal and Andrea Sikora, *Editors*

April 2027
Metabolic Emergencies in Critical Care
Guillermo Umpierrez and Andrew Demidowich, *Editors*

July 2027
Hematologic and Oncologic Emergencies
Monica Wattana and Molly Estes, *Editors*

RECENT ISSUES

July 2026
Infectious Diseases in the Intensive Care Unit
Sameer S. Kadri and Christina Yek, *Editors*

April 2026
Organization and Management of Critical Care Services
Stephen M. Pastores and John M. Oropello, *Editors*

January 2026
Cardiac Arrest and Cardiopulmonary Resuscitation
Sarah M. Perman, Robert A. Berg and Vinay M. Nadkarni, *Editors*

Preface

Beyond Syndromic Labels: Need for Molecular Mechanistic Reframing of Sepsis and Systemic Inflammatory Syndromes for Effective Translation

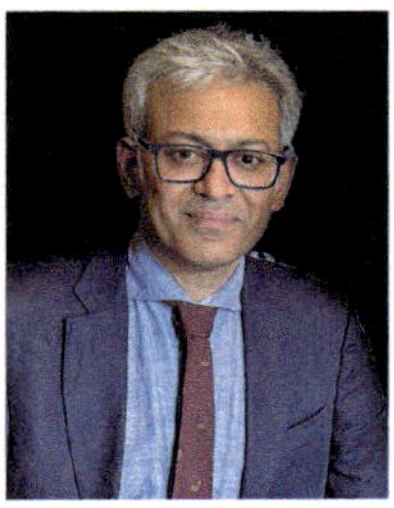

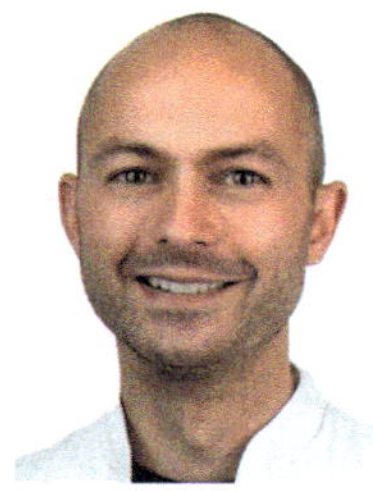

Manu Shankar-Hari, MSc, FFICM, MD, PhD, FRSE
Lieuwe D.J. Bos, MD, PhD
Editors

Sepsis and related systemic inflammatory syndromes are still defined more by clinical convenience than by biological clarity. Framed as a dysregulated host response to infection, the current model has improved recognition and early intervention, but it has not delivered effective host response–targeted therapies. This gap exposes a fundamental limitation: the syndromic label collapses biologically distinct processes into a single category, obscuring the mechanisms that drive outcomes and shape therapeutic response.

A consistent message across this issue is that heterogeneity in sepsis is not a nuisance, but an opportunity. Patients who meet identical clinical criteria can differ profoundly in host susceptibility, immune trajectories, pathogen features, and treatment responses. Early management therefore unfolds under unavoidable time pressure and incomplete mechanistic insight. The imperative for rapid antimicrobials and physiologic stabilization must be weighed against overtreatment, antimicrobial resistance, and downstream harm. This friction between speed and precision sits at the core of modern sepsis care.

The contributions in this issue support a broader and more integrated view of sepsis biology. Immune dysregulation, long considered central, is heterogeneous and dynamic, encompassing concurrent and evolving states of hyperinflammation and immunosuppression. However, immune pathways alone do not fully account for disease

Crit Care Clin 42 (2026) xiii–xv
https://doi.org/10.1016/j.ccc.2026.05.025
0749-0704/26/© 2026 Published by Elsevier Inc.

progression. Vascular, metabolic, neuroendocrine, and organ-specific processes interact with immune responses to determine whether the host maintains homeostasis or progresses to organ failure. These processes are interconnected, and responses that are initially adaptive may become maladaptive over time.

This system's perspective requires a shift from static descriptions to dynamic frameworks. Emerging approaches to subgrouping and phenotyping aim to identify reproducible patterns within this complexity using clinical, biomarker, and high-dimensional data. These approaches extend beyond classification. The goal is to define dominant mechanisms that are potentially modifiable. Complementary strategies, including the study of extreme phenotypes, emphasize that amplifying biological signal can reveal determinants of both susceptibility and resilience. Meaningful stratification will require integration across scales, from molecular networks to clinical trajectories.

A further implication is that sepsis is not confined to the acute phase. Organ-specific dysfunction, including brain injury, and the development of post–sepsis syndrome illustrate that the consequences of dysregulated host responses persist beyond initial resuscitation. Long-term outcomes reflect not only the severity of the acute insult but also the failure to restore physiologic and immunologic homeostasis. This temporal dimension reinforces the need to consider sepsis as a dynamic disease process with evolving therapeutic targets.

Several implications follow. Advancing sepsis care requires moving beyond syndromic definitions toward biologically informed models that capture heterogeneity and temporal evolution. Therapeutic strategies must account for the interplay between immune and nonimmune pathways rather than targeting isolated components. Implementation of precision approaches will depend not only on identifying subgroups but also on embedding reliable, real-time tools into clinical workflows.

This issue captures a field in transition. Sepsis is increasingly framed as a complex, dynamic disruption of host immune and nonimmune homeostasis, alongside impaired regulation. Turning that understanding into effective, mechanism-based care remains the defining challenge ahead of us.

DISCLOSURES

M. Shankar-Hari is supported by UK National Institute for Health and Care Research (NIHR) Senior Investigator Award (NIHR509126) from the NIHR, receives funding for his research from the NIHR, Wellcome Trust, the Medical Research Council, and Chief Scientist's Office Scotland and has done advisory board activity through the International Sepsis Forum with payments going either into the unrestricted institutional research funds or to the International Sepsis Forum. L.D.J. Bos is supported by grants from ZonMw and Health Holland, has consulted for AstraZeneca, Ambu, and has participated in a Data Safety Monitoring Board for an Aptarion-sponsored study. All fees were paid to the institution.

Manu Shankar-Hari, MSc, FFICM, MD, PhD, FRSE
Centre for Critical Illness Research
School of Immunology & Microbial Sciences
Kings College London
London, UK

Lieuwe D.J. Bos, MD, PhD
Department of Intensive Care
Amsterdam UMC
Amsterdam, The Netherlands

E-mail addresses:
manu.shankar-hari@kcl.ac.uk (M. Shankar-Hari)
L.d.bos@amsterdamumc.nl (L.D.J. Bos)

Post-Sepsis Syndrome after Critical Illness

Epidemiology and Long-term Outcomes

Hannah Wozniak, MD[a,b,*], Eleonora Balzani, MD[c],
Erminio Santangelo, MD[d], Margaret Herridge, MD, MSc[d]

KEYWORDS

- Sepsis survivorship • Post-sepsis syndrome • Long-term outcomes
- Patient-centered outcomes • Post-intensive care syndrome • Continuity of care

KEY POINTS

- Survival after sepsis has improved over recent decades, leading to a growing population of sepsis survivors with complex recovery needs.
- Sepsis survivorship is associated with substantial long-term morbidity, including physical, cognitive, and psychological impairments, recurrent hospitalization, excess long-term mortality and a significant burden on relatives and caregivers.
- Recovery after sepsis is heterogeneous, with patients following variable trajectories influenced by premorbid health, acute illness severity, organ dysfunction, complications, and postdischarge care.
- Immunologic profiling, biomarkers, and artificial intelligence–based approaches may help identify distinct recovery trajectories and support more personalized risk stratification.
- Structured post-sepsis follow-up is an essential component of the care continuum, aiming to detect persistent impairments, coordinate multidisciplinary care, and improve long-term patient-important outcomes.

INTRODUCTION

Sepsis is defined as life-threatening organ dysfunction caused by a dysregulated host response to infection.[1,2] Survival after sepsis has improved over recent decades, resulting in a growing population of sepsis survivors.[1,2] In the United States, sepsis accounts for an estimated 1.7 million adult hospitalizations annually, of which approximately 350,000 result in death in hospital or discharge to hospice, underscoring the

[a] Intensive Care Unit, Department of Acute Medicine, Geneva University Hospitals, Geneva, Switzerland; [b] Faculty of Medicine, University of Geneva, Geneva, Switzerland; [c] Centre for Medical Sciences-CISMed, University of Trento, Trento, Italy; [d] Interdepartmental Division of Critical Care Medicine, University of Toronto, Toronto, Ontario, Canada
* Corresponding author.
E-mail address: Hannah.Wozniak@hug.ch

Crit Care Clin 42 (2026) 683–700
https://doi.org/10.1016/j.ccc.2026.05.011 criticalcare.theclinics.com

Abbreviations	
AI	artificial intelligence
ICU	intensive care unit
PICS	post-intensive care syndrome
PSS	post-sepsis syndrome
PTSD	post-traumatic stress disorder
QoL	quality of life

substantial burden of organ injury.[3] Among intensive care unit (ICU) treated patients with sepsis, mortality remains high, and long-term recovery among survivors is variable. Survivorship after sepsis is frequently marked by significant long-term morbidity, including new functional dependence, cognitive impairment, anxiety, depression, post-traumatic stress symptoms, recurrent hospitalization, and excess long-term mortality.[4–7] In a recent prospective cohort of patients admitted to the ICU for sepsis, 38.7% of patients died before ICU discharge and 47.4% died before hospital discharge. Among ICU survivors, approximately 25% remained functionally dependent, 30% regained functional independence, and 45% had died by 3 years.[8]

Historically, sepsis research has focused predominantly on short-term outcomes, and much of the literature has centered on improving survival through acute care processes, such as timely antimicrobial administration, source control, hemodynamic resuscitation, treatment duration, and antibiotic de-escalation, with success measured primarily in terms of survival. Consistent with this, landmark interventional trials in sepsis have typically used in-hospital 28 day or 90 day mortality as their primary endpoint rather than longer-term patient-important outcomes, such as functional recovery or quality of life.[9–14] However, over the past decade, critical care and sepsis research have progressively shifted to enhanced risk stratification, phenotypic enrichment, prognostication, and granular patient-centered outcomes, recognizing the need to address heterogeneity to offer more tailored care and that survival alone is an incomplete and wholly inadequate measure of recovery.[1,7,8,15–17] This broader view of risk ascertainment and recovery is now reflected in contemporary guideline recommendations, which emphasize individualized post-sepsis treatment as an integral component of sepsis care.[18]

The aim of this article, therefore, is to present the current knowledge on the epidemiology of long-term outcomes among adult ICU sepsis survivors, with particular emphasis on patient-important outcomes, their prevalence, and contributing factors, and to discuss the emerging role of biomarkers, immunologic profiling, and artificial intelligence (AI) in prognostication, individualized prediction, and post-sepsis care pathways.

SEPSIS SURVIVORSHIP AFTER CRITICAL ILLNESS

ICU sepsis survivors represent a specific subgroup within the broader population of sepsis survivors. Sepsis may occur across a broad spectrum of severity, from patients treated for short periods of time in the community and on hospital wards to those requiring prolonged ICU stays with multiple organ support. Patients who survive sepsis after an ICU stay are therefore not only survivors of infection, but also survivors of critical illness, often exposed to mechanical ventilation, corticosteroids, immobility and deep coma related to paralytics and sedation, delirium, and prolonged hospitalization, each of which may contribute to long-term morbidity.[4–7]

From the perspective of patients and their families, the outcomes that matter most extend beyond survival alone. Recovery is often understood in terms of physical function, cognitive abilities, emotional well-being, social participation, return to work or prior activities, and the ability to regain an acceptable quality of life.[19,20] Family members may also experience psychological distress, caregiver burden, and disruption in social or professional roles. For this reason, survivorship after sepsis should be approached through a patient- and family-centered lens rather than focused on mortality alone.[18]

Within the ICU literature, the long-term consequences of critical illness are commonly conceptualized under the framework of post-intensive care syndrome (PICS), which encompasses new or worsening physical, cognitive, and mental health impairment arising after critical illness.[4–7] In the sepsis literature, the term post-sepsis syndrome (PSS) is often used to describe this multidimensional burden observed after sepsis.[1,21] Although PICS and PSS are not synonymous, they overlap substantially. PSS includes most of the physical, cognitive, and psychological sequelae captured by PICS, but further encompasses sepsis-specific features such as recurrent infection, rehospitalization, and persistent organ or immune dysfunction. In a multicenter prospective cohort study, mechanically ventilated ICU patients with sepsis had a higher risk of death than mechanically ventilated ICU patients admitted for nonsepsis diagnoses.[7] However, among survivors, 6 month outcomes were similar between groups, including new disability, health-related quality of life, mental health outcomes, cognitive function, and return to work. These findings suggest that many long-term sequelae of sepsis overlap with those of critical illness survivorship more broadly.

Importantly, recovery after ICU should be viewed as a trajectory rather than a fixed outcome assessed at a single time point.[16,22,23] Patients do not all follow the same path: some recover rapidly, some remain persistently impaired, and others develop new morbidity or die over subsequent months and years.[16] This dynamic nature of survivorship is reflected in studies showing heterogeneous trajectories, with disability and excess mortality persisting for up to 5 years or beyond after an ICU stay.[8,16,23,24]

MAJOR LONG-TERM OUTCOME DOMAINS

The long-term sequelae of sepsis represent a systemic health care burden requiring longitudinal care models beyond the traditional critical care boundaries.[15,17] Sepsis short-term mortality rates have significantly improved, and this has created an expanding population of survivors living with multidimensional long-term morbidity. The mechanisms underlying these chronic sequelae are multifactorial and may include persistent inflammation, prolonged immune dysregulation, persistent organ injury, and the progression of pre-existing comorbid disease.[1,25,26]

Functional disability represents one of the most prevalent domains of long-term morbidity among sepsis survivors. Recent meta-analytic data indicate that the prevalence of physical impairments exhibits significant heterogeneity, ranging from 25% to 80% across diverse patient populations.[27] A primary contributor to this profound functional decline is ICU-acquired weakness, defined as weakness that cannot be explained by a cause other than critical illness. ICU-acquired weakness has been reported in approximately 55% of assessable long-stay ICU patients. Sepsis is itself an important risk factor for ICU-acquired weakness, alongside other reported risk factors including greater severity of illness, multiple organ failure, prolonged immobilization, prolonged mechanical ventilation, hyperglycemia, and older age.[28,29] The pathophysiology encompasses critical illness polyneuropathy, myosin-depletion myopathy, disuse atrophy, and evident as muscle wasting, which may appear as early as the first week of an ICU stay.[30] Frailty, defined as a state of reduced physiologic reserve and increased vulnerability to stressors, is another important dimension of post-ICU functional disability. Baseline frailty is associated with worse ICU and post-ICU outcomes, including lower quality of life (QoL) and greater functional dependency, and frailty severity may further worsen during ICU hospitalization, with higher discharge frailty associated with poorer subsequent recovery.[31,32] Functional improvement is often greatest in the first 6 to 12 months after hospital discharge, but many patients do not fully regain their pre-illness functional baseline and may remain persistently disabled for years or indefinitely.[23,33] Longitudinal data suggest that severe sepsis survivors acquire approximately 1.5 new functional limitations after hospitalization, with these impairments persisting for years after the acute episode.[34] Moreover, the persistence of muscular weakness at the time of ICU discharge is independently associated with significantly elevated 1 year mortality and increased health care costs.[28] Lastly, survivors of sepsis may experience an increased long-term risk of cardiovascular events for up to 5 years after hospital discharge.[35] In a recent meta-analysis, the pooled cumulative incidence of myocardial infarction, stroke, and heart failure in sepsis survivors was as high as 9%, potentially contributing to impaired functional recovery.[35]

Cognitive impairment is an important and potentially disabling long-term sequela after critical illness, with up to 34% of patients presenting persistent cognitive impairment 1 year after an ICU stay.[36] The severity of this acquired dysfunction is considerable: one-quarter of post-ICU patients develop cognitive profiles comparable to early-stage Alzheimer's dementia, while 33% demonstrate severe neurocognitive profiles equivalent to those observed following traumatic brain injury.[36] Importantly, survivors of severe sepsis experience a greater increase in moderate-to-severe cognitive impairment than patients admitted for general, nonseptic hospitalizations, with an absolute increase of 10.6% points.[34] Implicated pathophysiological pathways include blood-brain barrier disruption, neuroinflammation, microvascular injury, neurotransmitter dysregulation, and hippocampal neuronal loss.[37] In the BRAIN-ICU study, which included patients admitted to the ICU for any reason, a longer duration of delirium in the hospital was independently associated with worse global cognition and executive function at 3 and 12 months after discharge.[36] In sepsis-specific studies, risk factors for poor cognitive outcomes included depressive symptoms, central nervous system infection, length of hospitalization due to infection, temporal proximity to the last period of infection, the time to first antibiotic dose, cumulative dose of haloperidol during the ICU stay, mean glycemia, severity scores on ICU admission scores, neuron-specific enolase, and IFN-γ levels at ICU discharge.[38,39] Although partial improvement may occur over the first year, these impairments often represent a major change, resulting in reduced autonomy and substantial caregiver dependence.[34,40]

The prevalence of psychological sequelae, including symptoms of anxiety, depression, and posttraumatic stress disorder (PTSD), is high after an ICU stay. In the year following critical illness, survivors have a median point prevalence of clinically significant depression of 28% to 33%, alongside substantial rates of PTSD and anxiety.[41,42] In a nation-wide population-based study, among 21,980 sepsis survivors, 54.8% were diagnosed with a new mental health issue in the 12-month postdischarge.[43] Reported risk factors for post-ICU psychological sequelae include pre-existing psychiatric illness, longer duration of mechanical ventilation or ICU stay, delirium, benzodiazepine exposure, and distressing ICU memories.[44,45] An elevated longitudinal risk of both self-harm and completed suicide has also been documented among survivors.[46] These psychological sequelae are often persistent, with up to one-third of patients still symptomatic at 12 months.[47] They are associated with long-term deficits in both mental and physical health-related quality of life.[42] Importantly, a recent study focused on PTSD symptoms found that a quarter of septic patients reported few symptoms at discharge, but an increase in symptoms in the subsequent 2 years, highlighting the importance of long-term follow-up.[48]

GENERAL IMPACT ON QUALITY OF LIFE AND RETURN TO WORK

QoL is consistently and significantly reduced among sepsis survivors. It has been reported that approximately one-third of septic survivors admitted to the ICU have not returned to independent living by 6 months, with frequent impairments in mobility, usual activities, and self-care.[49] Successful return to work often serves in the literature as a general surrogate for broader functional recovery, and approximately two-fifths of ICU survivors remain unemployed 1 year after an ICU stay.[50] Sepsis survivors frequently experience significant occupational disruption, manifesting as reduced working hours, involuntary career changes, and severe financial strain.[51] A recent nationwide Norwegian registry study of 12,260 previously employed survivors highlighted this important socioeconomic morbidity; 2 years following discharge, successful return to work was achieved by only 64.2% of ward-managed sepsis patients and only 52.2% of those requiring ICU admission.[52] The multidimensional disruption that persists after critical illness is particularly relevant for younger working-age survivors.

IMPACT ON FAMILIES AND CAREGIVERS

The sequelae of sepsis after critical illness are not isolated to the individual patient but also significantly affect their family members and caregivers. This has been described in the ICU literature as PICS-family. In most cases, caregiver support is provided by an informal family member, which may result in considerable psychological, social, and financial strain.[53] In the Canadian RECOVER cohort, 67% of the caregivers reported depressive symptoms at the time of the discharge and 43% remained symptomatic at 1 year.[53] In a French study from the FAMIREA group, PTSD symptoms were reported 3 months after an ICU stay in 33.1% of caregivers, reaching 81% among those who were involved in end-of-life decisions.[54] New mental illness has been reported in approximately one-quarter of spouses or partners of patients with sepsis or septic shock.[55,56] Importantly, worse patient outcomes have been shown to be associated with greater caregiver burden and with reduced mental health-related QoL.[55] Other reported risk factors for caregiver distress include younger patient age, history of mental illness, being a female, patient death and patient physical impairment.[57,58] Given this substantial and sustained burden, caregivers should be recognized as an essential component of post-sepsis care and integrated into the ICU care continuum. Moreover, as many patients with sepsis die during their hospital stay, caregivers and relatives of these patients should be considered. New mental health disorders, such as depression or generalized anxiety, have been reported in 34% of relatives of patients who died in the ICU, and complicated grief in up to 52% at 6 months after the event.[59,60]

Children of critically ill adults are also a vulnerable and often forgotten group. They are exposed to a disruption of family routine, altered parental relationship, and to the consequences of financial strain.[61] Although direct data are limited, they may also be at risk of internalizing symptoms, school underperformance, and psychological distress.[62] With an increase in patient comorbidity and complexity, a greater proportion of patients will sustain longer ICU stays and children may need specific additional psychological, social, and school support to navigate new physical and cognitive disability in a parent. This reality has not yet been broadly integrated into the design of current ICU follow-up care.

IMPACT ON HEALTH CARE WORKERS

Health care workers are also affected by the care of these patients. Critically ill sepsis patients often require prolonged ICU stays and undergo numerous invasive interventions and procedures. When care appears futile, when the treatment plan becomes uncertain, or when a patient is later seen after discharge with major disabilities and questions arise about the appropriateness of the care provided, health care workers may experience distress.[63,64] This can manifest as care-related regret, for which perceived futility has been highlighted as a major driver, and is associated with burnout and intention to change profession.[65] Although a direct link with patient long-term outcomes has not been clearly established, health care workers' well-being is relevant to the ICU care continuum because the delivery of sustained, patient- and family-centered care depends on a workforce that is adequately supported. This is especially relevant in the post-COVID-19 context, marked by substantial staff attrition, workforce shortages, and persistently high burnout rates.[64]

ECONOMIC OUTCOMES

Sepsis is one of the most costly conditions treated in hospital, with a substantial economic burden reported in Europe and in the United States.[66,67] In a systematic review of 26 studies, the median sepsis costs per stay were €36,191.[67] However, the economic burden of sepsis extends beyond the index admission and is driven by readmissions, recurrent hospitalization, ongoing rehabilitation needs related to persistent disabilities, and prolonged use of health care resources.[6,66] Recent data in the United States demonstrate that in the first year after discharge, the median total health care expenditure for sepsis survivors reached 28,719 USD, and these substantial costs continued into the second postdischarge year. Notably, the median cost associated with a single hospital readmission for this cohort was 20,320 USD. Resource utilization remains elevated for years, with sepsis survivors spending roughly 3 times more time in hospital or care facilities after the index episode than before their sepsis episode.[68]

DETERMINANTS OF LONG-TERM OUTCOMES

Long-term outcomes are the cumulative product of the interplay of multiple factors occurring across the trajectory of illness and recovery. These determinants can be broadly grouped into pre-existing patient vulnerability, severity, and management of the critical illness, and the quality of postdischarge recovery and follow-up.

Pre-existing health status is one of the strongest determinants of long-term outcomes. Older age, frailty, and burden of comorbid disease are consistently associated with mortality, poorer functional recovery, and lower health-related QoL after sepsis and critical illness.[15,69,70] Among these factors, frailty and sarcopenia are particularly relevant, as they independently predict both short- and long-term mortality, persistent functional impairment, and reduced quality of life.[71–75]

The severity of the acute sepsis episode is another main determinant. Critical illness severity, often captured by ICU severity scores, complicating shock, number of organ failures, and the need for invasive organ support including mechanical ventilation, renal replacement therapy, and vasopressors are all well-established risk factors for worse long-term outcome.[76] Among sepsis-specific factors, timely recognition, early, appropriate antimicrobial therapy adhering to antimicrobial stewardship tenets, adequate hemodynamic resuscitation, and prompt source control remain the most actionable in-ICU determinants of prognosis.[77–79] However, their association with longer-term patient-centered outcomes remains poorly studied. At the same time, prolonged or unnecessary broad-spectrum antimicrobial exposure may contribute to other complications, including the selection of multidrug-resistant organisms, gut microbiota dysbiosis and *Clostridium difficile* infections.[80,81] These downstream complications, in turn, may increase the likelihood of rehospitalization and greater long-term morbidity.[82]

CLINICAL IMPLICATIONS: SURVIVORSHIP CARE AND FOLLOW-UP

Critical illness due to sepsis does not end at ICU or hospital discharge; for many patients, recovery extends over months to years. This supports the concept of an ICU and sepsis care continuum, in which discharge represents a transition point rather than the end of care.[83] Contemporary guidelines reflect this perspective. In the 2026 Surviving Sepsis Campaign, clinicians are advised to provide survivors and their families with written and verbal information about sepsis, treatments received, and common post-sepsis impairments, while health systems are advised to facilitate post-discharge assessment and follow-up for physical, cognitive, and emotional problems.[18] The same guideline also suggests postcritical illness follow-up services for survivors of hospitalization with sepsis or septic shock, but acknowledges that the optimal format, timing, and intensity of follow-up remain uncertain. The transition from hospital to community is a vulnerable period during which multiple frequently neglected factors may shape long-term recovery. Medication reconciliation failures, underrecognized new impairments, the absence of structured follow-up, and fragmented communication with primary care represent the main challenges.[1,15] Access to rehabilitation might represent an important outcome modifiers: sepsis and septic shock survivors discharged to a rehabilitation facility had the best 5 year survival across severity strata, suggesting that structured postdischarge care may improve long-term recovery.[84]

A first practical implication is to identify patients at highest risk of poor long-term outcomes as early as possible. As discussed earlier, older age, baseline frailty, comorbidity burden, prolonged ICU stay, multiorgan failure, prolonged mechanical ventilation, delirium, and severe physical impairment at discharge are consistently associated with worse recovery trajectories after critical illness and sepsis.[15,69,70] These factors may help clinicians tailor information provided to patients and families, guide early discussions about likely recovery and potential sequelae, discuss goals of care, and flag high-risk survivors to primary care and rehabilitation services at the time of discharge.

A second implication is that some sequelae may be preventable, at least in part, through improvements in acute ICU care. Early mobilization has been associated with better physical recovery and, in a recent randomized trial, with lower long-term cognitive impairment 1 year after critical illness.[85] Delirium—common in patients with sepsis and a known risk factor for subsequent cognitive dysfunction—may be reduced through multicomponent approaches such as the ABCDEF bundle and through careful minimization of deep sedation and benzodiazepine exposure.[36,86] More recently, higher ABCDEF bundle compliance has also been associated with less disability in instrumental activities of daily living and better health-related QoL at 12 months after an ICU stay.[86] For mental health outcomes, family engagement, structured communication, and flexible visitation may improve the ICU experience and reduce distress, although evidence for durable long-term psychological benefit remains inconsistent. ICU diaries may also help reduce posttraumatic stress symptoms in patients and family members after critical illness, although their effects have not been consistent across studies.[87,88]

Across health systems, survivorship care pathways are highly heterogeneous. National initiatives in countries such as Australia and Switzerland have emphasized discharge planning, patient and family education, and improved transition from hospital to community care.[89,90] However, interventional studies of post-sepsis follow-up have produced mixed results. In the SMOOTH randomized trial, a structured primary care–focused aftercare program did not improve mental health–related QoL at 6 months after ICU discharge, although it informed subsequent work on sepsis aftercare.[91] In the recent ENCOMPASS trial, a navigator-led telehealth Sepsis Transition and Recovery program did not reduce the composite of 90 day readmission or death, despite a lower mortality signal in a secondary analysis.[92] A recent systematic review found that postacute interventions for sepsis survivors varied substantially in content, timing, and intensity, with inconsistent effects across outcomes.[93] Rehabilitation-oriented strategies showed some promise, whereas evidence for bundled follow-up, care coordination, and mental health interventions remained limited.[93]

Accordingly, future survivorship programs should move beyond a one-size-fits-all clinic model and instead use risk-stratified approaches that integrate discharge information, premorbid vulnerability, ICU exposures, and post-sepsis symptoms to guide referral toward rehabilitation, mental health support, medication review, or coordinated primary care follow-up. This approach is consistent with the 2026 Surviving Sepsis Campaign, which recommends physical rehabilitation services for selected survivors, mental health support after discharge, medication reconciliation at transitions of care, and improved communication with primary care and community services.[18] **Fig. 1** illustrates the trajectory of sepsis survivors and proposes a

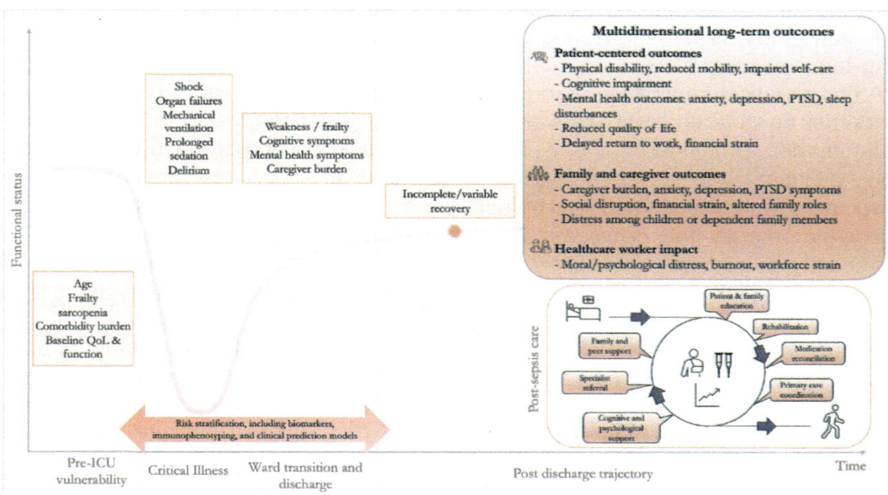

Fig. 1. Longitudinal determinants, consequences, and care model for post-sepsis recovery. The care continuum extends from pre-ICU status through the ICU stay, hospital ward, and rehabilitation, to community reintegration and return to previous social roles. Patient trajectories may be risk stratified and modified by factors arising at each stage, and further refined through biomarkers, immunophenotyping, and AI. The figure highlights outcomes at 3 levels: patients, family members/caregivers, and health care workers. Post-sepsis care includes family and peer support, specialist referral, cognitive and psychological support, patient and family education, rehabilitation, medication reconciliation, and coordination with primary care. (Developed by the authors based on concepts described by Herridge and Azoulay.[15])

longitudinal, multidisciplinary model of post-sepsis survivorship care, integrating pre-existing vulnerability, acute critical illness exposures, postdischarge outcomes, and coordinated follow-up needs across the recovery trajectory.

METHODOLOGICAL CHALLENGES IN STUDIES OF LONG-TERM OUTCOMES AFTER CRITICAL ILLNESS IN SEPTIC PATIENTS

Many studies of sepsis still focus on short-term outcomes, most commonly 28 day or 90 day mortality, without adequately assessing long-term outcomes.[94] Although 28 day mortality was long considered a pragmatic endpoint for evaluating acute treatment efficacy, it does not reflect meaningful recovery as studies have described persistent disabilities and excess mortality up to 5 years after an ICU stay.[24,95] As a result, studies restricted to short-term survival may substantially overestimate treatment success by failing to capture persistent disability and late death.

Another limitation is the inadequate characterization of patients before sepsis. Many studies summarize premorbid status using comorbidity counts or indices. While these are important predictors of poor long-term outcomes, they do not fully capture frailty, baseline functional status, or preadmission quality of life, which have all been highlighted as important determinants of long-term patient-centered outcomes.[74,96–98] Without this information, it can be difficult to determine whether impairments observed after sepsis are new or simply reflect pre-existing vulnerability.[94,99] Retrospective patient-reported or proxy-based assessments may partly address this issue, although both approaches have recognized limitations.[94,100,101]

Long-term follow-up studies are also vulnerable to several major sources of bias. First, attrition bias, resulting from differential loss to follow-up, is common because follow-up is often incomplete and nonrandom, with patients who are either most impaired or fully recovered being less likely to remain in the study.[102,103] Second, death is a competing risk for many patient-centered outcomes, and treating death as simple censoring may lead to overestimation of recovery.[102,103] Third, analyses restricted to survivors are vulnerable to collider bias, a form of selection bias that can occur when analyses condition on survival, potentially creating misleading associations between exposures and long-term outcomes.[103,104]

These limitations have important implications for study design and analysis. Follow-up should describe the nonsurvivors and extend beyond the early postdischarge period and ideally include repeated assessments over time, since recovery trajectories differ across physical, cognitive, and psychological domains. Outcome standardization is also needed, as the use of numerous different instruments has limited comparability across studies.[96,105,106] On the analytical side, methods that account for competing risks, nonrandom attrition, and heterogeneous recovery trajectories are likely to provide more valid estimates of long-term outcome than conventional complete-case or survivor-only approaches.

FUTURE DIRECTIONS: BIOMARKERS AND IMMUNOLOGIC PROFILING

In septic ICU patients, research on biomarkers and immunophenotyping is growing; however, this has mainly been studied in relation to short-term mortality. Examples include inflammatory markers such as IL-6 and procalcitonin, endothelial markers such as proadrenomedullin, and immune markers such as monocytic HLA-DR, all of which have been explored as predictors of early severity and death.[107–109] A useful biomarker for long-term outcomes would ideally serve 3 main functions.

First, early risk stratification: identifying which patients are most likely to develop poor long-term outcomes while there is still a window for intervention. NT-proBNP elevation within the first 24 hours, for example, has been associated with reduced physical function and muscle strength at 6 and 12 months.[110] NSE and IFN-γ levels at ICU discharge have been associated with poor cognitive outcomes in septic patients.[38,39] Dynamic profiling of angiogenic, metabolic, and immune markers may also help identify patients at risk of developing PICS.[25,111]

Second, mechanistic bridging: linking acute-phase biological disturbances with the sequelae that emerge months or years later. Some studies have moved beyond short-term survival and suggest that persistent biological dysregulation may contribute to adverse long-term trajectories. A study found that abnormalities in the host immune response persisted for up to 1 year after sepsis and were associated with a higher risk of readmission and long-term mortality.[25] Another study similarly reported prolonged immune disturbances 1 year after ICU discharge in septic shock survivors, while the FROG-ICU cohort linked sepsis-survivor heterogeneity to distinct biological profiles at ICU discharge and late adverse events.[26,112,113] Together, these findings suggest that failure to restore biological homeostasis may contribute to later morbidity and may help identify therapeutic targets capable of altering recovery trajectories.

Third, therapeutic targeting: biomarkers may enable predictive enrichment by matching the right intervention to the right patient. This approach is already emerging, with biomarkers being explored to identify biologically distinct subgroups that may benefit from more targeted interventions.[114] In a recent systematic review, biomarkers associated with successful enrichment strategies included suPAR, antithrombin, mHLA-DR, IL-6, and endotoxin activity assay.[115]

Importantly, most studies have evaluated the predictive utility of biomarkers on short-term endpoints, typically 28 day mortality. Few studies have investigated the association between biomarkers and patient-important outcomes and further studies are needed.

FUTURE DIRECTIONS: THE ROLE OF ARTIFICIAL INTELLIGENCE

Recent guidelines recommend postdischarge assessment and follow-up after sepsis or septic shock, but the evidence supporting specific follow-up models remains limited.[18] One major challenge is that sepsis survivors are heterogeneous, with substantial variation in premorbid vulnerability, ICU exposures, organ dysfunction, and postdischarge trajectories. As a result, patients are unlikely to derive equal benefit from the same intervention delivered at the same time point. A second challenge is that existing survivorship interventions differ widely in timing, intensity, and content, ranging from global transition-of-care programs to rehabilitation-focused strategies and ICU follow-up clinics.[93] Together, these observations argue against a one-size-fits-all model of post-sepsis care and support the need for individualized risk stratification.

AI may offer clinically useful tools to identify patients at highest risk of poor long-term outcomes and to guide more personalized follow-up. Several recent studies have developed prediction models for post-ICU or post-sepsis sequelae. A recent study using routinely collected data developed an interpretable machine-learning model to predict new functional impairment after critical illness, showing good discriminative performance with area under the ROC curve (AUROC) values up to 0.90.[116] This illustrates the feasibility of early prediction of functional decline using easily accessed clinical data. Similarly, a recent study developed and temporally validated an electronic health record–based machine-learning model to predict stressor-related psychiatric disorders within 1 year after hospitalization with sepsis.[117] In an independent test sample, patients in the highest-risk decile accounted for nearly one-third of subsequent psychiatric cases, suggesting that routinely available inpatient data may help identify survivors at risk for later psychological morbidity. For cognitive outcomes, a recently developed interpretable machine-learning model predicted post-sepsis cognitive impairment with good discrimination.[118] In this study, key predictors included age, education level, septic shock, benzodiazepine exposure, illness severity, and IL-10.[118] Similar work has extended prediction to family outcomes: a machine-learning model to predict PTSD in relatives of ICU patients has been developed, highlighting the possibility of stratifying risk not only for patients but also for family members.[58]

At present, most evidence in this field stops at prediction. There remains little evidence that implementing AI-based risk models to guide post-sepsis follow-up improves long-term patient-centered outcomes. The next step will therefore be to improve model performance and external validation, and in a second step to test whether AI-informed survivorship pathways can meaningfully alter recovery trajectories after septic critical illness.

SUMMARY

Survival after sepsis has improved significantly over time. Yet recovery extends far beyond survival alone. Survivors of sepsis-associated critical illness, together with their families, are forced to navigate a traumatic life event characterized by considerable physical, cognitive, psychological, social, and financial burden. ICU care should therefore be conceived as a continuum, aimed at mitigating the long-term burden borne by patients and families and improving outcomes that truly matter to them. This will require moving beyond short-term outcome measures in future trials, further refining risk stratification and leveraging machine learning and AI to better inform care pathways that optimally support survivorship and patient-centered recovery.

CLINICS CARE POINTS

- Sepsis survivorship is associated with substantial long-term morbidity, including physical, cognitive, and psychological impairments, recurrent hospitalization, excess long-term mortality, and a significant burden on relatives and caregivers.
- Recovery after sepsis is heterogeneous, with patients following variable trajectories influenced by premorbid health, acute illness severity, organ dysfunction, complications, and post discharge care.
- There is currently limited evidence to support one standardized model of post-sepsis follow-up; care should therefore be individualized according to patient risk, symptoms, and recovery trajectory, and should include multimodal assessment of physical function, cognition, mental health, comorbidities, medication review, and caregiver burden.
- Emerging approaches, including biomarkers, immunologic profiling, and artificial intelligence–based risk stratification, may help identify distinct recovery trajectories and support more personalized risk stratification.

DECLARATION OF AI AND AI-ASSISTED TECHNOLOGIES IN THE WRITING PROCESS

During the preparation of this work the authors used ChatGPT and OpenEvidence in order to support reference searches and to assist with language editing. After using this tool/service, the authors reviewed and edited the content as needed and take full responsibility for the content of the publication.

DISCLOSURES

The authors declare that they have no competing interests and no funding related to this research study.

REFERENCES

1. Prescott HC, Angus DC. Enhancing recovery from sepsis: a review. JAMA 2018; 319:62–75.
2. Singer M, Deutschman CS, Seymour CW, et al. The third international consensus definitions for sepsis and septic shock (Sepsis-3). JAMA 2016; 315:801–10.
3. Centers for disease control and prevention. Hospital sepsis program core elements. Available at: https://www.cdc.gov/sepsis/hcp/core-elements/index.html. Accessed May 4, 2026.
4. Pandolfi F, Brun-Buisson C, Guillemot D, et al. Care pathways of sepsis survivors: sequelae, mortality and use of healthcare services in France, 2015-2018. Crit Care 2023;27:441.
5. Shankar-Hari M, Harrison DA, Ferrando-Vivas P, et al. Risk factors at index hospitalization associated with longer-term mortality in adult sepsis survivors. JAMA Netw Open 2019;2:e194900.
6. Fleischmann-Struzek C, Rose N, Freytag A, et al. Epidemiology and costs of postsepsis morbidity, nursing care dependency, and mortality in Germany, 2013 to 2017. JAMA Netw Open 2021;4:e2134290.
7. Hodgson CL, Higgins AM, Bailey M, et al. Comparison of 6-month outcomes of sepsis versus non-sepsis critically ill patients receiving mechanical ventilation. Crit Care 2022;26:174.
8. Fleischmann-Struzek C, Born S, Kesselmeier M, et al. Functional dependence following intensive care unit-treated sepsis: three-year follow-up results from the prospective mid-German sepsis cohort. Lancet Reg Health Eur 2024;46: 101066.
9. Hernández G, Ospina-Tascón GA, Damiani LP, et al. Effect of a resuscitation strategy targeting peripheral perfusion status vs serum lactate levels on 28-day mortality among patients with septic shock: the ANDROMEDA-SHOCK randomized clinical trial. JAMA 2019;321:654–64.
10. ARISE Investigators, ANZICS Clinical Trials Group, Peake SL, Delaney A, Bailey M, et al. Goal-directed resuscitation for patients with early septic shock. N Engl J Med 2014;371:1496–506.
11. ProCESS Investigators, Yealy DM, Kellum JA, Huang DT, et al. A randomized trial of protocol-based care for early septic shock. N Engl J Med 2014;370: 1683–93.
12. Venkatesh B, Finfer S, Cohen J, et al. Adjunctive glucocorticoid therapy in patients with septic shock. N Engl J Med 2018;378:797–808.
13. National Heart, Lung, and Blood Institute Prevention and Early Treatment of Acute Lung Injury Clinical Trials Network, Shapiro NI, Douglas IS, Brower RG, et al. Early restrictive or liberal fluid management for sepsis-induced hypotension. N Engl J Med 2023;388:499–510.
14. Tabah A, Buetti N, Staiquly Q, et al. Epidemiology and outcomes of hospital-acquired bloodstream infections in intensive care unit patients: the EUROBACT-2 international cohort study. Intensive Care Med 2023;49:178–90.
15. Herridge MS, Azoulay É. Outcomes after critical illness. N Engl J Med 2023;388: 913–24.

16. Herridge MS, Chu LM, Matte A, et al. The RECOVER program: disability risk groups and 1-year outcome after 7 or more days of mechanical ventilation. Am J Respir Crit Care Med 2016;194:831–44.
17. Shankar-Hari M, Rubenfeld GD. Understanding long-term outcomes following sepsis: implications and challenges. Curr Infect Dis Rep 2016;18:37.
18.. Prescott HC, Antonelli M, Alhazzani W, et al. Surviving sepsis campaign: international guidelines for management of sepsis and septic shock 2026. Intensive Care Med 2026;52:863–936.
19. Auriemma CL, Harhay MO, Haines KJ, et al. What matters to patients and their families during and after critical illness: a qualitative study. Am J Crit Care 2021; 30:11–20.
20. Kerckhoffs MC, Kosasi FFL, Soliman IW, et al. Determinants of self-reported unacceptable outcome of intensive care treatment 1 year after discharge. Intensive Care Med 2019;45:806–14.
21. Mostel Z, Perl A, Marck M, et al. Post-sepsis syndrome: an evolving entity that afflicts survivors of sepsis. Mol Med 2020;26:6.
22.. Sahu R, Brown R, Bonavia AS. Longitudinal cognitive recovery after critical illness: trajectories in sepsis and non-sepsis survivors. J Intensive Care Med 2025;41:652–9.
23. Liu K, Watanabe S, Nakamura K, et al. One-year outcomes in sepsis: a prospective multicenter cohort study in Japan. J Intensiv Care 2025;13:23.
24. Cuthbertson BH, Elders A, Hall S, et al. Mortality and quality of life in the five years after severe sepsis. Crit Care 2013;17:R70.
25. Yende S, Kellum JA, Talisa VB, et al. Long-term host immune response trajectories among hospitalized patients with sepsis. JAMA Netw Open 2019;2: e198686.
26. Riché F, Chousterman BG, Valleur P, et al. Protracted immune disorders at one year after ICU discharge in patients with septic shock. Crit Care 2018;22:42.
27. Ayenew T, Gete M, Gedfew M, et al. Prevalence of post-intensive care syndrome among intensive care unit-survivors and its association with intensive care unit length of stay: systematic review and meta-analysis. PLoS One 2025;20: e0323311.
28. Hermans G, Van Mechelen H, Clerckx B, et al. Acute outcomes and 1-year mortality of intensive care unit-acquired weakness: a cohort study and propensity-matched analysis. Am J Respir Crit Care Med 2014;190:410–20.
29. Liu J, Xu Z, Luo S, et al. Risk factors for ICU-acquired weakness in sepsis patients: a retrospective study of 264 patients. Heliyon 2024;10:e32253.
30. Puthucheary ZA, Rawal J, McPhail M, et al. Acute skeletal muscle wasting in critical illness. JAMA 2013;310:1591–600.
31. Geense W, Zegers M, Dieperink P, et al. Changes in frailty among ICU survivors and associated factors: results of a one-year prospective cohort study using the Dutch clinical frailty scale. J Crit Care 2020;55:184–93.
32. Muscedere J, Bagshaw SM, Kho M, et al. Frailty, outcomes, recovery and care steps of critically ill patients (FORECAST): a prospective, multi-centre, cohort study. Intensive Care Med 2024;50:1064–74.
33. Puthucheary ZA, Gensichen JS, Cakiroglu AS, et al. Implications for post critical illness trial design: sub-phenotyping trajectories of functional recovery among sepsis survivors. Crit Care 2020;24:577.
34. Iwashyna TJ, Ely EW, Smith DM, et al. Long-term cognitive impairment and functional disability among survivors of severe sepsis. JAMA 2010;304:1787–94.

35. Kosyakovsky LB, Angriman F, Katz E, et al. Association between sepsis survivorship and long-term cardiovascular outcomes in adults: a systematic review and meta-analysis. Intensive Care Med 2021;47:931–42.
36. Pandharipande PP, Girard TD, Jackson JC, et al. Long-term cognitive impairment after critical illness. N Engl J Med 2013;369:1306–16.
37. Sekino N, Selim M, Shehadah A. Sepsis-associated brain injury: underlying mechanisms and potential therapeutic strategies for acute and long-term cognitive impairments. J Neuroinflammation 2022;19:101.
38. Calsavara AJC, Costa PA, Nobre V, et al. Factors associated with short and long term cognitive changes in patients with sepsis. Sci Rep 2018;8:4509.
39. Calsavara AJC, Barichello T, Teixeira AL, et al. Post-sepsis cognitive impairment and associated risk factors: a systematic review. Aust Crit Care 2018;31:242–53.
40. Honarmand K, Lalli RS, Priestap F, et al. Natural history of cognitive impairment in critical illness survivors: a systematic review. Am J Respir Crit Care Med 2020; 202:193–201.
41. Davydow DS, Gifford JM, Desai SV, et al. Posttraumatic stress disorder in general intensive care unit survivors: a systematic review. Gen Hosp Psychiatry 2008;30:421–34.
42. Davydow DS, Gifford JM, Desai SV, et al. Depression in general intensive care unit survivors: a systematic review. Intensive Care Med 2009;35:796–809.
43. Sell S, Fleischmann-Struzek C, Spoden M, et al. Mental health in the first year after ICU-treated sepsis: analysis of administrative diagnoses in German health claims data. Gen Hosp Psychiatry 2025;93:109–15.
44. Lee M, Kang J, Jeong YJ. Risk factors for post-intensive care syndrome: a systematic review and meta-analysis. Aust Crit Care 2020;33:287–94.
45. Parker AM, Sricharoenchai T, Raparla S, et al. Posttraumatic stress disorder in critical illness survivors: a meta-analysis. Crit Care Med 2015;43:1121–9.
46. Fernando SM, Ranzani OT, Herridge MS. Mental health morbidity, self-harm, and suicide in ICU survivors and caregivers. Intensive Care Med 2022;48:1084–7.
47. Marra A, Pandharipande PP, Girard TD, et al. Co-occurrence of post-intensive care syndrome problems among 406 survivors of critical illness. Crit Care Med 2018;46:1393–401.
48. Schmidt KFR, Gensichen JS, Schroevers M, et al. Trajectories of post-traumatic stress in sepsis survivors two years after ICU discharge: a secondary analysis of a randomized controlled trial. Crit Care 2024;28:65.
49. Yende S, Austin S, Rhodes A, et al. Long-term quality of life among survivors of severe sepsis: analyses of two international trials. Crit Care Med 2016;44: 1461–7.
50. Kamdar BB, Suri R, Suchyta MR, et al. Return to work after critical illness: a systematic review and meta-analysis. Thorax 2020;75:17–27.
51. Fleischmann-Struzek C, Ditscheid B, Rose N, et al. Return to work after sepsis: a German population-based health claims study. Front Med 2023;10:1187809.
52. Skei NV, Moe K, Nilsen TIL, et al. Return to work after hospitalization for sepsis: a nationwide, registry-based cohort study. Crit Care 2023;27:487.
53. Cameron JI, Chu LM, Matte A, et al. One-year outcomes in caregivers of critically ill patients. N Engl J Med 2016;374:1831–41.
54. Azoulay E, Pochard F, Kentish-Barnes N, et al. Risk of post-traumatic stress symptoms in family members of intensive care unit patients. Am J Respir Crit Care Med 2005;171:987–94.
55. Davydow DS, Hough CL, Langa KM, et al. Depressive symptoms in spouses of older patients with severe sepsis. Crit Care Med 2012;40:2335–41.

56. Chen HH, Lin CH, Wu CL, et al. Incidence and risk factors of mental illness among the spouses of patients with sepsis: a population-based cohort study. Intensive Care Med 2022;48:369–71.
57. Naef R, von Felten S, Ernst J. Factors influencing post-ICU psychological distress in family members of critically ill patients: a linear mixed-effects model. Biopsychosoc Med 2021;15:4.
58. Dupont T, Kentish-Barnes N, Pochard F, et al. Prediction of post-traumatic stress disorder in family members of ICU patients: a machine learning approach. Intensive Care Med 2024;50:114–24.
59. Kentish-Barnes N, Chaize M, Seegers V, et al. Complicated grief after death of a relative in the intensive care unit. Eur Respir J 2015;45:1341–52.
60. Siegel MD, Hayes E, Vanderwerker LC, et al. Psychiatric illness in the next of kin of patients who die in the intensive care unit. Crit Care Med 2008;36:1722–8.
61. Knutsson S, Samuelsson IP, Hellström AL, et al. Children's experiences of visiting a seriously ill/injured relative on an adult intensive care unit. J Adv Nurs 2008;61:154–62.
62. Kaasbøll J, Skokauskas N, Lydersen S, et al. Parental chronic illness, internalizing problems in young adulthood and the mediating role of adolescent attachment to parents: a prospective cohort study. Front Psychiatr 2021;12:807563.
63. Piers RD, Azoulay E, Ricou B, et al. Perceptions of appropriateness of care among European and Israeli intensive care unit nurses and physicians. JAMA 2011;306:2694–703.
64. Papazian L, Hraiech S, Loundou A, et al. High-level burnout in physicians and nurses working in adult ICUs: a systematic review and meta-analysis. Intensive Care Med 2023;49:387–400.
65. Wozniak H, Tejero-Aranguren J, Venkataraman V, et al. Care-related regret in the intensive care unit and its association with burnout and intention to change profession: a survey study. J Crit Care 2025;89:155159.
66. Paoli CJ, Reynolds MA, Sinha M, et al. Epidemiology and costs of sepsis in the United States: an analysis based on timing of diagnosis and severity level. Crit Care Med 2018;46:1889–97.
67. van den Berg M, van Beuningen FE, Ter Maaten JC, et al. Hospital-related costs of sepsis around the world: a systematic review exploring the economic burden of sepsis. J Crit Care 2022;71:154096.
68. Liu V, Lei X, Prescott HC, et al. Hospital readmission and healthcare utilization following sepsis in community settings. J Hosp Med 2014;9:502–7.
69. Lindström AC, Eriksson M, Mårtensson J, et al. Nationwide case-control study of risk factors and outcomes for community-acquired sepsis. Sci Rep 2021;11:15118.
70. Martin-Loeches I, Guia MC, Vallecoccia MS, et al. Risk factors for mortality in elderly and very elderly critically ill patients with sepsis: a prospective, observational, multicenter cohort study. Ann Intensive Care 2019;9:26.
71. Haas LEM, Boumendil A, Flaatten H, et al. Frailty is associated with long-term outcome in patients with sepsis who are over 80 years old: results from an observational study in 241 European ICUs. Age Ageing 2021;50:1719–27.
72. Wozniak H, Beckmann TS, Dos Santos Rocha A, et al. Long-stay ICU patients with frailty: mortality and recovery outcomes at 6 months. Ann Intensive Care 2024;14:42.
73. Wozniak H, Santangelo E, McInnis M, et al. Association of musculoskeletal indexes with 1-year outcomes after 7 days of mechanical ventilation. CHEST Crit Care 2025;3:100176.

74. Jaitovich A, Khan MMHS, Itty R, et al. ICU admission muscle and fat mass, survival, and disability at discharge: a prospective cohort study. Chest 2019;155: 322–30.
75. Darvall JN, Bellomo R, Bailey M, et al. Impact of frailty on persistent critical illness: a population-based cohort study. Intensive Care Med 2022;48:343–51.
76. Vincent JL, Marshall JC, Ñamendys-Silva SA, et al. Assessment of the worldwide burden of critical illness: the Intensive Care Over Nations (ICON) audit. Lancet Respir Med 2014;2:380–6.
77. Rüddel H, Rüddel DOT, Reinhart K, et al. Adverse effects of delayed antimicrobial treatment and surgical source control in adults with sepsis: results of a planned secondary analysis of a cluster-randomized controlled trial. Crit Care 2022;26:51.
78. Seymour CW, Gesten F, Prescott HC, et al. Time to treatment and mortality during mandated emergency care for sepsis. N Engl J Med 2017;376:2235–44.
79. PRISM Investigators, Rowan KM, Angus DC, Bailey M, et al. Early, goal-directed therapy for septic shock: a patient-level meta-analysis. N Engl J Med 2017;376: 2223–34.
80. Jernberg C, Löfmark S, Edlund C, et al. Long-term ecological impacts of antibiotic administration on the human intestinal microbiota. ISME J 2007;1:56–66.
81. Brown KA, Khanafer N, Daneman N, et al. Meta-analysis of antibiotics and the risk of community-associated Clostridioides difficile infection. Antimicrob Agents Chemother 2013;57:2326–32.
82. Chanderraj R, Baker JM, Kay SG, et al. In critically ill patients, anti-anaerobic antibiotics increase risk of adverse clinical outcomes. Eur Respir J 2023;61: 2200910.
83. Sehgal P, Piquette D, Detsky M, et al. Critical care education and the ICU care continuum. Am J Respir Crit Care Med 2024;209:360–1.
84. Rahmel T, Schmitz S, Nowak H, et al. Long-term mortality and outcome in hospital survivors of septic shock, sepsis, and severe infections: the importance of aftercare. PLoS One 2020;15:e0228952.
85. Patel BK, Wolfe KS, Patel SB, et al. Effect of early mobilisation on long-term cognitive impairment in critical illness in the USA: a randomised controlled trial. Lancet Respir Med 2023;11:563–72.
86. Boehm LM, Mart MF, LaNoue M, et al. Association between ABCDE bundle compliance and long-term outcomes: a secondary longitudinal analysis. Intensive Care Med 2026;52:466–75.
87. Nielsen AH, Angel S, Egerod I, et al. The effect of family-authored diaries on posttraumatic stress disorder in intensive care unit patients and their relatives: a randomised controlled trial (DRIP-study). Aust Crit Care 2020;33:123–9.
88. Jones C, Bäckman C, Capuzzo M, et al. Intensive care diaries reduce new onset post traumatic stress disorder following critical illness: a randomised, controlled trial. Crit Care 2010;14:R168.
89. Schlapbach LJ, Zimmermann EA, Meylan S, et al. Swiss sepsis national action plan: a coordinated national action plan to stop sepsis-related preventable deaths and to improve the support of people affected by sepsis in Switzerland. Front Med 2023;10:1114546.
90. Australian Commission on Safety and Quality in Health Care. National sepsis program. Available at: https://www.safetyandquality.gov.au/our-work/national-sepsis-program. Accessed May 4, 2026.

91. Schmidt K, Worrack S, von Korff M, et al. Effect of a primary care management intervention on mental health-related quality of life among survivors of sepsis: a randomized clinical trial. JAMA 2016;315:2703–11.
92. Taylor SP, Eaton T, Rios A, et al. Proactive telehealth-based sepsis transition and recovery support, hospital readmission, and mortality: a randomized clinical trial. JAMA Intern Med 2025;185:1238–46.
93. Bircak-Kuchtova B, Rose N, Geis C, et al. Effectiveness of targeted post-acute interventions and follow-up services for sepsis survivors: a systematic review. Crit Care 2025;29:351.
94. Dowdy DW, Needham DM, Mendez-Tellez PA, et al. Studying outcomes of intensive care unit survivors: the role of the cohort study. Intensive Care Med 2005; 31:914–21.
95. Cuthbertson BH, Roughton S, Jenkinson D, et al. Quality of life in the five years after intensive care: a cohort study. Crit Care 2010;14:R6.
96. Wilcox ME, Ely EW. Challenges in conducting long-term outcomes studies in critical care. Curr Opin Crit Care 2019;25:473–88.
97. Pietiläinen L, Hästbacka J, Bäcklund M, et al. Premorbid functional status as a predictor of 1-year mortality and functional status in intensive care patients aged 80 years or older. Intensive Care Med 2018;44:1221–9.
98. Muscedere J, Waters B, Varambally A, et al. The impact of frailty on intensive care unit outcomes: a systematic review and meta-analysis. Intensive Care Med 2017;43:1105–22.
99. Flaws D, Tronstad O, Fraser JF, et al. Tracking outcomes post intensive care: findings of a longitudinal observational study. Aust Crit Care 2025;38:101164.
100. Li M, Harris I, Lu ZK. Differences in proxy-reported and patient-reported outcomes: assessing health and functional status among medicare beneficiaries. BMC Med Res Methodol 2015;15:62.
101. Jeitziner M, Hantikainen V, Conca A, et al. Long-term consequences of an intensive care unit stay in older critically ill patients: design of a longitudinal study. BMC Geriatr 2011;11:52.
102. Sharafoddini A, Dubin JA, Maslove DM, et al. A new insight into missing data in intensive care unit patient profiles: observational study. JMIR Med Inform 2019; 7:e11605.
103. Powney M, Williamson P, Kirkham J, et al. A review of the handling of missing longitudinal outcome data in clinical trials. Trials 2014;15:237.
104. Colantuoni E, Scharfstein DO, Wang C, et al. Statistical methods to compare functional outcomes in randomized controlled trials with high mortality. Br Med J 2018;360:j5748.
105. Williamson PR, Altman DG, Blazeby JM, et al. Developing core outcome sets for clinical trials: issues to consider. Trials 2012;13:132.
106. Clarke M. Standardising outcomes for clinical trials and systematic reviews. Trials 2007;8:39.
107. Caironi P, Latini R, Struck J, et al. Circulating biologically active adrenomedullin predicts hemodynamic support requirement and mortality during sepsis. Chest 2017;152:312–20.
108. Drewry AM, Ablordeppey EA, Murray ET, et al. Comparison of monocyte human leukocyte antigen-DR expression and stimulated tumor necrosis factor alpha production as outcome predictors in severe sepsis: a prospective observational study. Crit Care 2016;20:334.
109. Song J, Park DW, Moon S, et al. Diagnostic and prognostic value of interleukin-6, pentraxin 3, and procalcitonin levels among sepsis and septic shock patients:

a prospective controlled study according to the Sepsis-3 definitions. BMC Infect Dis 2019;19:968.
110. Custodero C, Wu Q, Ghita GL, et al. Prognostic value of NT-proBNP levels in the acute phase of sepsis on lower long-term physical function and muscle strength in sepsis survivors. Crit Care 2019;23:230.
111.. Xu T, Lin C, Huang H, et al. Dynamic profiling of angiogenic, metabolic, and immune checkpoint biomarkers predicts chronic critical illness and long-term outcomes in abdominal sepsis. Shock 2026. https://doi.org/10.1097/SHK.0000000000002829.
112. Gayat E, Cariou A, Deye N, et al. Determinants of long-term outcome in ICU survivors: results from the FROG-ICU study. Crit Care 2018;22:8.
113. Soussi S, Sharma D, Jüni P, et al. Identifying clinical subtypes in sepsis-survivors with different one-year outcomes: a secondary latent class analysis of the FROG-ICU cohort. Crit Care 2022;26:114.
114. Shankar-Hari M, Calandra T, Soares MP, et al. Reframing sepsis immunobiology for translation: towards informative subtyping and targeted immunomodulatory therapies. Lancet Respir Med 2024;12:323–36.
115. Van Nynatten LR, Bokhary D, Wong MYS, et al. Predictive enrichment using biomarkers in studies of critically ill patients with sepsis: a systematic review. Crit Care 2025;29:504.
116. Xiao Z, Zeng L, Chen S, et al. Development and validation of early prediction models for new-onset functional impairment in patients after being transferred from the ICU. Sci Rep 2024;14:12447.
117. Papini S, Iturralde E, Lu Y, et al. Development and validation of a machine learning model using electronic health records to predict trauma- and stressor-related psychiatric disorders after hospitalization with sepsis. Transl Psychiatry 2023;13:400.
118. Liang G, Lu M, Pan Y. Development and validation of an interpretable machine learning model for predicting cognitive impairment in patients with sepsis. Front Med 2026;12:1753260.

Immune-Mediated Inflammatory Diseases and the Critically Ill

Jason Thomas, MBBCh, BAO, MCh[a,*],
Iain McInnes, PhD, FRCP(Gla), FRCP(Edin), FRSE, FMedSci[a],
Lucy McGeoch, MBChB, FRCP(UK)[b]

KEYWORDS

- Immune-mediated inflammatory disease (IMID)
- Inflammatory rheumatic musculoskeletal disease (iRMD) • Critical illness
- Critical care • Intensive care unit (ICU) • Rheumatoid arthritis (RA)

KEY POINTS

- Frailty and co-morbidity, which are highly prevalent in inflammatory rheumatic musculoskeletal disease (iRMD), play major roles in the intensive care unit (ICU) critical illness prognosis.
- Critical illness in iRMDs can pose challenges for diagnosis, disease assessment, and mortality prediction scoring tools.
- Understanding the safety profiles and indications for common anti-rheumatic therapeutics is a vital skill for clinicians in the ICU.

INTRODUCTION

Immune-mediated inflammatory diseases (IMIDs) comprise a range of conditions that share common underlying etiology manifest by dysregulated inflammation and variably, by the presence of autoimmunity.[1] IMIDs are clinically heterogeneous, usually associated with substantial morbidity and increased mortality, and impose a substantial burden on the individual, their families and wider society. IMIDs' estimated prevalence is around 10% of the global population and, as such, they are frequently represented in the critically ill hospital population. The range of IMIDs across disciplines is depicted in **Table 1**. IMIDs in general are associated with diminished effector immune-mediated defense, unstable immune homeostasis, with

[a] College of Medical, Veterinary and Life Sciences, University of Glasgow, Glasgow, UK; [b] Centre for Rheumatic Diseases, Glasgow Royal Infirmary, Glasgow, Scotland
* Corresponding author. College of Medical, Veterinary & Life Sciences, Wolfson Medical School Building, University of Glasgow, University Avenue, Glasgow, G12 8QQ.
E-mail address: jasonsamthomas@gmail.com

Crit Care Clin 42 (2026) 701–718
https://doi.org/10.1016/j.ccc.2026.05.001 **criticalcare.theclinics.com**

Abbreviations	
APACHE II	Acute Physiology and Chronic Health Evaluation II
APRs	acute phase reactants
CVD	cardiovascular disease
DMARDs	disease modifying anti-arthritic drugs
ECMO	extracorporeal membrane oxygenation
GCs	glucocorticoids
IMID	immune-mediated inflammatory disease
iRMD	inflammatory rheumatic musculoskeletal disease
ILD	interstitial lung disease
JAKi	Janus Kinase Inhibitors
LODS	Logistic Organ Dysfunction System
LN	lupus nephritis
MAS	Macrophage activation syndrome
SAPS	Simplified Acute Physiology Score
SOFA	Sequential Organ Failure Assessment

consequences for poor healing and delayed immune restitution after an infection induced immune response, and collectively are associated with poorer outcomes in the context of critical illness. They are usually chronic, exhibiting flare/remission patterns over time, with unpredictable trajectories, and as such accrued target tissue damage poses a further challenge in the context of critical illness. Consider for example, impaired renal function, pulmonary function, bone marrow reserve, mobility, sarcopenia. Finally, IMIDs are associated with substantial co-morbidity and multi-morbidity.

In addition to the challenges imposed by primary immune dysregulation, IMIDs share common risks inherent in immune suppression as a result of therapeutic interventions. The latter have been revolutionized in the last 2 decades. The field is quickly moving away from the use of broad-spectrum immune suppression, for example, methotrexate, gold, sulfasalazine, mesalazine, azathioprine, cyclosporin, and cyclophosphamide. Such medications offered some degree of efficacy across the range of IMIDs but were also associated with substantial toxicity and significant immune suppression, reducing host immune integrity with infectious consequences, and rendering vaccine and other prophylactic strategies suspect. Glucocorticoids (GCs) are of longest standing and represent perhaps the most perplexing of risk-benefit ratios in IMID management—overall their use is now focused on minimized dose administration for the shortest reasonable time.

The advent of biological therapeutics targeting pro-inflammatory cytokines, for example, TNF, IL-6, BlyS, IL-17A, IL-17F, IL-4, IL-5, type 1 interferons, and now upstream regulatory cytokines, for example, IL-23, has been transformative. To this armamentarium has been added cell targeting biological therapeutics, for example, B cell depleters that remove CD20, CD22, and CD19 cell subsets to variable degrees, and checkpoint regulators, for example, abatacept. Finally, an increasing array of oral selective immune modifiers are available, pioneered by the JAKinibs that inhibit proximal receptor Janus kinase family members, for example, JAK1, JAK3, TYK2. Remission can now often be achieved and maintained with long term drug administration and function and therefore tissue damage has been substantially reduced. This is a rich field of current drug development, and many more agents are anticipated in the next decade. Moreover, such immune selectivity has improved the tolerability and overall safety profile of immune suppression. However, the immune therapeutic revolution has not removed the primary risk of infection, usually with an odds ratio of

Table 1
List of IMIDs across disciplines[2]

Discipline	IMID
Rheumatology	Inflammatory arthropathies: (Rheumatoid arthritis, Spondyloarthropathies, Gout) Systemic lupus erythematosus (SLE) Scleroderma Vasculitis Myositis
Dermatology	Psoriasis (PsO) Atopic dermatitis Hidradenitis suppurativa
Gastroenterology	Crohn's Disease Ulcerative colitis (UC) Autoimmune hepatitis
Neurology	Multiple sclerosis (MS) Autoimmune neuropathies
Respiratory	Asthma Chronic obstructive pulmonary disease (COPD) Interstitial lung disease (ILD)
Ophthalmology	Uveitis
Renal	Immune mediated nephritides (e.g. SLE) IgA nephropathy Vasculitides

Abbreviation: IMRD, immune-mediated inflammatory diseases.

between 1.5 and 2, nor indeed the risk of immune dysregulation in response to such insult. It is timely therefore to briefly review the main considerations posed by IMIDs to those responsible for critical care. Whereas the principles of management of the IMID patient who is critically ill are similar across disciplines, herein we will focus our article to inflammatory rheumatic musculoskeletal diseases (iRMD). Our purpose is to summarize the literature surrounding etiology, prognosis, predisposing factors and management of iRMD and critical illness.

METHODS

A systematic search strategy was employed and implemented through Embase and Pubmed. The following search was undertaken: "(((Critically ill) OR (Intensive Care Unit) OR (High dependency unit) OR (Critical care unit) OR (sepsis) OR (septic) OR (life-threatening)) AND ((autoimmune) OR (immune mediated) OR (connective tissue disease) OR (Rheumatoid arthritis) OR (spondyloarthropathy)) AND ((DMARD) OR (Biologic)))." The inclusion criteria included meta-analyses, systematic reviews, standard approved guidelines and occasional high impact original articles/studies of relevance. The date range for the search was limited from January 2000 to February 2026. The research team also employed a systematic waterfall (cascade) approach to identify relevant studies.

Critical Illness and Immune-Mediated Inflammatory Diseases—Antecedent and Complicating Risk Factors?

Critical illness is a common complication of iRMDs. As many as one-third of hospitalized iRMD patients will require ICU admission.[3] It is notable however, that a majority of IMIDs are treated in the out-patient environment and as such the in-patient cohort represents a more severely afflicted patient subset. Sepsis (61.6%) and infection (47%) are the most common etiologies of critical illness and ICU admission in iRMDs. Flare of iRMD itself (32.8%–48%) and cardiovascular events (33.9%) account for a further tranche of admissions.[4–6]

Occasionally, critical illness can be the precipitating cause for diagnosing iRDs and be the primary clinical presentation (10.9% in one single-center retrospective study).[7] The purpose of this article is to compile the literature surrounding etiology, prognosis, predisposing factors and management of iRD critical illness, into a comprehensive and cohesive summary. Many factors might contribute to these admission rates. In particular, comorbidity, defined as the coexistence of at least 2 medical conditions occurring in one individual in which an index disease occurs first[8] is found in up to 92% of iRMD patients admitted to the ICU and is a major contributor to prognosis and etiology for iRD-related critical illness.[9] iRMDs are associated with numerous co-morbid conditions including increased risk of major adverse cardiac events, obesity, diabetes, mental health disorders, osteoporosis, and cancer incidence and prevalence. Accelerated immune system aging, or immunosenescence, is frequent in iRMDs and may also contribute (**Fig. 1**).[10]

In parallel, frailty is common in iRMDs, for example, occurring in as many as 23% of RA patients.[11] Frailty and co-morbidity are often mis-defined and used interchangeably. Frailty has a number of defining features, namely by phenotype and index definitions.[8] It can be defined as an indicator of aging and is linked to an increased risk of negative outcomes such as falls, injuries, and mortality with worse outcomes compared with their age-matched counterparts. Physiologic reserve significantly decreases in iRMD and is synonymous with the concept of frailty in this patient cohort.[12]

Specific attention should be paid to CVD risks. iRMDs are strongly linked with increased prevalence and early onset of cardiovascular disease (CVD). CVD-related complications arise from immune mediated acceleration of atherosclerotic plaque formation and subsequent rupture.[13] Circulating cytokines, acute phase reactants (APRs), immune complexes, and complement components are implicated. Moreover, lipoprotein assembly and composition are altered in iRMDs—for example, HDL loses its athero-protective properties, - as is cholesterol transport and metabolism. In parallel, acute CVD presentations such as pericardial disease, heart failure exacerbations and inflammatory cardiomyopathy may also represent a primary manifestation of

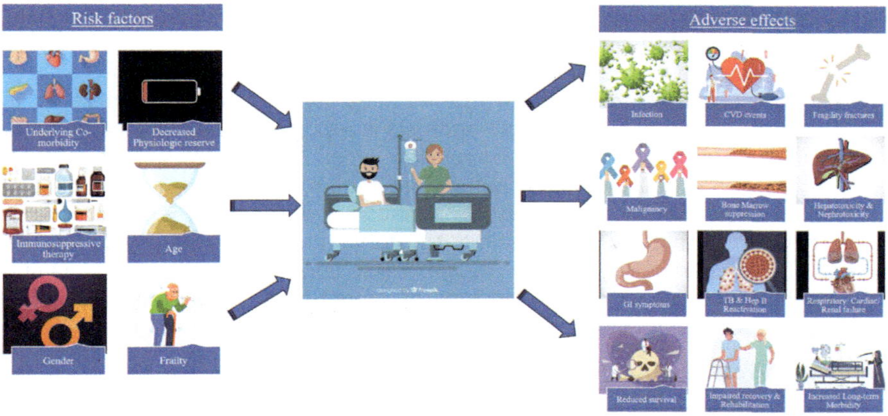

Fig. 1. Risk factors and adverse effects of critical illness in iRMD. Graphic depicting risk factors for developing critical illness in iRMD on the left side and adverse effects associated with critical illness in iRMD on the right side. iRMD, inflammatory rheumatic musculoskeletal disease. (Designed using Freepik.)

iRMD.[14,15] A further CVD risk is iRMD-induced anemia, arising from immune-mediated erythropoiesis impairment, shortened erythrocyte half-life and blunted erythropoietin activity.[16]

As an exemplar of the magnitude of risk, consider the COMORA trial that identified incidence rates of hypertension (40.4%) and hypercholesterolaemia in patients with RA (31.7%).[17] Rates are probably higher still in SLE and systemic sclerosis. By corollary, a high index of suspicion for the presence of compromised CV function in iRMDs should be assumed in the critically ill.

Cognitive dysfunction from iRMD can manifest as impaired orientation, attention/concentration, judgment/problem solving and memory, verbal, visual/spatial and executive functions.[18] Cognitive impairment as a comorbidity negatively impacts patient prognosis in critical care. Delirium leads to higher risk of mortality, length of stay, higher costs, poor mental health, and functional disability in ICUs.[19] RA with dementia shows poorer cognitive function and an increased mortality risk when compared with non-RA dementia cohorts.[20]

Other studies have linked the presence of iRDs with a higher rate of impairments across a range of cognitive domains.[21] Long-term treatment with disease modifying anti-arthritic drugs (DMARDs) such as MTX and GCs have been variously reported to contribute to this dysfunction both positively and negatively.[13] Recently, we proposed the existence of a brain joint axis that integrated immune, endocrine and neurologic pathways that combine to alter mental health and cognition in iRMDs.[22]

This axis is mediated by and number of effector mechanisms. Thus, excess levels of circulating proinflammatory cytokines (such as IL-6, IL-1β, TNF-α) may cross a vulnerable blood brain barrier to drive microglial activation and consequent neuronal dysfunction, altered neuroplasticity and altered nuclear connectivities. Migrating cell lineages, especially of myeloid origin may also migrate to the brain and participate in cognitive decline. Similarly, autoantibodies may be implicated in the pathogenesis of this cognitive decline through neuroinflammation and neurotoxicity driven in the cerebral parenchyma.[23] The critical consequence of this emerging and compelling component of IMID pathogenesis is that evaluation of cognitive function and consciousness in the critically ill patient should be considered to be challenging in the context of iRMDs and a high level of vigilance to the contribution of underlying inflammatory disease, as opposed to that driven by metabolic, fluid shift, hypoxic, and other ICU stressors should be maintained.

Finally, iRMD patients are particularly prone to osteopaenia, osteoporosis, fragility fractures and poor bone health.[24] Osteoporosis is reported to be twice as common in patients with RA as in the general population, presenting in 30% to 50% of all RA patients.[25,26] This is multifactorial in nature, but occurs more often in iRMD patients with high disease activity (increased inflammation), varying BMI, female predominance, decreased mobility, and treatment history with GCs.[27,28] Systemic iRMDs such as SLE are particularly at risk. Though of less importance in the acute setting, bone health becomes a critical element of longer-term rehabilitation post-ICU discharge, especially in the context of significant sarcopenia.

Factors that Predispose to Becoming Critically Ill

As noted, life-threatening illness in iRMD has a number of etiologies, including iRMD flares, superimposed infection from immunosuppression, adverse effects of therapeutics, malignancy secondary to medication and secondary illness unrelated to yet exacerbated by iRMDs.[3] RA and systemic inflammatory diseases (formerly connective tissue diseases) are considered to be the most common iRMDs to develop critical illness and necessitate ICU admission.[6,29] Rheumatologic specific emergencies include Pulmonary-Renal Syndrome, Sclerodermal renal crisis, Macrophage activation syndrome (MAS), and Catastrophic antiphospholipid syndrome, and all have a high associated mortality.[30]

Long-term effects of immune-mediated inflammatory diseases and physiologic reserve

The basis of IMID pathogenesis circulates around chronic inflammation and consequent accrual of progressive injury to multiple -organ systems. End organ damage is prevalent among all iRMDs and should be assumed to extend well beyond signature target organs to include major organs and their functional reserve. Thus, the respiratory system, kidneys, gastrointestinal tract/liver and blood/coagulation are most frequently affected systems at the time ICU admission and all should be considered potentially compromised a priori by coincident iRMD.[7]

Physiologic reserve is negatively affected by accrued end-organ damage. This decrease predisposes to acute decompensation when faced with stressors such as infection, inflammatory flares, and surgery. Impaired functional reserve increases the risk of ICU admission and worsens prognosis in iRMD.[31] Functional reserve also significantly decreases in iRMD patients following discharge from critical care. Some studies have reported, a 1 year mortality of ~30%.[4]

Cardio-pulmonary end-organ impairment

Pulmonary involvement encountered in patients with iRD bears clinical significance in terms of increased morbidity and mortality. Interstitial lung disease (ILD) is a major morbidity/mortality risk among the RA and SLE patient cohorts.[32] Restrictive lung conditions that stem from iRMDs significantly predispose to rapid deterioration of end-organ function. One multi-center study found respiratory failure to be the leading cause of ICU admission in critical iRMD patients (56.8%).[6] ILD may not be clinically obvious—for example, up to 58% of RA patients have been reported to suffer from RA-ILD at some level, usually sub-clinical and undetected, but nevertheless carrying potential for functional significance in the event of ICU admission[33]

In addition to the accelerated CVD morbidity described above, iRMDs, best exemplified in RA and SLE, typically may manifest cardiac impairment as part of the primary disease syndrome, through valvular impairment, cardiac arrhythmia, cardiomyopathy, pericardial disease, and heart failure.[34] The most numerous causes of ICU admission and critical illness in this population are coronary events linked with iRMDs.[35] At the coronary artery level, endothelial dysfunction in large and small vessels can lead to ischemic heart disease, either secondary or not, to atherosclerosis.[34]

Renal end-organ impairment

Renal disease is common in iRMDs and carries adverse prognostic implication in the critical care setting. However, variations are apparent in reported prevalence of renal disease in iRMDs, with older studies showing higher rates and newer evidence showing improvement (likely from tighter DMARD control and monitoring enhancements).[36] One study states that 18% of iRMD patients have stage 3 CKD or poorer, in comparison to 5% in the general population.[37,38] The MATRIX study showed that RA patients present with stage 2 (20%–20.3%) and stage 3 (15%–24.1%) kidney disease.[39] Some studies report as low as 5% prevalence in RA patients.[40] Some reports state that acute renal failure is the most common organ failure among the critically ill iRMD patients in ICU.[5]

The etiology of renal end-organ impairment stems from a wider range of factors including the use of NSAIDs, DMARDs and other immune modulator therapeutics that have nephrotoxic adverse events, secondary renal amyloidosis, progressive glomerulonephritis, immune complex deposition and others.[41] Consider that lupus nephritis (LN) will develop within 10 years of SLE diagnosis and in turn, 5% to 20% of patients with LN develop end-stage kidney disease.[42]

Effects of therapeutics on the likelihood of becoming critically ill

The therapeutic protocols used most widely for iRMDs are defined in international recommendations and guidelines published by international societies such as EULAR and ACR. Such approaches, combined with the strategic evolution of iRMD treatment to embrace "Treat to Target," whereby therapeutics are escalated until disease activity is minimized, has on balance driven a more aggressive use of DMARDs, biologics, corticosteroids and other immunosuppressants. This has had beneficial impact on clinical outcomes for the iRMDs, and indeed reduces attendant co-morbidities associated with iRMDs. However, these approaches modify host defense immunologic pathways and may in the 'wrong context' predispose to accelerated critical care presentation and progression. In one analysis, iRMD patients in ICU settings were found to be on GCs (66%), DMARDs (18%), immunosuppressants (16%), and anti-TNF drugs (6%), respectively.[5,43]

Conventional use of immunosuppressants (eg, azathioprine, cyclosporin, mycophenolate, cyclophosphamide), are associated with opportunistic pathogens potentially resulting in critical illnesses secondary to infection.[3]

GCs are very effective in treating iRDs, specifically in acute flares, but significantly increase the likelihood of becoming critically ill by masking inflammatory symptoms. GCs risks accrue especially in patients receiving long-term oral doses above 7 mg/day (prednisone equivalent).[44,45]

Biological and targeted synthetic DMARDs (**Table 2**) are variously associated with increased infection risk and as such will increase the likelihood of critical illness. There is however a curious relationship for TNFi whereby the risk of ICU admission is increased by this drug class, but survival once admitted is better in those on TNFi at admission.[46] These data emphasize the ying-yang of immune mediated tissue damage and organ failure balanced with essential immune defense.

Table 2
Summary of the most commonly used anti-rheumatic medications for the management of iRDs and their associated drug class, indications, and adverse effects[83–87]

Drug Class	Medication	Indication for Use	Indication for Stopping	Common Adverse Effects
Glucocorticoids (GCs)	Prednisone Prednisolone Dexamethasone Hydrocortisone Methylprednisolone Betamethasone	Bridging therapy Flare management RA, SLE, PMR, and other iRDs	Sustained remission	Infections, CVD events, HTN, Diabetes Osteoporosis/fractures, GI effects, Psychological/ behavioural changes, Dermatological effects, Cataracts/ glaucoma, Weight gain, oedema
TNF Inhibitors (bDMARD)	Adalimumab Certolizumab Etanercept Golimumab Infliximab	RA, PsA, AS, axSpA	Active serious infection, TB, Demyelinating disease, Severe heart failure, Malignancy	Serious infections, TB & hepatitis B reactivation, injection site/infusion reactions, Malignancy, Demyelinating disorders, Lupus-like syndrome, Heart failure exacerbation
Anti-IL-1 (bDMARD)	Anakinra	RA, NOMID, DIRA, AOSD	Active serious infection	Injection site reactions, infections, neutropenia, headache
Anti-IL-6/IL-6R (bDMARD)	Tocilizumab Sarilumab	RA, GCA, PMR, polyarticular	Active serious infection, Diverticulitis/GI	Serious infections, GI perforation, Neutropenia, thrombocytopenia, Elevated liver enzymes,
		JIA, systemic JIA	perforation risk, Severe neutropenia, Severe thrombocytopenia, Elevated transaminases	Hyperlipidemia, Injection site reactions
Anti-IL-12/23 (bDMARD)	Ustekinumab	PsA, PsO, Crohn's disease, UC	Active serious infection, tuberculosis	Infections, nasopharyngitis, Headache, fatigue
Anti-IL-23 (bDMARD)	Guselkumab Risankizumab Tildrakizumab	PsA, PsO, Crohn's disease, UC	Active serious infection	Infections, URTIs, nasopharyngitis, Headache
Anti-IL-17A Anti- IL-17AF (bDMARD)	Secukinumab Ixekizumab Bimekizumab	PsA, AS, axSpA, PsO, enthesitis-related arthritis	Active serious infection, inflammatory bowel disease (relative contraindication)	Infections, nasopharyngitis, URTI, candida infections, IBD exacerbation
Anti-Interferon (bDMARD)	Anifrolumab	SLE	Active serious infection, tuberculosis	Infections, infusion reactions, herpes zoster
Anti-B Cell (bDMARD)	Rituximab Belimumab	Rituximab: RA, vasculitis Belimumab: SLE, lupus nephritis	Active serious infection, hepatitis B, Progressive multifocal leukoencephalopathy (PML)	Rituximab: Serious infections, hepatitis B reactivation, PML, cardiac reactions, infusion reactions, cytopenias Belimumab: Infections, infusion reactions, depression

(*continued on next page*)

Table 2
(*continued*)

CD28 Inhibitor (bDMARD)	Abatacept	RA, polyarticular JIA, PsA	Active serious infection, TB, COPD exacerbation	Infections, nasopharyngitis, COPD exacerbation, headache, Infusion/injection reactions
csDMARDs	Methotrexate	1st line DMARD for RA, PsA, JIA, and other inflammatory arthritides	Pregnancy, severe liver or kidney disease, bone marrow suppression, active infection, pneumonitis	Nausea, stomatitis, alopecia, hepatotoxicity, bone marrow suppression, pneumonitis (rare), diarrhea, fatigue, headache
csDMARDs	Sulfasalazine (SFZ)	RA, PsA, AS, axSpA	Hypersensitivity to sulfonamides/salicylates, Active infection	Rash, N+V+D, anorexia, Hypersensitivity reactions, agranulocytosis, Hepatotoxicity, azoospermia
csDMARDs	Hydroxychloroquine	RA, SLE, mild inflammatory arthritis	Retinopathy, hypersensitivity to 4-aminoquinoline compounds	Retinal toxicity, GI upset, rash, myelosuppression (rare), cardiomyopathy (rare), QT prolongation
csDMARDs	Leflunomide (LEF)	RA, PsA	Pregnancy (requires elimination protocol), severe liver disease, active infection	Diarrhea, nausea, alopecia, HTN, hepatotoxicity, bone marrow suppression, peripheral neuropathy
csDMARDs	Azathioprine	SLE, vasculitis, myositis, other inflammatory rheumatic diseases	Pregnancy (relative), severe bone marrow suppression, active infection	Bone marrow suppression, hepatotoxicity, GI upset, infections, increased malignancy risk
csDMARDs	Cyclophosphamide	Severe SLE, vasculitis, severe organ-threatening disease	Active infection, severe bone marrow suppression, hemorrhagic cystitis	Bone marrow suppression, hemorrhagic cystitis, infections, infertility, malignancy, alopecia, nausea
csDMARDs	Ciclosporin Voclosporin	RA (rarely), SLE, lupus nephritis	Uncontrolled hypertension, severe renal impairment, active infection	Nephrotoxicity, hypertension, hirsutism, gingival hyperplasia, tremor, infections
csDMARDs	Mycophenolate mofetil or Mycophenolic acid	SLE, lupus nephritis, vasculitis, myositis	Pregnancy, active serious infection	GI upset (diarrhea, nausea), bone marrow suppression, infections, hepatotoxicity
JAK Inhibitors	Tofacitinib Baricitinib Upadacitinib Filgotinib	RA, PsA, AS, axSpA, JIA	Active serious infection, age ≥65 years with CVD RFs, malignancy, VTE risk	Infections (herpes zoster), MACE, VTE, malignancy, elevated liver enzymes, hyperlipidaemia, cytopenias (anaemia, neutropenia, lymphopenia), GI perforation, headache, nasopharyngitis, elevated creatine kinase

Abbreviations: AOSD, adult-onset Still's disease; axSpA, axial spondyloarthritis; DIRA, deficiency of the interleukin-1 receptor antagonist; JIA, juvenile idiopathic arthritis; MACE, major adverse cardiovascular events; NOMID, neonatal-onset multisystem inflammatory disease; PMR, polymyalgia rheumatica; VTE, venous thromboembolism.

There are interactions also between the pathogenetic effector pathways of iRMDs and relevant therapeutics. For example, RA is associated with developing septic arthritis; greater than 35 times greater likelihood. This is attributed to joint damage, immune defense vulnerability arising from RA pathogenesis, treatment with corticosteroids, DMARDs and biological therapies.[47]

Side effects of treatment may also be idiosyncratic, for example, methotrexate (MTX) can induce MAS in RA.[48]

Finally, there is an indirect relationship between biological and tsDMARD therapeutics via altered vaccine efficacy, which, in turn, increase infection risks a priori. The most remarkable effects are those mediated by rituximab. However, MTX, abatacept, JAKinibs and TNFi reduce vaccine induced protective antibody titers, though this correlates poorly with protection.[49]

Impact of Inflammatory Rheumatic Musculoskeletal Diseases on Disease/Mortality Evaluation

Mortality rates in critically ill iRMD patients vary across studies. One retrospective study found that the 5 year survival in RA patients after ICU admission was 47%, and 30 day, 90 day, and 1 year mortality rates were 22%, 27%, and 37%, respectively.[50] However, other studies suggested either no prognostic difference,[51] or an increased mortality rate.[29]

Sepsis and systemic autoimmune inflammatory disease flares share very similar clinical presentations and can be difficult to distinguish in critical care settings. Even with extensive use of conventional clinical, blood-based and imaging tools, it can be a challenge to accurately come to a definitive diagnosis.

Critical illness scoring systems

Clinical severity tools such as Sequential Organ Failure Assessment (SOFA), Simplified Acute Physiology Score (SAPS), National Early Warning Score (NEWS), Acute Physiology and Chronic Health Evaluation II (APACHE II), Mortality Probability Model, and Mortality in Emergency Department Sepsis are all utilized in the ICU to evaluate mortality risks and prognoses. The most common validated severity scoring systems used in unwell ICU patients are designed for the general population as opposed to those with iRD.

Common scoring systems such as APACHE II, have demonstrated high score correlation with a higher predictive estimation of mortality in iRD patients.[29,52] ODIN and APACHE II are good predictors for iRD patient mortality in the ICU.[9] SOFA scores can be unreliable, as one study found some accurate correlation with crude mortality, but underestimated short term mortality overall.[6] Another study showed that the mortality rates (16%) observed were in alignment with expected mortality rates associated with their values on their SAPS2 and Logistic Organ Dysfunction System (LODS) scores.[5] The LODS score assesses organ failure severity in ICU patients and may be a useful predictor of 30 day mortality in the critically ill iRMD patient.[5]

Specific but less commonly used tools exist that are only of tangential value as they do not directly address the prognostic challenge. The Rheumatic Disease Comorbidity Index measures mortality with co-morbidity in iRMD.[53]

The CORAL score has shown promising results to identify high risk serious infection in iRMD patients, in those with prolonged high-dose GCs.[54]

Specific scoring systems depicting iRMD disease activity at a given timepoint, such as the Disease Activity Score with 28-Joint Counts, SS Disease Damage Index, and Systemic Lupus Erythematosus Disease Activity Index are widely available but evolved to support clinical trial and clinical monitoring of iRMD disease activity.[55]

These are not specifically used for assessing prognosis or mortality.[56]

Acute phase reactants

APRs such as CRP, SAA, and ESR are standard biomarkers for assessing inflammatory responses in critically unwell and septic patients. Skewed interpretation of severity scores that utilize these APRs can occur, leading to misrepresentation, especially in the critically ill in which either infection or iRMD activity could theoretically drive their elevation.[57] IL-6 levels are associated with iRMD flares. Combining SAPS with IL-6 concentrations may offer more accurate risk stratification in iRMDs.[58] Caution should be exercised in the interpretation of APRs in patients receiving drugs that inhibit IL-6R, for example, tocilizumab or its proximal signaling, for example, JAKinibs. They may normalize APRs as a pharmacodynamic effect of hepatic IL-6R signal inhibition, independent of true clinical improvement.[57,59]

Procalcitonin is a proposed differentiator between disease flare and bacterial sepsis, particularly in comparison with general inflammatory markers like CRP and ESR. It has greater specificity and sensitivity in JIA and SLE.[60] Additionally, procalcitonin with presepsin may offer strong diagnostic potential for differentiating iRMD flare from bacterial sepsis.[61] Albumin has long been considered a prognostic indicator of mortality, length of stay, and re-admission in ICU patients. Although serum albumin levels inversely correlate to IMID activity, they also correlate with septic and critically unwell ICU patients, so it is not recommended as a reliable differentiator.[62]

Therapeutic Mx of iRDs in Context of the Critically Ill

Diagnostic challenges

Determining whether critical illness is co-existent with iRMD, or directly arising from iRMD exacerbation, is a fundamental step in management planning. Understanding that these presentations can occur simultaneously is a valuable insight for responsible clinicians. Early identification and admission to ICU, with multidisciplinary management for these patients allows for a more favorable outcome.[63]

General considerations around immune modulators

Guidelines surrounding immunomodulatory agent use in iRMD-associated infection is generally to withhold these agents temporarily, unless there is a pressing iRD flare that is coincident. Balancing the benefits of immunosuppressive therapy for iRMD flare management, with the risk of superimposed infection is a major challenge faced by in ICU, and best practice is still debated. However, 30 day mortality in those treated with immunosuppressive therapy has been shown to be acceptable in this cohort and not consistent with an increased risk of severe infection, matching the expected mortality rate.[5]

An argument can be made that organ failure associated with acute flare is the main driver of acquired infection in ICU admitted iRMD patients, as opposed to immunosuppressive treatments. Secondary organ failure predisposes to acquired infection through impaired immune function. In one retrospective study, fear of acquired infection should not prompt withholding in-ICU use of immunosuppressants.[64] There are however conflicting approaches, and further research is required. At present therefore clinical judgment is vital and communication between ICU and iRMD specialists essential. There are extensive recommendations and points to consider offered by EULAR (https://www.eular.org/recommendations-home) and ACR (https://rheumatology.org/clinical-practice-guidelines).

Glucocorticoids

GCs are a significant concern in the ICU setting. One study showed that 92.2% of patients were already receiving steroids at the time of ICU admission, in a median dose of 20 mg/day (prednisone equivalent).[5] Meta-analysis shows that the use of GCs in septic patients has been associated with significant improvement in 28 day mortality.[65] However, immunomodulatory drugs that have the greatest immunosuppressant effects, including cyclophosphamide and GCs, are considered to have the highest risk of serious infection.[66] Understanding their high risk and benefit profile is important for clinical guidance. The use of steroids and its associated dosing are highly dependent on disease severity as opposed to specific iRMD indications.[67] iRMD patients may require higher dosing and longer durations of GC administration for effective management.[7]

Given chronic GC use, a proportion of iRMD patients are adrenal insufficient and at risk of adrenal crisis.[68] Iatrogenic adrenal insufficiency secondary occurs in up to 48% of RA patients.[69] Management as per the European Society of Endocrinology guidelines for adrenal crisis in iRMD is advised and includes parenteral GC in critical illness.[70] The reader is also referred to a variety of EULAR recommendations concerning GC use and risks (www.eular.org).

Janus kinase inhibitors (tsDMARDs)

JAKinibs, tsDMARDs, are increasingly used across a range of iRMDs.[71]

A comprehensive meta-analysis of Janus Kinase Inhibitors (JAKi) showed that tofacitinib, baricitinib, and upadacitinib all exhibited a significantly increased risk of serious infections compared with placebo.[72] Dose-dependent differences have been observed with varying infection risks from a recent expert consensus statement.[73] In this statement, no current JAKi displayed a higher infection risk compared with the others, though filgotinib had a lower risk of herpes zoster.[73] In RA patients, the use of tofacitinib compared with non-TNF biologics, though not definitive, did not demonstrate differences in hospitalized infections or effectiveness.[74] Given the high rate of overlap in iRMD patients with renal failure, caution should be taken when prescribing JAKis as they are contraindicated for patients with creatinine clearance of less than 15 mL/min.[73] Overall, therefore the use of JAKinibs in the ICU setting is uncertain. Short cessation may be helpful given their short half-life in the context of overwhelming sepsis. Some JAKinibs reduced mortality when used in critical COVID-19 infection and ventilatory support.[75] We can learn more about the safety of these and similar medications through upcoming trials such as the PANTHER trial.[76]

Biologics (bDMARD)

Meta-analysis findings comparing biologics versus csDMARDS have shown that high-dose biologics have a higher risk of associated infection, whereas low dose biologics do not show a difference.[77]

Newer evidence however suggests that biologics/bDMARDs have either no difference in infective rates, or perhaps even a preferable and lower risk of recurrent serious infection.[78,79] bDMARDs are often therefore withheld in ICU with infection, though, in some context, IL-6R inhibitors may offer beneficial outcomes, for example, in COVID-19.[80–82]

Extracorporeal membrane oxygenation, ventilation, renal replacement therapy (RRT)

Extracorporeal membrane oxygenation (ECMO) therapy has been shown to be used in treatment more frequently in patients with iRMD related critical illness (16.1% vs 5.2%, $P = .019$).[7] A benefit/risk ratio of immunosuppressant administration should be undertaken for patients receiving mechanical ventilation, renal replacement therapy, or

ECMO, as these treatments for end-organ failure have a higher risk of acquired infection when given simultaneously.[64]

SUMMARY

Many challenges arise when iRMDs are encountered in the ICU. Attention to the patient as a whole in terms of functional reserve, frailty, and co-morbidities are vital. Recognizing the potential for rapid progression from disease flare and sepsis to multi-organ failure should permit earlier focused management, and will significantly improve outcomes. Therapeutics in iRMD management including csDMARDS, tsDMARDs/JAKis, bDMARDS, immunosuppressants, and GC have been transformative in the iRMD field but carry risk. Physicians should be aware of the protocols and recommendations for therapeutic alterations in critical illnesses. And these are sign-posted in this article. Employing a multidisciplinary approach to managing iRMD in the ICU and, reciprocally, critical illness in the iRMDs is vital.

CLINICS CARE POINTS

- Understanding the aetiology, risk factors, co-morbidities and management of iRMDs is a vital skill for clinicians in the ICU.
- Critical illness in iRMDs can pose challenges for diagnosis, disease assessment, and mortality prediction scoring tools, so caution with interpretation should be used.
- Early intervention can have significant effects on the high mortality rates associated with iRMDs.

DISCLOSURES

The authors have no financial disclosures or conflicts of interest to disclose.

REFERENCES

1. McInnes IB, Gravallese EM. Immune-mediated inflammatory disease therapeutics: past, present and future. Nat Rev Immunol 2021;21(10):680–6.
2. Monteleone G, Moscardelli A, Colella A, et al. Immune-mediated inflammatory diseases: common and different pathogenic and clinical features. Autoimmun Rev 2023;22(10):103410.
3. Janssen NM, Karnad DR, Guntupalli KK. Rheumatologic diseases in the intensive care unit: epidemiology, clinical approach, management, and outcome. Crit Care Clin 2002;18(4):729–48.
4. Chabert P, Danjou W, Mezidi M, et al. Short- and long-term prognosis of acute critically ill patients with systemic rheumatic diseases: a retrospective multicentre study. Medicine 2021;100(35).
5. Faguer S, Ciroldi M, Mariotte E, et al. Prognostic contributions of the underlying inflammatory disease and acute organ dysfunction in critically ill patients with systemic rheumatic diseases. Eur J Intern Med 2013;24(3):e40–4.
6. Dumas G, Géri G, Montlahuc C, et al. Outcomes in critically ill patients with systemic rheumatic disease: a multicenter study. Chest 2015;148(4):927–35.
7. Schneeweiss-Gleixner M, Hillebrand C, Jaksits S, et al. Characteristics and outcome of critically ill patients with systemic rheumatic diseases referred to the intensive care unit. RMD Open 2023;9(4):e003287. https://doi.org/10.1136/rmdopen-2023-003287.

8. Espinoza SE, Quiben M, Hazuda HP. Distinguishing comorbidity, disability, and frailty. Curr Geriatr Rep 2018;7(4):201–9.
9. Camargo JF, Tobón GJ, Fonseca N, et al. Autoimmune rheumatic diseases in the intensive care unit: experience from a tertiary referral hospital and review of the literature. Lupus 2005;14(4):315–20.
10. Salaffi F, Di Matteo A, Farah S, et al. Inflammaging and frailty in immune-mediated rheumatic diseases: how to address and score the issue. Clin Rev Allergy Immunol 2023;64(2):206–21.
11. Hanlon P, Morton F, Siebert S, et al. Frailty in rheumatoid arthritis and its relationship with disease activity, hospitalisation and mortality: a longitudinal analysis of the Scottish early rheumatoid arthritis cohort and UK biobank. RMD Open 2022; 8(1):e002111. https://doi.org/10.1136/rmdopen-2021-002111.
12. Motta F, Sica A, Selmi C. Frailty in rheumatic diseases. Front Immunol 2020;11: 576134. https://doi.org/10.3389/fimmu.2020.576134.
13. Buch MH, Mallat Z, Dweck MR, et al. Current understanding and management of cardiovascular involvement in rheumatic immune-mediated inflammatory diseases. Nat Rev Rheumatol 2024;20(10):614–34.
14. Weber BN, Garshick M, Abbate A, et al. Acute cardiovascular complications of immune-mediated systemic inflammatory diseases. European Heart Journal Acute Cardiovascular Care 2023;12(11):792–801.
15. Wassif H, Saad M, Desai R, et al. Outcomes following acute coronary syndrome in patients with and without rheumatic immune-mediated inflammatory diseases. J Am Heart Assoc 2022;11(18):e026411.
16. Weiss G, Schett G. Anaemia in inflammatory rheumatic diseases. Nat Rev Rheumatol 2013;9(4):205–15.
17. Dougados M, Soubrier M, Antunez A, et al. Prevalence of comorbidities in rheumatoid arthritis and evaluation of their monitoring: results of an international, cross-sectional study (COMORA). Ann Rheum Dis 2014;73(1):62–8.
18. Meade T, Manolios N, Cumming SR, et al. Cognitive impairment in rheumatoid arthritis: a systematic review. Arthritis Care Res 2018;70(1):39–52.
19. Haddad DN, Mart MF, Wang L, et al. Socioeconomic factors and intensive care unit-related cognitive impairment. Ann Surg 2020;272(4):596–602.
20. Mo M, Eriksdotter M, Ajeganova S, et al. Association of rheumatoid arthritis with progression of cognitive impairment and risk of mortality in people with dementia. Neurology 2025;104(5):e213405. https://doi.org/10.1212/wnl.0000000000213405.
21. Gwinnutt JM, Toyoda T, Barraclough M, et al. Cognitive impairment in the immune-mediated inflammatory diseases compared with age-matched controls: systematic review and meta-regression. Semin Arthritis Rheum 2023;58:152131.
22. Brock J, Basu N, Schlachetzki JCM, et al. Immune mechanisms of depression in rheumatoid arthritis. Nat Rev Rheumatol 2023;19(12):790–804.
23. Basile MS, Ciurleo R, Bramanti A, et al. Cognitive decline in rheumatoid arthritis: insight into the molecular pathogenetic mechanisms. Int J Mol Sci 2021;22(3). https://doi.org/10.3390/ijms22031185.
24. Bultink IEM, Lems WF, Kostense PJ, et al. Prevalence of and risk factors for low bone mineral density and vertebral fractures in patients with systemic lupus erythematosus. Arthritis Rheum 2005;52(7):2044–50.
25. Hauser B, Riches PL, Wilson JF, et al. Prevalence and clinical prediction of osteoporosis in a contemporary cohort of patients with rheumatoid arthritis. Rheumatology 2014;53(10):1759–66.
26. Ashai S, Harvey NC. Rheumatoid arthritis and bone health. Clin Med 2020;20(6): 565–7.

27. Bultink IE, Vis M, van der Horst-Bruinsma IE, et al. Inflammatory rheumatic disorders and bone. Curr Rheumatol Rep 2012;14(3):224–30.
28. Staa TPV, Geusens P, Bijlsma JWJ, et al. Clinical assessment of the long-term risk of fracture in patients with rheumatoid arthritis. Arthritis Rheum 2006;54(10): 3104–12.
29. Moreels M, Mélot C, Leeman M. Prognosis of patients with systemic rheumatic diseases admitted to the intensive care unit. Intensive Care Med 2005;31(4): 591–3.
30. Paudel A, Bhandari S, Jha S, et al. Rheumatological emergencies – perspective of an intensivist. Journal of Nepalese Society of Critical Care Medicine 2023; 1(2):22–8.
31. Dostanko N, Yagur V, Dostanko V. AB0245 functional reserves decline index and severity status of rheumatoid arthritis patients. Ann Rheum Dis 2013;72:A861–2.
32. Akiyama M, Kaneko Y. Pathogenesis, clinical features, and treatment strategy for rheumatoid arthritis-associated interstitial lung disease. Autoimmun Rev 2022; 21(5):103056.
33. Ha Y-J, Lee YJ, Kang EH. Lung involvements in rheumatic diseases: update on the epidemiology, pathogenesis, clinical features, and treatment. BioMed Res Int 2018;2018(1):6930297.
34. Pan S-Y, Tian H-M, Zhu Y, et al. Cardiac damage in autoimmune diseases: target organ involvement that cannot be ignored. Review. Front Immunol 2022;13. https://doi.org/10.3389/fimmu.2022.1056400.
35. Owlia MB, Mostafavi Pour Manshadi SM, Naderi N. Cardiac manifestations of rheumatological conditions: a narrative review. ISRN Rheumatol 2012;2012: 463620. https://doi.org/10.5402/2012/463620.
36. Couderc M, Tatar Z, Pereira B, et al. Prevalence of renal impairment in patients with rheumatoid arthritis: results from a cross-sectional multicenter study. Arthritis Care Res 2016;68(5):638–44.
37. Hill A, Thomson R, Hunter J, et al. The prevalence of chronic kidney disease in rheumatology outpatients. Scott Med J 2009;54(2):9–12.
38. Oweis AO, Alawneh KM, Alshelleh SA, et al. Renal dysfunction among rheumatoid arthritis patients: a retrospective cohort study. Ann Med Surg 2020;60:280–4.
39. Karie S, Gandjbakhch F, Janus N, et al. Kidney disease in RA patients: prevalence and implication on RA-related drugs management: the MATRIX study. Rheumatology 2008;47(3):350–4.
40. Mantilla Ribero MJ, Sarmiento Monroy JC, Villota-Eraso C, et al. AB0304 chronic kidney disease in patients with rheumatoid arthritis: a retrospective cohort study. Ann Rheum Dis 2022;81(Suppl 1):1277–8.
41. Anders H-J, Vielhauer V. Renal co-morbidity in patients with rheumatic diseases. Arthritis Res Ther 2011;13(2):222.
42. Anders H-J, Saxena R, Zhao M-H, et al. Lupus nephritis. Nat Rev Dis Primers 2020;6(1):7.
43. Bernal-Macías S, Reyes-Beltrán B, Molano-González N, et al. Outcome of patients with autoimmune diseases in the intensive care unit: a mixed cluster analysis. Lupus Science & Medicine 2015;2(1):e000122. https://doi.org/10.1136/lupus-2015-000122.
44. Hysa E, Vojinovic T, Gotelli E, et al. The dichotomy of glucocorticosteroid treatment in immune-inflammatory rheumatic diseases: an evidence-based perspective and insights from clinical practice. Reumatologia 2023;61(4):283–93.
45. Bijlsma JWJ, Saag KG, Buttgereit F, et al. Developments in glucocorticoid therapy. Rheum Dis Clin N Am 2005;31(1):1–17.

46. Richter A, Listing J, Schneider M, et al. Impact of treatment with biologic DMARDs on the risk of sepsis or mortality after serious infection in patients with rheumatoid arthritis. Ann Rheum Dis 2016;75(9):1667–73.
47. Favero M, Schiavon F, Riato L, et al. Rheumatoid arthritis is the major risk factor for septic arthritis in rheumatological settings. Autoimmun Rev 2008;8(1):59–61.
48. Kato H, Suzuki M, Misumi K, et al. Macrophage activation syndrome triggered by methotrexate-related lymphoproliferative disease in a patient with rheumatoid arthritis. Immunological Medicine 2023;46(4):191–5.
49. Friedman MA, Curtis JR, Winthrop KL. Impact of disease-modifying antirheumatic drugs on vaccine immunogenicity in patients with inflammatory rheumatic and musculoskeletal diseases. Ann Rheum Dis 2021;80(10):1255–65.
50. Fujiwara T, Tokuda K, Momii K, et al. Prognostic factors for the short-term mortality of patients with rheumatoid arthritis admitted to intensive care units. BMC Rheumatol 2020;4(1):64.
51. Beil M, Sviri S, de la Guardia V, et al. Prognosis of patients with rheumatic diseases admitted to intensive care. Anaesth Intensive Care 2017;45(1):67–72.
52. Brünnler T, Susewind M, Hoffmann U, et al. Outcomes and prognostic factors in patients with rheumatologic diseases admitted to the ICU. Intern Med 2015;54-(16):1981–7.
53. Dolomisiewicz A, Ali H, Roul P, et al. Updating and validating the rheumatic disease comorbidity index to incorporate ICD-10-CM diagnostic codes. Arthritis Care Res 2023;75(10):2199–206.
54. Choi SR, Kim JY, Ha Y-J, et al. Development and validation of a risk score for serious infection in patients with rheumatic diseases receiving prolonged high-dose glucocorticoids. Arthritis Res Ther 2026;28(1):72.
55. Del Papa N, Minniti A, Maglione W, et al. Instruments for outcome evaluation of specific domains in primary sjögren's syndrome. Biomolecules 2021;11(7). https://doi.org/10.3390/biom11070953.
56. Johnson TM, Michaud K, England BR. Measures of rheumatoid arthritis disease activity. Arthritis Care Res 2020;72(Suppl 10):4–26.
57.. Smolen JS, Edwards CJ, Konzett V, et al. EULAR recommendations for the management of rheumatoid arthritis with synthetic and biologic disease-modifying antirheumatic drugs: 2025 update. Ann Rheum Dis 2026;85(6):991–1009.
58. Jahn M, Rekowski J, Jánosi RA, et al. Score performance of SAPS 2 and SAPS 3 in combination with biomarkers IL-6, PCT or CRP. PLoS One 2020;15(9): e0238587. https://doi.org/10.1371/journal.pone.0238587.
59. Narazaki M, Kishimoto T. Current status and prospects of IL-6–targeting therapy. Expert Rev Clin Pharmacol 2022;15(5):575–92.
60. Majumder S, Nandi M, Mondal S, et al. Role of serum procalcitonin in differentiating disease flare and systemic bacterial infection among febrile children with known chronic rheumatic diseases: a cross-sectional study. Turk J Pediatr 2024;66(6):681–9.
61. Ichimura Y, Kawaguchi Y, Tochimoto A, et al. SAT0667 presepsin and procalcitonin are of diagnostic value for bacterial infection in patients with connective tissue diseases. Ann Rheum Dis 2017;76:1026–7.
62. Gremese E, Bruno D, Varriano V, et al. Serum albumin levels: a biomarker to be repurposed in different disease settings in clinical practice. J Clin Med 2023;12-(18):6017.
63. Mustafa M, Gladston Chelliah E, Hughes M. Patients with systemic rheumatic diseases admitted to the intensive care unit: what the rheumatologist needs to know. Rheumatol Int 2018;38(7):1163–8.

64. Assan F, Bay P, Mathian A, et al. In-ICU-acquired infections in flare-up systemic rheumatic disease patients receiving immunosuppressant. Clin Rheumatol 2022; 41(9):2845–54.
65. Fang F, Zhang Y, Tang J, et al. Association of corticosteroid treatment with outcomes in adult patients with sepsis: a systematic review and meta-analysis. JAMA Intern Med 2019;179(2):213–23.
66. Bernatsky S, Hudson M, Suissa S. Anti-rheumatic drug use and risk of serious infections in rheumatoid arthritis. Rheumatology 2007;46(7):1157–60.
67. Florescu A, Mușetescu AE, Criveanu C, et al. Applications of corticosteroid therapy in inflammatory rheumatic diseases. In: Pereira C, editor. Corticosteroids - a paradigmatic drug class. IntechOpen; 2021.
68. Ornetti P, Bouillet B, Denimal D. New guidelines on glucocorticoid-induced adrenal insufficiency: the end of short synacthen test in rheumatology? RMD Open 2025;11(1):e005251. https://doi.org/10.1136/rmdopen-2024-005251.
69. Filippa MG, Tektonidou MG, Mantzou A, et al. Adrenocortical dysfunction in rheumatoid arthritis: α narrative review and future directions. Eur J Clin Invest 2022; 52(1):e13635.
70. Beuschlein F, Else T, Bancos I, et al. European society of endocrinology and endocrine society joint clinical guideline: diagnosis and therapy of glucocorticoid-induced adrenal insufficiency. J Clin Endocrinol Metab 2024; 109(7):1657–83.
71. Giollo A, Fuzzi E, Doria A. Methotrexate in early rheumatoid arthritis: is the anchor drug still holding? Autoimmun Rev 2022;21(4):103031.
72. Li X, Hu Q, Xu T. Janus kinase inhibitors and the risk of infections: a network meta-analysis across disease indications. Expert Opin Drug Saf 2025;1–13. https://doi.org/10.1080/14740338.2025.2502037.
73. Nash P, Kerschbaumer A, Konzett V, et al. Expert consensus statement on the treatment of immune-mediated inflammatory diseases with janus kinase inhibitors: 2024 update. Ann Rheum Dis 2025;84(5):664–79.
74. Machado MADÁ, Moura CSD, Guerra SF, et al. Effectiveness and safety of tofacitinib in rheumatoid arthritis: a cohort study. Arthritis Res Ther 2018;20(1):60.
75. Amstutz A, Schandelmaier S, Ewald H, et al. Effects of Janus kinase inhibitors in adults admitted to hospital due to COVID-19: a systematic review and individual participant data meta-analysis of randomised clinical trials. Lancet Respir Med 2025;13(6):530–44.
76. The PRACTICAL P, TRAITS, INCEPT, Investigators R-C. The rise of adaptive platform trials in critical care. Am J Respir Crit Care Med 2024;209(5):491–6. https://doi.org/10.1164/rccm.202401-0101CP.
77. Singh JA, Cameron C, Noorbaloochi S, et al. Risk of serious infection in biological treatment of patients with rheumatoid arthritis: a systematic review and meta-analysis. Lancet 2015;386(9990):258–65.
78. Subesinghe S, Rutherford AI, Byng-Maddick R, et al. Biologic prescribing decisions following serious infection: results from the British Society for Rheumatology Biologics Register-Rheumatoid arthritis. Rheumatology 2018;57(12):2096–100.
79. Opdam MAA, den Broeder N, van Crevel R, et al. Continuation versus temporary interruption of immunomodulatory agents during infections in patients with inflammatory rheumatic diseases: a randomized controlled trial. Clin Infect Dis 2025; 82(3):420–6.
80. Cooksey R, Kennedy J, Rahman M, et al. The pattern of anti-IL-6 versus non-anti-IL-6 biologic disease modifying anti-rheumatic drugs use in patients with

rheumatoid arthritis in Wales, UK: a real-world study using electronic health records. Rheumatol Adv Pract 2025;9(1):rkae140. https://doi.org/10.1093/rap/rkae140.
81. Kalyoncu U, Pehlivan Y, Akar S, et al. Preferences of inflammatory arthritis patients for biological disease-modifying antirheumatic drugs in the first 100 days of the COVID-19 pandemic. Turk J Med Sci 2021;51(4):1615–23.
82. Okada M, Kita Y, Kanamaru N, et al. Anti-IL-6 receptor antibody causes less promotion of tuberculosis infection than anti-TNF-α antibody in mice. Clin Dev Immunol 2011;2011:404929. https://doi.org/10.1155/2011/404929.
83.. Joint Formulary Committee. British national formulary. Available at: https://bnf.nice.org.uk/. Accessed April 15, 2026.
84. Aletaha D, Smolen JS. Diagnosis and management of rheumatoid arthritis: a review. JAMA 2018;320(13):1360–72.
85. Mikuls TR, Johnson SR, Fraenkel L, et al. American College of rheumatology guidance for the management of rheumatic disease in adult patients during the COVID-19 pandemic: version 3. Arthritis Rheumatol 2021;73(2):e1–12.
86. Fragoulis GE, Brock J, Basu N, et al. The role for JAK inhibitors in the treatment of immune-mediated rheumatic and related conditions. J Allergy Clin Immunol 2021;148(4):941–52.
87. Wang F, Sun L, Wang S, et al. Efficacy and safety of tofacitinib, baricitinib, and upadacitinib for rheumatoid arthritis: a systematic review and meta-analysis. Mayo Clin Proc 2020;95(7):1404–19.

Early Management of Sepsis

Elizabeth S. Munroe, MD, MSc[a,*], Ithan D. Peltan, MD, MSc[a], Hallie C. Prescott, MD, MSc[b]

KEYWORDS

- Sepsis • Septic shock • Antimicrobial therapy • Resuscitation • IV fluids • Vasopressors

KEY POINTS

- Early sepsis management has 2 major goals: (1) infection control and (2) hemodynamic resuscitation.
- Infection management should focus on prompt and appropriate antimicrobial therapy and source control. Clinicians should re-evalaute for adequacy of infection control if patients do not improve.
- Patients with hypoperfusion benefit from a fluid bolus, followed by personalized fluid resuscitation guided by dynamic assessments of fluid responsiveness.
- Patients with persistent hypotension despite fluid resuscitation should be started on norepinephrine, with vasopressin and corticosteroids added for worsening shock.
- Noninvasive hemodynamic management, with peripheral vasopressors and noninvasive blood pressure measurements, is feasible for many patients.

INTRODUCTION

Sepsis is a leading cause of morbidity and mortality, resulting in over 11 million deaths globally in 2017 and accounting for 1 in every 2 to 3 hospital deaths in the United States.[1–3] Sepsis is defined as life-threatening acute organ dysfunction due to a dysregulated host response to infection.[4] In practice, sepsis diagnosis is based on presence of both infection and acute organ dysfunction.[4] Prompt recognition and appropriate early management are associated with reduced mortality.[5] There are 2 major goals of early sepsis management, which should be pursued urgently and in parallel: (1) treatment of the infection and (2) hemodynamic resuscitation. Achieving these goals helps halt the damaging host response and prevent progressive organ

[a] Department of Pulmonary and Critical Care Medicine, Intermountain Medical Center, Murray, UT, USA; [b] Department of Internal Medicine, University of Michigan, VA Center for Clinical Management Research, Ann Arbor, MI, USA
* Corresponding author. Department of Pulmonary and Critical Care, 5121 Cottonwood Street, Murray, UT 84107.
E-mail address: elizabeth.munroe@imail.org

Crit Care Clin 42 (2026) 719–743
https://doi.org/10.1016/j.ccc.2026.05.002 **criticalcare.theclinics.com**
0749-0704/26/

Abbreviations	
AngII	angiotensin II
CKD	chronic kidney disease
CO	cardiac output
CRT	capillary refill time
CVC	central venous catheter
ED	emergency department
HFrEF	heart failure with reduced ejection fraction
IR	interventional radiology
IV	intravenous
LR	Lactated Ringer's
MAP	mean arterial pressure
NS	normal saline
SBP	systolic blood pressure
SSC	Surviving Sepsis Campaign
SV	stroke volume

dysfunction. In this article, we review key aspects of early sepsis management related to both infection management and resuscitation.

SCOPE

While early sepsis recognition is essential for timely and effective treatment, approaches to sepsis diagnosis are outside the scope of this article.

CASE

A 62-year-old woman with hypertension, heart failure with reduced ejection fraction (HFrEF), and chronic kidney disease (CKD) presents to the emergency department (ED) with 3 days of pain with urination, 2 days of bloody urine, and 1 day of fevers, chills, and left flank pain. On presentation, blood pressure is 84/52 mm Hg, heart rate is 110 beats per minute, and respiratory rate is 24 breaths per minute. On examination, she is confused and has trouble following commands. Based on the clinical presentation consistent with urinary infection and acute organ dysfunction (altered mental status, hypotension), you diagnose sepsis. What should you do next?

Treating Infection

Antimicrobial therapy

Early initiation of appropriate antimicrobial therapy is a core tenet of sepsis management, which has consistently been linked to decreased mortality.[5–7] The Surviving Sepsis Campaign (SSC) guidelines recommend administering antimicrobial therapy within 1 hour of recognition for patients with definite or probable sepsis, as well as in patients with shock and possible sepsis.[8,9] For patients with possible sepsis without shock, the guidelines suggest a rapid assessment of infectious and noninfectious causes of illness, with antibiotic administration within 3 hours if concern for sepsis persists. While the 1- and 3-hour thresholds are helpful to guide management and drive performance improvement, antibiotic timing is a continuous measure without a clear threshold effect. The absolute increase in mortality with each hour of delay is greater in patients with shock,[10,11] though earlier antibiotic administration is associated with reduced mortality for all patients with sepsis.[12] Clinicians should therefore evaluate possible sepsis urgently, and start antibiotic therapy as soon as possible after sepsis is deemed likely, ideally within 1 hour (**Fig. 1**).

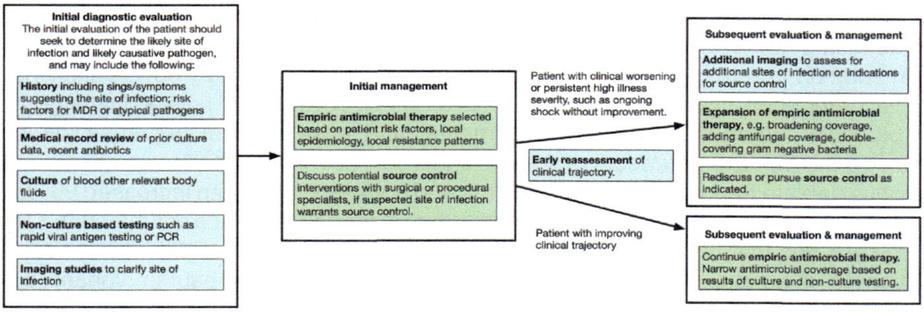

Fig. 1. Approach to infection management in patients with suspected sepsis. This figure outlines the approach to infection management in patients with suspected sepsis. Blue boxes indicate clinical evaluation and diagnostic testing. Green boxes indicate treatments and interventions. MDR, multi-drug resistance; PCR, polymerase chain reaction.

Timely antibiotic initiation is a complex, multidisciplinary process—the clinician must order the antibiotics, the pharmacist must prepare the drugs (or have it available on the unit), and the nurse must see the order, get the medication, ensure available intravenous (IV) access, and start the infusion.[13] Even with this complex process, antibiotic delays are often driven by delayed sepsis recognition and antibiotic ordering rather than delays between ordering and administration. Indeed, in a large study of Veteran Affairs hospitals, the median time from ED antibiotic order to administration was 23 minutes (interquartile range 15 to 34 minutes).[14] Therefore, initiatives aimed at decreasing time-to-antibiotics should focus on sepsis recognition and expedited antibiotic ordering, in addition to streamlining postorder processes and ensuring that new antibiotic orders default to immediate administration.[15]

While some experts have raised concern that efforts to shorten time to antibiotic administration in sepsis may worsen antimicrobial stewardship, such effects have not been demonstrated. In a study of over 1 million patients at 152 hospitals, as time to antimicrobial administration for sepsis decreased over time, there were concurrent reductions in overall antimicrobial use and broad-spectrum antibiotics.[16] Furthermore, in a large multicenter study of physician variation in door-to-antibiotic time, faster antibiotic prescribing was not associated with overtreatment.[17] These findings indicate that timely antibiotic initiation can be balanced with antimicrobial stewardship.

Blood culture timing

Blood cultures should be drawn before initiating antibiotic therapy[8,9,18] since cultures collected after antibiotic initiation have lower yield and reduced ability to detect blood stream infection.[19] However, the mortality benefit of prompt antibiotic therapy outweighs the potential benefit of increased blood culture yield, especially given culture-negative sepsis is common.[20] Therefore, in the event that blood cultures cannot be drawn in a timely manner (eg, due to limited resources or difficult access), clinicians should proceed with antibiotic therapy.[21]

Antibiotic selection

Prompt antibiotic therapy can reduce mortality only if it is effective—ie, the therapy adequately covers the inciting pathogen.[22] Given the inciting pathogen is rarely known at time of initial treatment, clinicians should aim to maximize the likelihood that antibiotic therapy will be effective by selecting empiric antibiotics to cover likely potential pathogens based on (1) suspected site of infection, (2) patient-specific risk factors for resistant or atypical pathogens, (3) the patient's prior culture results, and (4) local epidemiology of resistance.[23]

In addition to ensuring that the selected empiric antibiotic therapy covers likely potential pathogens, it is also important to avoid or limit coverage of unlikely pathogens. In particular, there is mounting experimental and observational human evidence showing the detrimental effects of empiric anaerobic coverage.[24,25] Antianaerobic antibiotics deplete the healthy gut microbiome and are associated with increased 90-day mortality—likely mediated by increased risk for secondary or recurrent infection.[24,25] In the ACORN trial comparing empiric antibiotics, mortality did not differ by randomization to cefepime (anaerobe-sparing) versus piperacillin-tazobactam (anaerobe-depleting).[26] However, this trial was not designed to test the impact of anaerobic coverage, since many patients in the cefepime arm received cotreatment with metronidazole. Furthermore, the trial examined outcomes to only 14 days, before mortality benefit with anaerobe-sparing regimens would be expected.[25,26] In general, unnecessary antianaerobic coverage should be avoided for sites of infection where anaerobic pathogens are unlikely, such as respiratory or urinary tract.

Other antimicrobial therapy

While we have focused on antibiotics, sepsis can be caused by pathogens other than bacteria, including fungi, particularly *Candida* species, and viruses.[27] In retrospective analyses of patients with *Candida* infections, delays in time-to-antifungal therapy have been associated with higher mortality.[28,29] However, prospective trials have not found benefit of empiric antifungal therapy. The EMPIRICUS trial randomized 260 patients with empirical antifungal treatment in ICUS-acquired sepsis to addition of empiric micafungin versus placebo and found no difference in fungal infection–free survival to day 28.[30] However, few patients ended up having confirmed fungal infection (5%), which limited the power of this trial to detect potential benefit of empiric micafungin and highlights the challenge of predicting fungal infection in practice. Empiric antifungal therapy should be considered on a case-by-case basis in high-risk patients, particularly those not showing clinical improvement with initial antibiotic therapy, but should not be used across the board for empiric treatment of hospital-onset sepsis.[8,31] Given the rise of azole-resistant *Candida* species, echinocandins (eg, micafungin or anidulafungin) are the preferred empiric antifungal agents in many regions.[31]

Viruses can also cause sepsis. Antiviral therapy has been associated with reduced mortality in some viral infections (eg, oseltamivir in influenza).[32,33] However, empiric antiviral therapy is rarely indicated since rapid diagnostic testing can identify viral infections quickly and guide initiation of antiviral therapy in a timely manner.[34] Instead, a common clinical challenge for patients with positive viral testing is determining whether to treat with empiric antibiotic therapy for possible concomitant bacterial infection. Given there is little room for error in omitting antibiotics in critically ill patients with potential bacterial coinfection,[35] empiric antibiotic therapy should be considered in patients with positive viral testing and shock or severe respiratory failure if there is any concern for concomitant bacterial infection.[36,37] However, antibiotic therapy should be reassessed daily and discontinued if subsequent testing (eg, serial procalcitonin) suggest bacterial coinfection is unlikely.

Source control

Even with appropriate antibiotic therapy, some infections require source control interventions for timely cure. Source control encompasses surgical and procedural interventions to drain or remove the nidus of infection (eg, appendectomy or removal of infected hardware) or correct anatomic blockages that impede infection clearance (eg, endoscopic retrograde cholangiopancreatography for biliary stricture). Many infections require source control, including intrabdominal infections (eg, appendicitis), infections proximal to an obstruction (eg, obstructive kidney stone, cholangitis), infected devices (eg, infected central lines), empyema, and abscesses.[23] Delayed source control in these scenarios is associated with increased risk of mortality, particularly among patients with shock.[38,39] For example, in a multicenter study of nearly 5000 patients with sepsis who underwent source control procedures, later source control (after 6 hours) was associated with higher mortality than early source control, particularly for abdominal and soft tissue infections.[39] Given the importance of source control, the initial diagnostic workup for infection should seek to clarify the site of infection and assess whether source control should be prioritized after initial stabilization of the patient.

Re-evaluation: missed bug? Missed source?

Most patients with sepsis begin to show signs of clinical improvement after resuscitation and initiation of appropriate antimicrobial therapy. When a patient does not stabilize or improve during the initial hours of treatment, it is essential to consider whether the initial infection control measures were sufficient. For patients with worsening clinical trajectories or persistent clinical instability (eg, ongoing shock without improvement), clinicians should consider the following questions: (a) Was the initial antimicrobial therapy appropriate? Or should it be broadened to cover additional pathogens (eg, methicillin-resistant *Staph aureus*) or expanded to include double coverage[40] for potential resistant gram-negative bacteria? (b) Is there an additional site of infection beyond what has been identified? (c) Is there an indication for source control? Or, has the need for source control been adequately ruled out?

Back to the Case (Infection management): We ordered blood cultures, urine culture, and urinalysis to evaluate the suspected source of infection urinary tract infection (UTI) and completed a history, physical examination, and chart review with particular attention to prior culture data and risk factors for resistant organisms, which were not present. We started empiric antibiotic therapy with Ceftriaxone to cover likely urinary pathogens. We started antibiotics as quickly as possible by ordering them promptly and coordinating with pharmacy and nursing to ensure timely initiation (goal <1 hour). The patient had worsening shock despite initial treatment, which prompted re-evaluation and a computed tomography scan (CT scan) of the abdomen. CT revealed an obstructing left kidney stone with proximal hydronephrosis and evidence of associated left pyelonephritis. Interventional radiology (IR) was consulted emergently for the placement of a percutaneous nephrostomy tube. The patient's shock improved within a few hours of this source control procedure.

Restoring Organ Perfusion (Resuscitation)

In sepsis, systemic inflammation can lead to vasodilation, which decreases preload, causes hypotension, and eventually impairs organ perfusion. Patients with sepsis also often have concomitant hypovolemia from dehydration and fluid losses (eg, diarrhea, insensible losses from fever).[41] Patients with sepsis-induced hypoperfusion require prompt resuscitation to restore organ perfusion and prevent progressive organ damage. Initial clinical evaluation should focus on identifying evidence of hypotension and hypoperfusion (eg, delayed capillary refill), while initial laboratory evaluation should include lactate measurement to evaluate for occult hypoperfusion (**Fig. 2**).

Case: Let's come back to the beginning of our case to focus on the patient's hemodynamic resuscitation. In the case, the patient is presenting with sepsis due to a

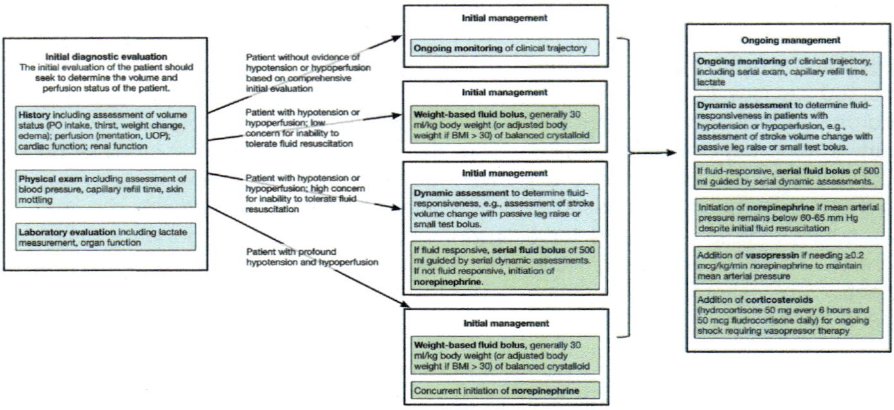

Fig. 2. Approach to hemodynamic resuscitation in sepsis. This figure outlines the approach to hemodynamic resuscitation in patients with sepsis-induced hypoperfusion or shock. Blue boxes indicate clinical evaluation and diagnostic testing. Green boxes indicate treatments and interventions. PO, oral; UOP, urine output.

urinary source and has an initial blood pressure of 84/52 mm Hg (mean arterial pressure [MAP] 63 mm Hg). How should we resuscitate this patient?

Fluid resuscitation

Initial fluid resuscitation. IV fluids are a key component of sepsis resuscitation, as they help correct intravascular volume depletion, restore preload, and improve organ perfusion. Fluid resuscitation is indicated for patients with sepsis who have hypotension (eg, systolic blood pressure [SBP]<90 mm Hg or MAP<65 mm Hg) or lactate greater than 4 mmol/L. Fluid resuscitation should also be considered in patients with relative hypotension (ie, SBP below known baseline), intermediate lactate elevation (lactate 2–4 mmol/L), and other measures of end-organ dysfunction (eg, abnormal capillary refill time [CRT]).

The goal of resuscitation is to improve blood pressure and restore organ perfusion as soon as possible. The optimal fluid volume to support this goal varies across patients. Both under-resuscitation and over-resuscitation are associated with worse outcomes,[42–44] so clinical status should be monitored closely to guide ongoing resuscitation.

The 2026 SSC guidelines suggest an initial bolus of 30 mL/kg body weight (or adjusted body weight if obese[45]) as the default practice, which translates to between 1.5 and 4L for most adult patients.[9] This pragmatic recommendation is based on observational studies[46–50] and pre-enrollment fluid volumes in major trials[51–53]—not trials directly comparing 30 mL/kg versus other initial fluid volumes. Observational studies suggest optimal outcomes with an initial volume around 30 mL/kg, with both lower and higher volumes (typically >5L or >70 mL/kg) associated with worse outcomes.[42,44,48–50,54] However, by issuing a conditional (rather than strong) recommendation on initial fluid volume, the SSC guidelines acknowledge the importance of considering the clinical context when selecting initial fluid bolus volume. For patients at very high risk of harm from fluid overload or a clinical evaluation concerning for mixed shock, a smaller initial bolus and sooner transition to personalized resuscitation guided by serial dynamic assessments may be warranted (see **Fig. 2**).

The initial fluid bolus should be given rapidly to restore perfusion as quickly as possible. *Stuttering* resuscitation approaches—whereby smaller volumes are given intermittently over longer time periods—are suboptimal and can delay time to achieving intravascular repletion (**Fig. 3**). Likewise, *aborted* resuscitation approaches—where fluid is capped at an arbitrary volume due to risk for fluid overload—are also suboptimal because clinical history (eg, history of HFrEF or CKD) and physical examination features (eg, edema) are unreliable in determining fluid responsiveness.[55] Instead, patients with hypoperfusion but high risk for fluid-related harms should be transitioned more quickly to personalized resuscitation approaches guided by serial assessment of fluid responsiveness, as discussed in the next section.

Ongoing fluid resuscitation. After initial fluid resuscitation with a weight-based fluid bolus, clinicians should use dynamic assessments of fluid responsiveness to guide ongoing resuscitation.

Prior trials comparing *fluid-liberal* versus *fluid-restrictive* approaches to ongoing resuscitation yielded neutral results, suggesting that neither approach is optimal as a general strategy (**Table 1**). The CLOVERS trial randomized 1563 patients with sepsis-induced hypotension to restrictive fluids (paired with early vasopressors) versus liberal fluids (up to 5 L) in the first 24 hours of presentation.[56] The CLASSIC trial randomized 1554 patients with septic shock to a restrictive approach to ICU fluid management (no maintenance fluids, boluses for only limited clinical criteria) versus usual care for the duration of ICU admission.[57] Both studies found no difference in mortality.

By contrast, trials evaluating personalized approaches to resuscitation that include serial assessments of fluid responsiveness have resulted in improved outcomes.[58,73]

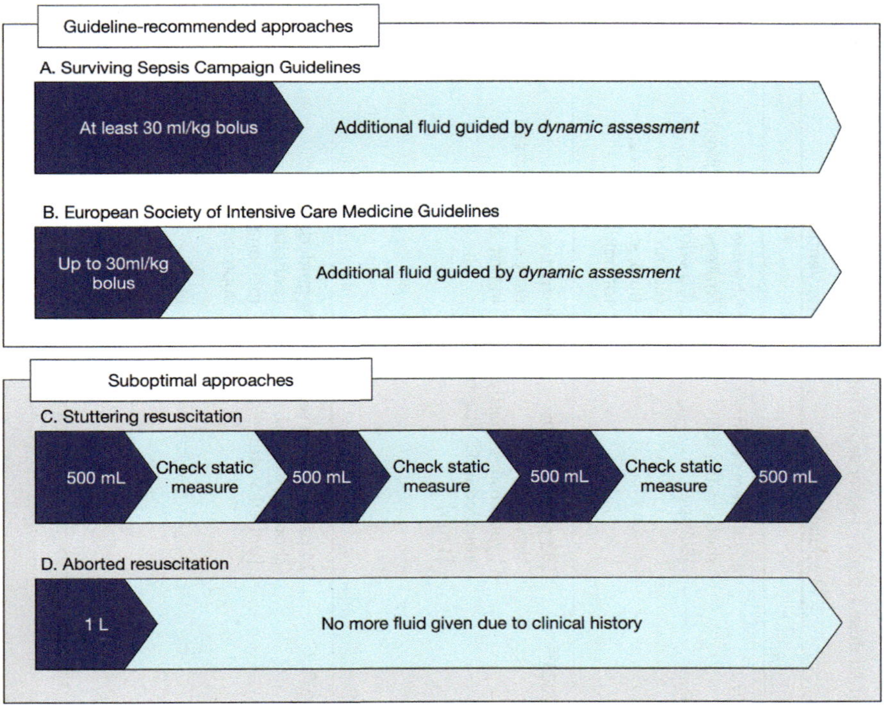

Fig. 3. Approaches to initial fluid resuscitation. Panels *A* and *B* represent the Surviving Sepsis Campaign and European Society of Intensive Care Medicine guidelines for initial fluid resuscitation, respectively. Panels *C* and *D* represent common alternative, but suboptimal, approaches to initial fluid resuscitation used in practice.

Table 1
Summary of landmark trials in early sepsis resuscitation

Trial	Population	Intervention	Comparator	Outcome[a]	Takeaway
Fluid resuscitation					
CLASSIC, 2022[57]	1554 patients with septic shock in the ICU [Europe]	Restrictive fluid strategy throughout ICU admission (no maintenance fluid, strict criteria for boluses)	Usual care	*90-d mortality:* 42.3% vs 42.1%, *P* = .96	Restrictive strategies to managing fluid in the ICU do not reduce mortality. Patients received a median of 3L of fluid before enrollment.
CLOVERS, 2023[56]	1563 patients with sepsis-induced hypotension, mostly enrolled in ED [United States]	Restrictive fluid, early vasopressors in first 24 h	Liberal fluid (up to 5 L) in first 24 h	*Death before discharge home by day 90:* 14.0% vs 14.9%, *P* = .61	Generalized restrictive vs liberal strategies for ongoing fluid resuscitation in the first 24 h result in similar outcomes. Patients received a median 2L of IV fluid before enrollment.
FRESH, 2020[58]	124 patients with septic shock in the ICU [United States]	SV-guided fluid resuscitation (personalized approach)	Usual care	*72-h fluid balance:* 0.65 vs 2.02 L RRT: 5.1% vs 17.5%, *P* = .04. Mechanical ventilation: 17.7% vs 34.1%, *P* = .04	Personalizing ongoing fluid resuscitation based on SV assessments may decrease fluid overload and improve patient outcomes. Patients received a median of 2.5 L fluid before enrollment.

Fluid choice					
SMART, 2018[59]	7942 patients in the ICU [United States]	Balanced fluid	NS	*Major adverse kidney event:* 14.3% vs 15.4%, *P* = .04	Balanced fluid may improve patient outcomes. In secondary analyses, larger effects were seen in sicker patients, patients with sepsis, and when balanced fluid was used from the onset of resuscitation (starting in the ED).[60,61]
PLUS, 2022[62]	5037 patients in the ICU [Australia/New Zealand]	Balanced fluid	NS	*90-d mortality*: 21.8% vs 22.0%, *P* = .90	No difference in mortality with fluid choice, though all patients were enrolled in the ICU, potentially missing the effects of starting balanced fluid in the ED that was seen in secondary analyses of SMART.
BaSICs, 2023[63]	11,052 patients in the ICU [Brazil]	Balanced fluid	NS	*90-d mortality*: 26.4% vs 27.2%, *P* = .47	No difference in mortality with fluid choice, though secondary analysis suggest benefit with balanced fluids for patients with sepsis and when balanced fluid was used from the onset of resuscitation (starting in the ED).[61]

(*continued on next page*)

Table 1
(*continued*)

Trial	Population	Intervention	Comparator	Outcome[a]	Takeaway
Vasopressor selection					
SOAP II, 2010[64]	1679 patients with septic, cardiogenic, or hemorrhagic shock [Europe]	Norepinephrine	Dopamine	*28-d mortality: 48.5% vs* 52.5%, *P* = .10. Results were statically significant favoring norepinephrine in patients with cardiogenic shock. Arrhythmias: 12.4% vs 24.1%, *P*<.001	First-line norepinephrine carries less risk of arrhythmias than dopamine and may be associated with lower mortality. Based on this trial, norepinephrine became widely adopted as the preferred first-line vasopressor in shock, including septic shock.
VASST, 2008[65]	778 patients with septic shock in the ICU [Canada, Australia, United States]	Norepinephrine + Vasopressin	Norepinephrine	*28-d mortality*: 35.4% vs 39.3%, *P* = .26. Results were statistically significant in patients with less severe shock (norepinephrine doses of 5–14 mcg/min): 26.5% vs 35.7%, *P* = .05.	Based on the VASST trial, many clinicians favor earlier vasopressin initiation in patients with less severe shock.

Adjunctive therapies—corticosteroids					
ADRENAL, 2018[66]	3800 patients with septic shock on mechanical ventilation and vasopressors at any dose for ≥4 h [Europe, Australia, Saudi Arabia]	Hydrocortisone (continuous, 200 mg/day)	Placebo	*90-d mortality:* 27.9% vs 28.8%, *P* = .50. Resolution of shock: 3 vs 4 d, *P*<.001.	Taken together, these trials suggest that corticosteroids reduce the duration of septic shock and in patients on higher doses of vasopressors (≥0.25 mcg/kg/min norepinephrine, as in APROCCHSS), may also improve mortality.
APROCCHSS, 2018[67]	1241 patients with septic shock on vasopressor dose ≥0.25 mcg/kg/min of norepinephrine or equivalent for ≥6 h [France]. This trial included a factorial design with activated protein C.	Hydrocortisone + Fludrocortisone	Placebo	*90-d mortality:* 43.0% vs 49.1%, *P* = .03. Vasopressor-free days: 17 vs 15, *P*<.001	
Resuscitation Targets					
SEPSISPAM, 2014[68]	776 patients with septic shock [France]	MAP target: 65–70 mm Hg	MAP target: 80–85 mm Hg	*28-d mortality*: 34.0% vs 36.6%, *P* = .57 Atrial fibrillation: 2.8% vs 6.7%, *P* = .02	MAP ≥65 mm Hg became the accepted target for resuscitation.
The 65 Trial, 2020[69]	2600 patients ≥ 65 year old with vasodilatory hypotension [UK]	MAP target: 60–65 mm Hg	MAP target: ≥65 mm Hg	*90-d mortality:* 41.0% vs 43.8%, *P* = .15	Lower MAP targets (60–65 mm Hg) are safe in older patients.
ANDROMEDA-SHOCK, 2019[70]	424 patients with septic shock [South America]	Resuscitation protocol aimed at normalizing CRT	Resuscitation protocol aimed at normalizing lactate	*28-d mortality:* 34.9% vs 43.4%, *P* = .06. Among patients with lower APACHE II, HR 0.61 (0.39–0.96).	Targeting resuscitation to normalizing peripheral perfusion (CRT) may improve outcomes compared to targeting lactate clearance.

(*continued on next page*)

Table 1
(*continued*)

Trial	Population	Intervention	Comparator	Outcome[a]	Takeaway
ANDROMEDA-SHOCK 2, 2025[71]	1467 patients with septic shock [Americas, Europe, Asia]	Personalized resuscitation protocol targeted to CRT	Usual care	*WIN ratio of death, duration of vital support, and hospital length of stay:* 1.16 (95% CI: 1.02–1.33), favoring intervention	Personalized hemodynamic resuscitation targeted to normalizing peripheral perfusion (CRT) may improve patient outcomes.
Hemodynamic monitoring					
EVERDAC, 2025[72]	1010 ICU patients on vasopressors [France]	Invasive strategy: insertion of arterial catheter within 4 h of randomization	Noninvasive strategy: delayed insertion of arterial catheter. Arterial catheter only placed for key *safety criteria*.	*28-d mortality:* 36.9% vs 34.3%, $P = .006$ for noninferiority	A noninvasive strategy involving placing an arterial catheter only for certain safety criteria is noninferior to an early invasive strategy where arterial catheters are routinely placed in all patients with shock.

Abbreviations: CI, confidence interval; ED, emergency department; EGDT, early goal-directed therapy; HR, hazard ratio; RRT, renal replacement therapy; SEPSIS-PAM, Assessment of Two Levels of Arterial Pressure on Survival in Patients With Septic Shock.

[a] Outcomes are listed for intervention group versus comparator group. The primary outcome is italicized. Selected secondary outcomes are presented when relevant.

Dynamic assessments of fluid responsiveness are superior to static measures (eg, central venous pressure, inferior venous cava collapsibility), which reflect the patient's volume status but not their potential to respond to fluid.[55] Dynamic assessments involve 2 steps: (1) a fluid challenge, which can be performed with either passive leg raise or small 250 to 500 mL *test* bolus and (2) measurement of change in cardiac output (CO) or stroke volume (SV) with the fluid challenge.[55] There are several validated tools for measuring change in CO and SV, which range from noninvasive technologies like bioreactance (Starling [Baxter]; formerly NICOM [Cheetah Medical]) to technologies that require central venous catheters [CVCs] and/or arterial catheters (transpulmonary thermodilution, PiCCO [Getinge]; pulse contour analysis, Flotrac [Edwards]) or a clinician trained in ultrasound.[55,73] A recent meta-analysis of several smaller studies found fluid resuscitation guided by dynamic assessments performed using any of these validated tools was associated with reduced mortality.[73] For example, the FRESH trial randomized 124 patients with sepsis-induced hypotension to SV-guided fluid resuscitation, using bioreactance-based serial dynamic assessments, versus usual care (see **Table 1**).[58] Patients randomized to SV-guided resuscitation had less intubation (17.7% vs 34.1%, $P = .04$), less dialysis (5.1% vs 17.5%), and numeric decreases in mortality and ICU length of stay.[58] Further supporting the value of serial dynamic assessments, the ANDROMEDA-SHOCK 2 trial, discussed below in the *Resuscitation Targets* section, found that a hemodynamic-guided resuscitation protocol that included dynamic assessments of fluid responsiveness improved patient outcomes compared to usual care.[71]

In the FRESH trial, SV-guided fluid resuscitation was started after initial fluid resuscitation (approximately 2.5 L or around 25 mL/kg). However, this strategy can be used earlier, particularly in patients at high risk of fluid-related harms. Earlier use of personalized fluid strategies may be particularly helpful in patients with hospital-onset sepsis, who have different characteristics[74] and for whom there are little trial data to guide resuscitation (many landmark sepsis trials have focused on patients presenting to the ED with community-onset sepsis.[75])

Type of fluid. Balanced solutions, such as Lactated Ringer's (LR), should be used for resuscitation based on accruing data indicating a likely mortality benefit with balanced solutions versus 0.9% normal saline (NS). In the cluster-randomized SMART trial, critically ill patients randomized to balanced solutions had a lower incidence of major adverse kidney events (the primary composite outcome) (see **Table 1**).[59] In the prespecified subgroup of 1641 patients with sepsis, patients randomized to balanced solutions had lower 30-day mortality (26.3% vs 31.1%, $P = .01$), which was consistent in both unadjusted and adjusted analyses.[60] The effect was strongest (and only detectable) when balanced solutions were used throughout resuscitation—suggesting that resuscitation should start with LR and not merely convert to LR in the event of metabolic derangements with NS.[60] Secondary analyses of the individually randomized BaSICs trial comparing NS versus LR and the CLOVERS trial of fluid resuscitation strategies likewise suggest the importance of using LR throughout resuscitation.[61,63,76,77]

Subsequent large-scale implementation studies have confirmed the feasibility and benefit of using LR in real-world practice.[78,79] LR is also associated better outcomes in other conditions beyond sepsis, such as diabetic ketoacidosis and sickle cell vaso-occlusive episodes—suggesting that LR can be the default IV fluid for most conditions, simplifying implementation.[80,81] The only exception is for patients with traumatic brain injury, where balanced solutions are associated with harm, likely due to their hypotonicity and risk for increased intracranial pressures.[59] Pragmatic algorithms for addressing drug incompatibilities with LR can help to improve implementation (**Fig. 4**).

Vasopressors

The goal of sepsis resuscitation is to restore organ perfusion. This is initially achieved with IV fluids, as discussed above. However, some patients have persistent hypoperfusion despite restoration of intravascular volume and require vasopressor therapy to increase systemic vascular resistance and raise blood pressure.

Vasopressor Timing

Vasopressors should generally be started if a patient remains hypotensive after initial weight-based fluid resuscitation. However, in patients who present with unstable shock and profound hypotension, vasopressors may need to be started concurrently with initial fluids. While that delayed vasopressor initiation is associated with increased mortality in retrospective cohorts, these studies are subject to selection bias and confounding by indication given they often exclude patients who never received vasopressors.[82,83] Trial data on timing of vasopressor initiation have been mixed. The single-center CENSER trial of 310 patients with sepsis-induced hypotension found that starting fixed, low-dose norepinephrine was associated with decreased time to

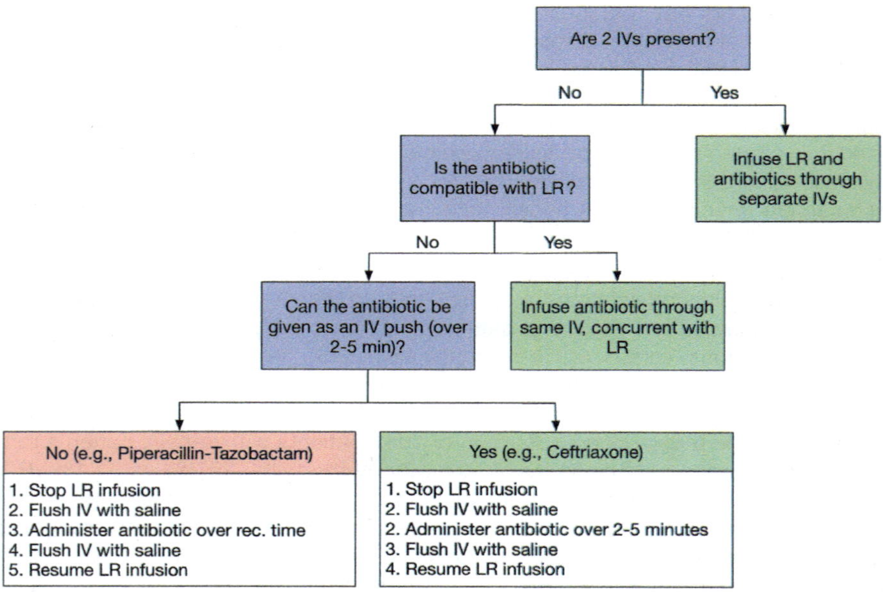

Fig. 4. Implementing LR for patients with septic shock. This figure outlines an approach to implementing LR and balancing potential incompatibilities with antibiotics used by the Michigan Hospital Medicine Safety sepsis initiative. Most common antibiotics are compatible with LR, with the exception of Ceftriaxone, Piperacillin-Tazobactam without ethylenediaminetetraacetic acid (EDTA), and Ciprofloxacin. Ceftriaxone can be given as an IV push over 3 to 5 minutes. However, Piperacillin-Tazobactam and Ciprofloxacin must be given as slower infusions, requiring pausing of LR during administration. Of note, most Piperacillin-Tazobactam is formulated with EDTA, a chelator that helps improve compatibility and makes the antibiotic safe to administer concurrently with LR. Pausing LR infusion for Piperacillin-Tazobactam administration is only necessary when it is formulated without EDTA.

shock control versus placebo.[84] However, these findings were not supported by the larger, multicenter CLOVERS trial,[56] which found no difference in mortality despite time to vasopressor initiation of 1.8 versus 3.2 hours between arms.

Vasopressor Selection—First-line

Norepinephrine is the first-line vasopressor of choice in sepsis. The use of norepinephrine over dopamine is a strong recommendation in the 2026 SSC guidelines,[9] informed by evidence of the superiority of norepinephrine over dopamine in the SOAP II trial (see **Table 1**).[64] The guidelines include a conditional recommendation for the use of norepinephrine over other vasopressors.[9] A quasiexperimental study leveraging drug shortages found a 3.7% absolute mortality increase during shortage periods, when phenylephrine was used as the primary vasopressor instead of norepinephrine.[85] Trials directly comparing norepinephrine with phenylephrine are limited, though there is an ongoing trial comparing first-line phenylephrine versus norepinephrine for patients with shock (NCT 02118467), which will provide additional information.

Vasopressor Selection—Second-line

In patients requiring escalating doses of norepinephrine, clinicians should add vasopressin, as suggested in the SSC guidelines.[8,9] Vasopressin is a noncatecholamine vasopressor that works by increasing vascular smooth muscle contraction and renal free water retention.[86] Based on currently available data, vasopressin should typically be started at norepinephrine doses around 0.2 mcg/kg/minute. This practice balances the potential benefit of vasopressin with cost and the resource utilization of adding a second vasopressor (eg, potential need to place a CVC, see below). Vasopressin may have more benefit in less severe shock based on a secondary analysis of the VASST trial[65] and the OVISS study,[87] which found lower mortality associated with starting vasopressin based on the recommendations of a machine learning model, which suggested adding vasopressin more often and at lower doses of norepinephrine (0.2 vs 0.37 mcg/kg/minute) than clinicians used in practice.[87] Two trials comparing thresholds for vasopressin initiation are ongoing. The Vasopressin in Septic Shock Pragmatic trial is a United States–based trial comparing vasopressin initiation at 0.1 versus 0.4 mcg/kg/minute norepinephrine.[88] The Norepinephrine and Vasopressin for Rescue versus Early Vasopressin for Vasopressor Dependent Sepsis (NoVa; NCT06464510) is comparing immediate vasopressin initiation versus delayed initiation at 0.5 mcg/kg/minute of norepinephrine.

Beyond vasopressin, angiotensin II (AngII) offers another potential catecholamine-sparing vasopressor option. AngII acts through the renin–angiotensin–aldosterone system to cause vasoconstriction and renal sodium resorption. In the AngII for the Treatment of High Output Shock (ATHOS-3) trial, AngII improved blood pressure when added to norepinephrine.[89] However, there have been no trials evaluating the effect of AngII on clinical outcomes or comparing AngII to common alternative agents, including vasopressin and other catecholamines. Interestingly, secondary analyses of the ATHOS-3 trial found that the blood pressure effects of AngII were more pronounced in certain patients, for example, patients with acute kidney injury or high renin levels.[90,91] Such findings have piqued interest in novel approaches to vasopressor management, with calls for the use of multimodal therapy (eg, low doses of multiple vasopressors simultaneously) and personalized approaches (eg, guiding vasopressor choice based on clinical characteristics and/or biomarkers).[87] However, trials are needed to prospectively validate such approaches, and for now, AngII remains a third-line vasopressor.

Adjuvant therapy—corticosteroids

Corticosteroids can also help increase blood pressure, in addition to providing potential benefit by decreasing inflammation.[92] Stress-dose corticosteroids should be added for patients with sepsis who have persistent vasopressor requirements despite fluid resuscitation and antibiotics, as suggested in the 2026 SSC guidelines.[9] Typically, IV hydrocortisone is used at a dose of 200 mg/day, either as a continuous infusion or in divided doses (50 mg every 6 hours).[8] Use of corticosteroids in septic shock is supported by 2 large trials: APROCCHSS and ADRENAL (see **Table 1**).[66,67] In APROCCHSS, among 1241 patients with septic shock on $\geq$0.25 mcg/kg/minute norepinephrine, addition of hydrocortisone and fludrocortisone reduced mortality versus placebo (43.0% vs 49.1%, P = .03).[67] While no mortality difference was observed in ADRENAL, which evaluated a less severely ill population, there was faster resolution of shock among patients randomized to continuous hydrocortisone versus placebo (3 vs 4 days).[66] Taken together, these trials suggest that corticosteroids shorten the duration of shock and, in patients on higher doses of norepinephrine, may also improve mortality.

It is worth highlighting that APROCCHSS used hydrocortisone plus fludrocortisone while ADRENAL used hydrocortisone alone. Fludrocortisone has a stronger mineralocorticoid effect than hydrocortisone, and thus may provide additional benefit for raising blood pressure and shortening shock duration.[93] In an observational target trial emulation, addition of fludrocortisone to hydrocortisone was associated with a 3.7% decrease in mortality compared to hydrocortisone alone,[94] similar to the magnitude of benefit estimated in a recent meta-analysis.[93] Given available evidence and the low cost and low risk of fludrocortisone, fludrocortisone should be prescribed alongside hydrocortisone in patients with enteral access.

Resuscitation targets

Hemodynamic resuscitation should be guided by holistic clinical assessment, including monitoring of MAP and serial assessments of CRT and lactate.

MAP should be used as a target for titrating vasopressors in real time. Historically, higher MAP goals were thought to improve perfusion. However, the 2014 Assessment of Two Levels of Arterial Pressure on Survival in Patients With Septic Shock trial compared MAP targets of 75 to 85 versus $\geq$65 mm Hg and found no difference in mortality, but less vasopressor use and less atrial fibrillation among patients randomized to the lower MAP target (see **Table 1**).[68] This led the SSC to recommend a MAP goal of $\geq$65 mm Hg over higher targets.[8] More recently, the 65 trial compared a MAP goal of $\geq$65 mm Hg to *permissive hypotension* (MAP goal 60–65 mm Hg) among 2600 patients aged greater than or equal to 65 year old with vasodilatory shock and found no difference in mortality, with a point estimate favoring permissive hypotension and significant mortality benefit in adjusted secondary analyses.[69] While both groups in the 65 trial overshot their MAP targets, in combination with a meta-analysis, these findings suggest using permissive targets in older patients is safe.[95] Data on using permissive hypotension (MAP 60–65 mm Hg) in younger patients are lacking.

While MAP is a practical and easily measurable resuscitation target, it does not fully capture a patient's perfusion status. MAP measures perfusion at the macrovascular level, but patients in septic shock can have ongoing organ hypoperfusion due to microvascular dysfunction despite a normal MAP.[96] While there has been interest in using microvascular resuscitation targets, methods of measuring microvascular perfusion are not well validated and often require special equipment not routinely available, such as sublingual microscopes.[97]

However, readily available tissue perfusion markers—CRT and lactate—can augment the use of MAP during resuscitation. Using these measures as targets for resuscitation was evaluated in the ANDROMEDA-SHOCK trial, which compared resuscitation guided to lactate clearance versus normalizing CRT among 424 patients with septic shock. While this trial found no difference in mortality overall, CRT-guided resuscitation was associated with lower mortality among patients with lower illness severity and a secondary Bayesian analysis found a 90% probability that a CRT-guided strategy was superior to lactate (see **Table 1**).[70,98] In practice, both CRT, which can be measured quickly at the bedside, and lactate, which may have better inter-rater reliability, provide a more comprehensive view of a patient's perfusion status than MAP alone.

Being able to detect hypoperfusion is insufficient on its own. Rather, clinicians must be able to respond to this information and administer interventions that improve perfusion. The ANDROMEDA-SHOCK 2 trial evaluated a complex resuscitation protocol that involved hourly CRT assessments (hours 1–6) and provided a multilevel algorithm for responding to abnormal CRT, including serial dynamic assessments of fluid responsiveness and bedside echocardiograms with the potential to test the impact of increasing MAP or adding inotropes.[71] This resuscitation protocol was carried out by a dedicated member of the research team, who was present at bedside for the first 6 hours in addition the clinical care team. In the trial, among 1467 patients with septic shock, the CRT-guided resuscitation protocol led to improvement in a hierarchical composite outcome of death and organ support compared to usual care.[71] There are many aspects of this protocol that could explain its benefit: (a) CRT could allow clinicians to better detect hypoperfusion than other markers; (b) integrating multiple assessment indicators to determine resuscitation could help tailor treatment to each patient's needs; or (c) more intense early monitoring could be beneficial regardless of what resuscitation algorithm is used.[99] Unfortunately, the ANDROMEDA-SHOCK 2 algorithm is complex and resource intensive, making it difficult to implement at many institutions. However, clinicians can take away that using markers of tissue perfusion (ie, CRT) likely augment the use of MAP targets and personalizing hemodynamic resuscitation and performing hourly bedside reassessments early in a patient's course may improve outcomes.

Hemodynamic monitoring

Patients with septic shock require close monitoring during resuscitation. Traditionally, such monitoring necessitated a CVC to monitor central venous pressure and administer vasopressors and an arterial catheter to monitor blood pressure. However, recent studies have suggested that many patients with septic shock may be managed effectively without CVCs or arterial catheters.

Vasopressors can be administered via peripheral IVs as long as there is frequent monitoring of the IV site and treatment protocols for extravasation. Incidence of peripheral vasopressor extravasation is low (3%–5%), and risk of tissue injury is minimal when monitoring and treatment protocols are in place (0 cases in adults in meta-analyses).[100–102] Based on this evidence, the SSC guidelines suggest initiating vasopressors peripherally rather than delaying initiation for CVC placement,[8] and recent multicenter studies indicate peripheral vasopressor use is common in practice.[103–105] While peripheral vasopressors are practical and safe, there is wide variation in hospital policies and clinician practices for when to place a CVC in patients on vasopressors.[106,107] In general, CVCs should be placed for patients with worsening shock requiring high dose or multiple vasopressors (typically at a norepinephrine dose around 0.2–0.3 mcg/kg/minute), who have poor peripheral intravenous (PIV) access, or have other indications for central access.

The use of arterial catheters also varies widely and is not necessary for all patients.[108] While rates of complications from arterial catheters are lower than from CVCs, arterial catheters still pose a risk of ischemia, hematoma, and infection.[47] The recent EVERDAC trial was a large, multicenter trial comparing invasive versus noninvasive strategies of blood pressure monitoring among 1010 patients with shock (see **Table 1**).[72] Patients in the invasive arm had arterial catheters inserted within 4 hours of randomization, whereas patients in the noninvasive arm had arterial catheters inserted only for predefined safety criteria (inability to obtain a blood pressure or pulse oximetry noninvasively, 5 failed arterial puncture attempts, need for extracorporeal membrane oxygen therapy or high-risk surgery, or escalation to a vasopressor dose more than the equivalent of 2.5 mcg/kg/minute of norepinephrine plus epinephrine). Only 14.7% of patients in the noninvasive arm received an arterial catheter, and 28-day mortality was similar between arms. However, there are trade-offs for these strategies to consider in practice. Patients assigned to the invasive arm had higher rates of hematoma or hemorrhage (8.2% vs 1.0%), whereas patients assigned to the noninvasive arm required more arterial blood draws (total 742 vs 269) and experienced more patient-reported discomfort from blood pressure monitoring (13.1% vs 9.0%). Overall, a conservative strategy of inserting arterial catheters when noninvasive monitoring measures fail or a patient has escalating shock is reasonable.

Back to the Case (Resuscitation)

Our patient received a 30 mL/kg bolus of LR over an hour. She remained hypotensive with prolonged CRT, so was initiated on norepinephrine. A passive leg raise was performed and SV change was 15% as measured using noninvasive bioreactance technology, suggesting the patient was fluid responsive (≥10% SV change indicates fluid responsiveness). She was given another 500 mL of LR. While her vasopressor requirement initially improved, over the next hour norepinephrine had to be increased to 0.25 mcg/kg/minute. Repeat passive leg raise (PLR) showed SV change of 5% (not fluid responsive); no additional fluid was given. Vasopressin was added. At this time, as discussed above, infectious etiologies and sources were revisited and she was sent to IR for a percutaneous nephrostomy tube for source control. After coming back from the procedure, her vasopressors were quickly weaned. She never required a CVC or arterial catheter, though if she had not improved with the IR procedure, placing a CVC and arterial catheter and starting stress-dose steroids may have been warranted.

SUMMARY

Sepsis is a life-threatening emergency. Early recognition and treatment are essential to improve survival. Initial management should focus on treating infection with prompt antimicrobial therapy and source control and resuscitation using personalized approaches to tailor fluid and vasopressor therapy to patient needs. In patients who do not improve with initial antibiotic therapy and resuscitation, clinicians must continue to re-evaluate antibiotic coverage, the potential source of infection, and adequacy of resuscitation using dynamic assessments.

CLINICS CARE POINTS

- Prompt recognition and treatment improve survival for patients with sepsis.
- Early sepsis management should focus on both treatment of the infection and hemodynamic resuscitation, which should be pursued urgently and in parallel.

- Infection management should focus on early, appropriate antimicrobial therapy and source control, when needed.
- If patients do not improve with initial treatment, clinicians should re-evaluate for missed organisms or sources.
- Hemodynamic management should focus on fluid resuscitation with an initial bolus of balanced crystalloids with additional fluid guided by serial dynamic assessments of fluid-responsiveness.
- Vasopressors may be needed in addition to fluid resuscitation to maintain blood pressure.

DISCLOSURE

E. Munroe reports support from NHLBI (K23HL177175, L30HL170379). I.D. Peltan reports support from NIGMS (R35GM151147), and outside the present work, payments to his institution for research enrollments from Regeneron, Bluejay Diagnostics, and Novartis. H.C. Prescott reports payments from Aurobac Therapeutics for scientific consulting and from DynaMed for editorial services; and serving as co-Chair of the Surviving Sepsis Campaign guidelines. This material is the result of work supported with resources and use of facilities at the Ann Arbor VA Medical Center. This article does not represent the views of the Department of Veterans Affairs or the US government.

REFERENCES

1. Rudd KE, Johnson SC, Agesa KM, et al. Global, regional, and national sepsis incidence and mortality, 1990–2017: analysis for the global burden of disease study. Lancet 2020;395(10219):200–11.
2. Liu V, Escobar GJ, Greene JD, et al. Hospital deaths in patients with sepsis from 2 independent cohorts. JAMA 2014;312(1):90.
3. Rhee C, Jones TM, Hamad Y, et al. Prevalence, underlying causes, and preventability of sepsis-associated mortality in US acute care hospitals. JAMA Netw Open 2019;2(2):e187571. https://doi.org/10.1001/jamanetworkopen.2018.7571.
4. Singer M, Deutschman CS, Seymour CW, et al. The third international consensus definitions for sepsis and septic shock (Sepsis-3). JAMA 2016; 315(8):801.
5. Seymour CW, Gesten F, Prescott HC, et al. Time to treatment and mortality during mandated emergency care for sepsis. N Engl J Med 2017;376(23):2235–44.
6. Leung LY, Huang HL, Hung KK, et al. Door-to-antibiotic time and mortality in patients with sepsis: systematic review and meta-analysis. Eur J Intern Med 2024; 129:48–61.
7. Johnston ANB, Park J, Doi SA, et al. Effect of immediate administration of antibiotics in patients with sepsis in tertiary care: a systematic review and meta-analysis. Clin Ther 2017;39(1):190–202.e6.
8. Evans L, Rhodes A, Alhazzani W, et al. Surviving sepsis campaign: international guidelines for management of sepsis and septic shock 2021. Crit Care Med 2021;49(11):e1063–143.
9. Prescott HC, Antonelli M, Alhazzani W, et al. Surviving sepsis campaign: international guidelines for management of sepsis and septic shock 2026. Crit Care Med 2026;54(4):725–812.
10. Hechtman RK, Kipnis P, Cano J, et al. Heterogeneity of benefit from earlier time-to-antibiotics for sepsis. Am J Respir Crit Care Med 2024;209(7):852–60.

11. Han X, Spicer A, Carey KA, et al. Identifying high-risk subphenotypes and associated harms from delayed antibiotic orders and delivery. Crit Care Med 2021; 49(10):1694–705.
12. Peltan ID, Brown SM, Bledsoe JR, et al. ED door-to-antibiotic time and long-term mortality in sepsis. Chest 2019;155(5):938–46.
13. Tarrant C, O'Donnell B, Martin G, et al. A complex endeavour: an ethnographic study of the implementation of the sepsis six clinical care bundle. Implement Sci IS 2016;11(1):149.
14. Wayne MT, Seelye S, Molling D, et al. Temporal trends and hospital variation in time-to-antibiotics among veterans hospitalized with sepsis. JAMA Netw Open 2021;4(9):e2123950. https://doi.org/10.1001/jamanetworkopen.2021.23950.
15. Kashiouris MG, Zemore Z, Kimball Z, et al. Supply chain delays in antimicrobial administration after the initial clinician order and mortality in patients with sepsis. Crit Care Med 2019;47(10):1388–95.
16. Prescott HC, Seelye S, Wang XQ, et al. Temporal trends in antimicrobial prescribing during hospitalization for potential infection and sepsis. JAMA Intern Med 2022;182(8):805.
17. Peltan ID, Groat D, Butler J, et al. Physician variation in early sepsis management. JAMA Netw Open 2026;9(2):e2556945. https://doi.org/10.1001/jamanetwork open.2025.56945.
18. Levy MM, Evans LE, Rhodes A. The surviving sepsis campaign bundle: 2018 update. Intensive Care Med 2018;44(6):925–8.
19. Hirosawa T, Sakamoto T, Hanai S, et al. Effect of prior antibiotic treatment on blood culture in an outpatient department of general internal medicine: a retrospective cCase aControl Analysis. Int J Gen Med 2023;16:2709–17.
20. Shappell CN, Klompas M, Ochoa A, et al, CDC Prevention Epicenters Program. Likelihood of bacterial infection in patients treated with broad-spectrum IV antibiotics in the emergency department. Crit Care Med 2021;49(11):e1144–50.
21. Rhodes A, Evans LE, Alhazzani W, et al. Surviving sepsis campaign: international guidelines for management of sepsis and septic shock: 2016. Crit Care Med 2017;45(3):486–552.
22. Kumar A, Ellis P, Arabi Y, et al. Initiation of inappropriate antimicrobial therapy results in a fivefold reduction of survival in human septic shock. Chest 2009; 136(5):1237–48.
23. Meyer NJ, Prescott HC. Sepsis and septic shock. In: Hardin CC, editor. N Engl J Med 2024;391(22):2133–46.
24. Chanderraj R, Baker JM, Kay SG, et al. In critically ill patients, anti-anaerobic antibiotics increase risk of adverse clinical outcomes. Eur Respir J 2023;61(2): 2200910. https://doi.org/10.1183/13993003.00910-2022.
25. Chanderraj R, Admon AJ, He Y, et al. Mortality of patients with sepsis administered piperacillin-Tazobactam vs cefepime. JAMA Intern Med 2024;184(7): 769–77.
26. Qian ET, Casey JD, Wright A, et al. Cefepime vs piperacillin-tazobactam in adults hospitalized with acute infection: the ACORN randomized clinical trial. JAMA 2023;330(16):1557.
27. Prescott HC. The epidemiology of sepsis. In: Wiersinga WJ, Seymour CW, editors. Handbook of sepsis. Springer International Publishing; 2018. p. 15–28. https://doi.org/10.1007/978-3-319-73506-1_2.
28. Morrell M, Fraser VJ, Kollef MH. Delaying the empiric treatment of candida bloodstream infection until positive blood culture results are obtained: a

potential risk factor for hospital mortality. Antimicrob Agents Chemother 2005;49(9):3640–5.
29. Garey KW, Rege M, Pai MP, et al. Time to initiation of fluconazole therapy impacts mortality in patients with candidemia: a multi-institutional study. Clin Infect Dis Off Publ Infect Dis Soc Am 2006;43(1):25–31.
30. Timsit JF, Azoulay E, Schwebel C, et al. Empirical micafungin treatment and survival without invasive fungal infection in adults with ICU-acquired sepsis, candida colonization, and multiple organ failure: the EMPIRICUS randomized clinical trial. JAMA 2016;316(15):1555–64.
31. Pappas PG, Kauffman CA, Andes DR, et al. Clinical practice guideline for the management of candidiasis: 2016 update by the infectious diseases society of America. Clin Infect Dis 2016;62(4):e1–50.
32. Pott H, Andrew MK, Shaffelburg Z, et al. Oseltamivir reduces 30-Day mortality in older adults with influenza: a pooled analysis from the 2012-2019 serious outcomes surveillance network of the Canadian immunization research network. Open Forum Infect Dis 2025;12(2):ofaf058.
33. Lewis NM, Harker EJ, Grant LB, et al. Benefit of early oseltamivir therapy for adults hospitalized with influenza A: an observational study. Clin Infect Dis 2025;81(1):190–7.
34. S Pavia C, M Plummer M. The evolution of rapid antigen detection systems and their application for COVID-19 and other serious respiratory infectious diseases. J Microbiol Immunol Infect Wei Mian Yu Gan Ran Za Zhi 2021;54(5):776–86.
35. Prescott HC, Iwashyna TJ. Improving sepsis treatment by embracing diagnostic uncertainty. Ann Am Thorac Soc 2019;16(4):426–9.
36. Klompas M, Al-Hasan M, Al Mohajer M, et al. Infectious Diseases Society of America (IDSA) position statement: why IDSA did not endorse the community-acquired pneumonia guidelines 2025 update. Clin Infect Dis 2026;82(4):622–4.
37. Jones BE, Ramirez JA, Oren E, et al. Diagnosis and management of community-acquired pneumonia: an official American Thoracic Society Clinical Practice Guideline. Am J Respir Crit Care Med 2026;212(1):24–44.
38. Rüddel H, Thomas-Rüddel DO, Reinhart K, et al. Adverse effects of delayed antimicrobial treatment and surgical source control in adults with sepsis: results of a planned secondary analysis of a cluster-randomized controlled trial. Crit Care 2022;26(1):51.
39. Reitz KM, Kennedy J, Li SR, et al. Association between time to source control in sepsis and 90-Day mortality. JAMA Surg 2022;157(9):817–26.
40. Strich JR, Heil EL, Masur H. Considerations for empiric antimicrobial therapy in sepsis and septic shock in an era of antimicrobial resistance. J Infect Dis 2020;222(Suppl 2):S119–31.
41. Warren JL, Bacon WE, Harris T, et al. The burden and outcomes associated with dehydration among US elderly, 1991. Am J Publ Health 1994;84(8):1265–9.
42. Marik PE, Linde-Zwirble WT, Bittner EA, et al. Fluid administration in severe sepsis and septic shock, patterns and outcomes: an analysis of a large national database. Intensive Care Med 2017;43(5):625–32.
43. Sadaka F, Juarez M, Naydenov S, et al. Fluid resuscitation in septic shock: the effect of increasing fluid balance on mortality. J Intensive Care Med 2014;29(4):213–7.
44. Boyd JH, Forbes J, Nakada T-A, et al. Fluid resuscitation in septic shock: a positive fluid balance and elevated central venous pressure are associated with increased mortality. Crit Care Med 2011;39(2):259–65.

45. Taylor SP, Karvetski CH, Templin MA, et al. Initial fluid resuscitation following adjusted body weight dosing is associated with improved mortality in obese patients with suspected septic shock. J Crit Care 2018;43:7–12.
46. The PRISM investigators. Early, goal-directed therapy for septic shock — a patient-level meta-analysis. N Engl J Med 2017;376(23):2223–34. https://doi.org/10.1056/NEJMoa1701380.
47. Munroe ES, Hyzy RC, Semler MW, et al. Evolving management practices for early sepsis-induced hypoperfusion: a narrative review. Am J Respir Crit Care Med 2023;207(10):1283–99.
48. Liu V, Morehouse JW, Soule J, et al. Fluid volume, lactate values, and mortality in sepsis patients with intermediate lactate values. Ann Am Thorac Soc 2013;10(5):466–73.
49. Liu VX, Morehouse JW, Marelich GP, et al. Multicenter implementation of a treatment bundle for patients with sepsis and intermediate lactate values. Am J Respir Crit Care Med 2016;193(11):1264–70.
50. Wang HL, Shao J, Liu WL, et al. Initial fluid resuscitation (30 mL/kg) in patients with septic shock: more or less? Am J Emerg Med 2021;50:309–15.
51. Mouncey PR, Osborn TM, Power GS, et al. Trial of early, goal-directed resuscitation for septic shock. N Engl J Med 2015;372(14):1301–11.
52. The ProCESS Investigators, Yealy DM, Kellum JA, Huang DT, et al. A randomized trial of protocol-based care for early septic shock. N Engl J Med 2014;370(18):1683–93.
53. ARISE Investigators, ANZICS Clinical Trials Group, Peake SL, Delaney A, Bailey M, et al. Goal-directed resuscitation for patients with early septic shock. N Engl J Med 2014;371(16):1496–506.
54. Andrews B, Muchemwa L, Kelly P, et al. Simplified severe sepsis protocol: a randomized controlled trial of modified early goal–directed therapy in Zambia. Crit Care Med 2014;42(11):2315–24.
55. Bentzer P, Griesdale DE, Boyd J, et al. Will this hemodynamically unstable patient respond to a bolus of intravenous fluids? JAMA 2016;316(12):1298.
56. Shapiro NI, Douglas IS, Brower RG, et al, National Heart, Lung, and Blood Institute Prevention and Early Treatment of Acute Lung Injury Clinical Trials Network. Early restrictive or liberal fluid management for sepsis-induced hypotension. N Engl J Med 2023;388(6):499–510.
57. Meyhoff TS, Hjortrup PB, Wetterslev J, et al. Restriction of intravenous fluid in ICU patients with septic shock. N Engl J Med 2022;386(26):2459–70.
58. Douglas IS, Alapat PM, Corl KA, et al. Fluid response evaluation in sepsis hypotension and shock. Chest 2020;158(4):1431–45.
59. Semler MW, Self WH, Wanderer JP, et al. Balanced crystalloids versus saline in critically ill adults. N Engl J Med 2018;378(9):829–39.
60. Jackson KE, Wang L, Casey JD, et al. Effect of early balanced crystalloids before ICU admission on sepsis outcomes. Chest 2021;159(2):585–95.
61. Zampieri FG, Machado FR, Biondi RS, et al. Association between type of fluid received prior to enrollment, type of admission, and effect of balanced crystalloid in critically ill adults: a secondary exploratory analysis of the BaSICS clinical trial. Am J Respir Crit Care Med 2022;205(12):1419–28.
62. Finfer S, Micallef S, Hammond N, et al. Balanced multielectrolyte solution versus saline in critically ill adults. N Engl J Med 2022;NEJMoa2114464. https://doi.org/10.1056/NEJMoa2114464.

63. Zampieri FG, Machado FR, Biondi RS, et al. Effect of intravenous fluid treatment with a balanced solution vs 0.9% saline solution on mortality in critically ill patients: the BaSICS randomized clinical trial. JAMA 2021;326(9):818.
64. De Backer D, Biston P, Devriendt J, et al. Comparison of dopamine and norepinephrine in the treatment of shock. N Engl J Med 2010;362(9):779–89.
65. Russell JA, Walley KR, Singer J, et al. Vasopressin versus norepinephrine infusion in patients with septic shock. N Engl J Med 2008;358(9):877–87.
66. Venkatesh B, Finfer S, Cohen J, et al. Adjunctive glucocorticoid therapy in patients with septic shock. N Engl J Med 2018;378(9):797–808.
67. Annane D, Renault A, Brun-Buisson C, et al. Hydrocortisone plus fludrocortisone for adults with septic shock. N Engl J Med 2018;378(9):809–18.
68. Asfar P, Meziani F, Hamel JF, et al. High versus low blood-pressure target in patients with septic shock. N Engl J Med 2014;370(17):1583–93.
69. Lamontagne F, Richards-Belle A, Thomas K, et al. Effect of reduced exposure to vasopressors on 90-Day mortality in older critically ill patients with vasodilatory hypotension: a randomized clinical trial. JAMA 2020;323(10):938.
70. Hernández G, Ospina-Tascón GA, Damiani LP, et al. Effect of a resuscitation strategy targeting peripheral perfusion status vs serum lactate levels on 28-Day mortality among patients with septic shock: the ANDROMEDA-SHOCK randomized clinical trial. JAMA 2019;321(7):654.
71. The ANDROMEDA-SHOCK-2 Investigators for the ANDROMEDA Research Network, Spanish Society of Anesthesiology, Reanimation and Pain Therapy (SEDAR), and Latin American Intensive Care Network (LIVEN). Personalized hemodynamic resuscitation targeting capillary refill time in early septic shock: the ANDROMEDA-SHOCK-2 randomized clinical trial. JAMA 2025;334(22):1988.
72. Muller G, Contou D, Ehrmann S, et al. Deferring arterial catheterization in critically ill patients with shock. N Engl J Med 2025;393(19):1875–88.
73. Wang J, Blake LM, Orozco N, et al. Dynamic measures of fluid responsiveness to guide resuscitation in patients with sepsis and septic shock: a systematic review and meta-analysis. Crit Care Explor 2025;7(9):e1303. https://doi.org/10.1097/CCE.0000000000001303.
74. Rhee C, Wang R, Zhang Z, et al, CDC Prevention Epicenters Program. Epidemiology of hospital-onset versus community-onset sepsis in U.S. hospitals and association with mortality: a retrospective analysis using electronic clinical data. Crit Care Med 2019;47(9):1169–76.
75. Munroe E, Kenana RB, Capellini A, et al. Understanding the prevalence of community-onset vs hospital-onset sepsis in sepsis trials: a scoping review. Chest 2025;168(4):A2192–3.
76. Gelbenegger G, Shapiro NI, Zeitlinger M, et al. Lactated ringer's or normal saline for initial fluid resuscitation in sepsis-induced hypotension. Crit Care Med 2025;53(5):e1140–4.
77. Khan A, Munroe E, Koike S, et al. Impact of balanced crystalloids vs saline by resuscitation strategy in sepsis A secondary analysis of the crystalloid liberal or vasopressor early resuscitation in sepsis trial. CHEST Crit Care 2025;4(2):100226. https://doi.org/10.1016/j.chstcc.2025.100226.
78. Bledsoe J, Peltan ID, Bunnell RJ, et al. Order substitutions and education for balanced crystalloid solution use in an integrated health care system and association with major adverse kidney events. JAMA Netw Open 2022;5(5):e2210046. https://doi.org/10.1001/jamanetworkopen.2022.10046.

79. McIntyre L, Fergusson D, McArdle T, et al. A crossover trial of hospital-wide lactated ringer's solution versus normal saline. N Engl J Med 2025;393(7):660–70.
80. Alwang AK, Law AC, Klings ES, et al. Lactated ringer vs normal saline solution during sickle cell vaso-occlusive episodes. JAMA Intern Med 2024;184(11):1365.
81. Szabó GV, Szigetváry C, Turan C, et al. Fluid resuscitation with balanced electrolyte solutions results in faster resolution of diabetic ketoacidosis than with 0.9% saline in adults - a systematic review and meta-analysis. Diabetes Metab Res Rev 2024;40(5):e3831. https://doi.org/10.1002/dmrr.3831.
82. Ospina-Tascón GA, Hernandez G, Alvarez I, et al. Effects of very early start of norepinephrine in patients with septic shock: a propensity score-based analysis. Crit Care 2020;24(1):52.
83. Yeo HJ, Lee YS, Kim TH, et al. Vasopressor initiation within 1 hour of fluid loading is associated with increased mortality in septic shock patients: analysis of national registry data. Crit Care Med 2021;50(4):e351–60.
84. Permpikul C, Tongyoo S, Viarasilpa T, et al. Early use of norepinephrine in septic shock resuscitation (CENSER). A randomized trial. Am J Respir Crit Care Med 2019;199(9):1097–105.
85. Vail E, Gershengorn HB, Hua M, et al. Association between US norepinephrine shortage and mortality among patients with septic shock. JAMA 2017;317(14):1433–42.
86. Wieruszewski PM, Khanna AK. Vasopressor choice and timing in vasodilatory shock. Crit Care 2022;26(1):76.
87. Kalimouttou A, Kennedy JN, Feng J, et al. Optimal vasopressin initiation in septic shock: the OVISS reinforcement learning study. JAMA 2025;333(19):1688–98.
88. Peltan ID, Groat D, Jacobs JR, et al. Protocol and statistical analysis plan for the vasopressin for septic shock pragmatic (VASSPR) cluster-crossover randomized trial. CHEST Crit Care 2025;3(4):100178. https://doi.org/10.1016/j.chstcc.2025.100178.
89. Khanna A, English SW, Wang XS, et al. Angiotensin II for the treatment of vasodilatory shock. N Engl J Med 2017;377(5):419–30.
90. Bellomo R, Forni LG, Busse LW, et al. Renin and survival in patients given angiotensin II for catecholamine-resistant vasodilatory shock. A clinical trial. Am J Respir Crit Care Med 2020;202(9):1253–61.
91. Chaba A, Zarbock A, Forni LG, et al. Angiotensin II for catecholamine-resistant vasodilatory SHOCK IN patients with acute kidney injury: a post HOC analysis of the ATHOS-3 trial. Shock 2025;63(1):88–93.
92. Werumeus Buning J, Van Faassen M, Brummelman P, et al. Effects of hydrocortisone on the regulation of blood pressure: results from a randomized controlled trial. J Clin Endocrinol Metab 2016;101(10):3691–9.
93. Teja B, Berube M, Pereira TV, et al. Effectiveness of fludrocortisone plus hydrocortisone versus hydrocortisone alone in septic shock: a systematic review and network meta-analysis of randomized controlled trials. Am J Respir Crit Care Med 2024;209(10):1219–28.
94. Bosch NA, Teja B, Law AC, et al. Comparative effectiveness of fludrocortisone and hydrocortisone vs hydrocortisone alone among patients with septic shock. JAMA Intern Med 2023;183(5):451–9.

95. Angriman F, Momenzade N, Adhikari NKJ, et al. Blood pressure targets for adults with vasodilatory shock — an individual patient data meta-analysis. NEJM Evid 2025;4(1). https://doi.org/10.1056/EVIDoa2400359.
96. Hinshaw LB. Sepsis/septic shock: participation of the microcirculation. Crit Care Med 1996;24(6):1072–8.
97. Damiani E, Carsetti A, Casarotta E, et al. Microcirculation-guided resuscitation in sepsis: the next frontier? Front Med 2023;10:1212321. https://doi.org/10.3389/fmed.2023.1212321.
98. Zampieri FG, Damiani LP, Bakker J, et al. Effects of a resuscitation strategy targeting peripheral perfusion status versus serum lactate levels among patients with septic shock. A bayesian reanalysis of the ANDROMEDA-SHOCK trial. Am J Respir Crit Care Med 2020;201(4):423–9.
99. Machado FR, Semler MW. Capillary refill time in sepsis—searching for the holy grail. JAMA 2025;334(22):1983.
100. Tian DH, Smyth C, Keijzers G, et al. Safety of peripheral administration of vasopressor medications: a systematic review. Emerg Med Australas 2020;32(2):220–7.
101. Tran QK, Mester G, Bzhilyanskaya V, et al. Complication of vasopressor infusion through peripheral venous catheter: a systematic review and meta-analysis. Am J Emerg Med 2020;38(11):2434–43.
102. Owen VS, Rosgen BK, Cherak SJ, et al. Adverse events associated with administration of vasopressor medications through a peripheral intravenous catheter: a systematic review and meta-analysis. Crit Care 2021;25(1):146.
103. Munroe ES, Heath ME, Eteer M, et al. Use and outcomes of peripheral vasopressors in early sepsis-induced hypotension across Michigan hospitals: a retrospective cohort study. Chest 2024;165(4):847–57.
104. Munroe ES, Co IN, Douglas I, et al. Peripheral vasopressor use in early sepsis-induced hypotension. JAMA Netw Open 2025;8(8):e2529148. https://doi.org/10.1001/jamanetworkopen.2025.29148.
105. Shyu D, Ingraham NE, Linke CA, et al. Overview of peripheral vasopressor usage in an academic health system. Ann Am Thorac Soc 2025;24:24.
106. Munroe E, Claar D, Tamae-Kakazu M, et al. Hospital policies on intravenous vasopressor administration and monitoring: a survey of Michigan hospitals. Ann Am Thorac Soc 2022;19(10):1769–72.
107. Munroe ES, Weinstein J, Gershengorn HB, et al. Understanding how Clinicians personalize fluid and vasopressor decisions in early sepsis management. JAMA Netw Open 2024;7(4):e247480. https://doi.org/10.1001/jamanetworkopen.2024.7480.
108. Gershengorn HB, Garland A, Kramer A, et al. Variation of arterial and central venous catheter use in United States intensive care units. Anesthesiology 2014;120(3):650–64.

Post-Sepsis Syndrome

From Pathogenesis Toward Novel Management Strategies

Daphne Schouten, MD, PhD Candidate[a,*],
W. Joost Wiersinga, MD, PhD[b], Lonneke van Vught, MD, PhD[c]

KEYWORDS

- Post-sepsis syndrome • Sepsis survivorship • Readmission
- Post-acute infection syndrome • Immune dysregulation • Primary care

KEY POINTS

- Post-sepsis syndrome (PSS) is common after sepsis regardless of severity, but remains underrecognized and poorly standardized.
- Long-term morbidity and mortality are not confined to critically ill patients, and all sepsis survivors show substantial risk of rehospitalization, new disease, and long-term health impairments.
- Emerging evidence in PSS points to persistent immune dysregulation involving immunosuppression, (neuro)inflammation, mitochondrial/endothelial dysfunction, and microbiome disruption.
- Overlap with post-acute infection syndromes, including long COVID, suggests shared features in pathogenesis and thus opportunities for cross-field learning.
- A pragmatic, primary-care–centered, risk-stratified follow-up model could be feasible, but needs further evaluation.

INTRODUCTION

The global burden of sepsis, known as a dysregulated host response to an infection leading to organ dysfunction,[1] is rising. Recent estimates report 166 million sepsis cases annually, accounting for approximately 31.5% of all global deaths.[2] With

[a] Center for Infection and Molecular Medicine (CIMM), Amsterdam Institute for Infection and Immunity (AII), Amsterdam UMC, University of Amsterdam, Amsterdam, The Netherlands; [b] Division of Infectious Diseases, Department of Medicine, Center for Infection and Molecular Medicine (CIMM), Amsterdam Institute for Infection and Immunity (AII), Amsterdam UMC, University of Amsterdam, Amsterdam, The Netherlands; [c] Department of General Practice and Nursing Science, Julius Center for Health Sciences and Primary Care, University Medical Center Utrecht, Utrecht University, Utrecht, Netherlands
* Corresponding author. Meibergdreef 9, 1105 AZ, Amsterdam.
E-mail address: d.schouten2@amsterdamumc.nl

Crit Care Clin 42 (2026) 745–761
https://doi.org/10.1016/j.ccc.2026.05.003 criticalcare.theclinics.com
0749-0704/26/

Abbreviations	
ADL	activities of daily living
AKI	acute kidney injury
BBB	blood–brain barrier
CLP	cecal ligation and puncture
DAMP	damage-associated molecular pattern
GP	general practitioner
HMGB1	high-mobility group box 1
ICU	intensive care unit
IL	interleukin
MDSC	myeloid-derived suppressor cell
PAIS	post-acute infection syndrome
PPI	proton pump inhibitor
PSS	post-sepsis syndrome
PTSD	post-traumatic stress disorder
SAE	septic-associated encephalopathy

medical advancements in quality of care, in-hospital mortality from sepsis has declined, substantially increasing the number of sepsis survivors.[3] Due to the aging population, a rise in chronic conditions, and increased antibiotic resistance, this number is expected to increase even further in the coming years.[4] Patients who survive their initial sepsis episode frequently experience long lasting medical, cognitive, and psychological sequelae.[5] These complications following sepsis have long been underrecognized, despite their substantial impact on long-term health and quality of life. So far, standardized care pathways and coordinated approaches to support patients after sepsis and improve long-term outcomes have not been widely implemented.

Patients surviving their initial sepsis episode face an increased long-term risk of rehospitalization and mortality after hospital discharge.[6–10] Approximately 1 in 5 sepsis patients are readmitted within 30 days after discharge,[9] increasing up to three-quarters within the first year.[10] Compared to patients hospitalized for infection without organ dysfunction, sepsis survivors have a 10.4% higher absolute risk of late mortality, with excess mortality persisting up to 1 year.[8] Although these sequelae are often discussed as part of post–intensive care syndrome (PICS), many affected sepsis survivors were never admitted to the intensive care unit (ICU).[8,10–12] After adjustment for prior health status, the association between sepsis and subsequent disabilities persists, suggesting that sepsis itself may initiate or accelerate a process of long-term health deterioration rather than merely unmask pre-existing disease.[8,13]

Although post-sepsis syndrome (PSS) currently lacks a standardized case definition, it refers to the constellation of physical, cognitive, and/or psychological impairments that develop after survival from sepsis, persist beyond the acute recovery phase, and cannot be explained by pre-existing conditions.[14,15] The underlying mechanisms of long-term sequalae after sepsis remain poorly understood and are hypothesized as a complex interplay between a patient's pre-sepsis health status, the individual clinical course of the disease, severity and source of the infection, comorbidities, availability of health care resources care, and so on.[16] The recently updated surving sepsis campaign guidelines have stressed the urgent need for post hospital evaluation, management and rehabiliation after hospitalization for sepsis.[17] To date, the lack of evidence-based treatment guidelines for PSS is regarded as one of the most urgent research priorities in sepsis.[18] This article synthesizes current evidence and key knowledge gaps on long-term sequelae specifically attributable to PSS rather than critical illness survivorship more broadly. It proposes a primary care–oriented framework for postdischarge follow-up and identifies priorities for prevention and targeted intervention.

CLINICAL SEQUELAE

A considerable proportion of readmissions are for diagnoses that may be preventable with earlier outpatient recognition and management,[6] implying that hospital readmissions alone underestimate the overall burden, as emerging sequelae may be managed in primary care or outpatient settings. Consistent with this, up to three-quarters of sepsis survivors develop at least one new medical, cognitive, or psychological diagnosis after discharge,[13] and approximately 1 in 6 develop severe, persistent long-term impairments[5] (**Fig. 1**). While clinical outcomes are primarily derived from observational studies rather dan randomized controlled trials (RCTs), possibly resulting in residual confounding, the association between sepsis and clinical sequelae is firmly established across international literature.

Sepsis Survivors Are More Prone to Disease and Rehospitalization

Reinfection

Recurrent sepsis is reported as the leading readmission diagnosis, accounting for approximately 29% to 52% of early readmission across studies on sepsis survivors.[6,19,20] In an age-matched and sex-matched analysis, individuals who survived a severe sepsis admission had over 8 times higher risk of experiencing recurrent severe sepsis compared to the general population.[21] A French nationwide study further showed that readmission with recurrent sepsis regardless of severity is strongly associated with 1-year mortality, alongside age and comorbidity burden.[10] In this study, factors associated with recurrent sepsis included malignancy, renal disease, older age, and longer length of hospital stay, whereas rehospitalization for recurrent sepsis was lower in ICU admitted patients without septic shock.[10] Approximately two-thirds of patients readmitted for sepsis within 90 days experience sepsis recurrence at the same site of infection as their initial hospitalization.[19] However, microbiological data indicate that in roughly half of these cases the episode represents a newly acquired infection rather than an ongoing primary infection.[19]

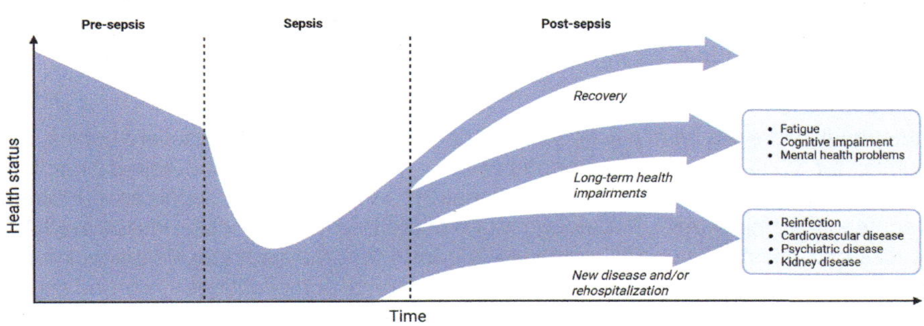

Fig. 1. Conceptual model of post-sepsis clinical trajectories. Many sepsis survivors do not return to their pre-sepsis health status. Instead, they may follow overlapping trajectories of partial recovery, persistent long-term impairment, and/or new disease with rehospitalization. Arrow thickness reflects the relative clinical burden of each trajectory based on representative estimates from the literature. Estimates are illustrative, derived from heterogeneous study designs and follow-up periods. (Created in BioRender. Appelman, B. (2026) https://BioRender.com/8zy7c4p.)

Cardiovascular disease

Sepsis is a clinically meaningful, nontraditional cardiovascular risk factor as shown in pooled results from several studies.[22,23] Rehospitalization for cardiovascular disease has been reported in approximately 3.5% of sepsis survivors within 30 days, while heart failure-related readmissions occur in 1.5% by 30 days and 2.9% by 90 days.[24] New-onset heart failure after sepsis is the most common cardiovascular complication (8.6%), followed by stroke (4.9%) and myocardial infarction (2.4%).[23] One in 4 ICU sepsis survivors without pre-existing cardiovascular disease developed new, acute cardiovascular events.[25] This corresponds to a 1.9 fold increased risk compared to matched controls, a risk magnitude similar to traditional factors such as smoking, diabetes, and hypercholesterolemia.[14]

Large population-based cohorts consistently show sustained long-term cardiovascular risk after sepsis, regardless of ICU admission. An US administrative cohort of more than 8 million sepsis survivors showed higher cardiovascular mortality and rehospitalization than propensity score–matched, hospitalized non-sepsis controls over up to 12 years of follow-up, with the strongest association for heart failure hospitalization (adjusted hazard ratio [HR] 1.51).[12] Consistently, a Taiwanese cohort of more than 93,000 sepsis survivors showed increased risks of cardiovascular events ranging from HR 1.14 to HR 1.42, compared to propensity score-matched, hospitalized non-sepsis controls.[26] Risk of all-cause mortality (HR, 1.95) and major adverse events (HR 1.27) were highest within 1 year and persisted for more than 5 years.[26] Notably, ICU admission was associated with higher all-cause mortality, but did not increase the risk of major cardiovascular disease.[26]

Psychiatric disease

Post-sepsis psychiatric disease represents a frequent and clinically relevant component of PSS, encompassing depression, anxiety, and posttraumatic stress disorder (PTSD).[27] Approximately one-quarter of sepsis survivors develop a new psychiatric diagnosis, with depression being the most common disorder, affecting 16.2% of patients without a prior history of depression.[28] While longitudinal data suggest that the prevalence of PTSD and anxiety tend to decrease over time, depressive symptoms often persist or increase, indicating divergent recovery trajectories.[29] Persistent post-sepsis depression is independently associated with excess long-term mortality, as shown across multiple cohorts.[30,31] Notably, a nationwide cohort study in Korea reported a 5-year all-cause mortality of 46.2% among patients with post-sepsis depression, corresponding to a 1.29 fold increased risk compared to matched controls.[30]

Kidney disease

Acute renal failure is a relatively frequent readmission diagnosis after severe sepsis, accounting for 3.3% of readmissions compared to 1.2% in matched non-sepsis hospitalizations.[6] Approximately 4.5% of early unplanned readmissions after sepsis are attributed to acute kidney injury (AKI).[24] Although much of the literature on sepsis-associated AKI focuses on critically ill cohorts, evidence supports that the pathophysiological impact of sepsis on renal function contributes to sustained renal complications in a broad sepsis population.[32] A retrospective cohort study of 1636 patients with sepsis admitted to the ward and ICU reported a high AKI incidence of 61% at admission.[33] Among survivors with sepsis-associated AKI and available follow-up, 19% progressed to chronic kidney disease within 1 year, unrelated to AKI stage at presentation.[33]

Cancer

Cancer increases the risk of sepsis, but growing evidence suggests this relationship may be bidirectional.[34,35] Beyond malignancy as a predisposing factor, sepsis has been linked to a higher subsequent cancer incidence than in the general population.[35] In a Swedish nationwide study of 18,550 one-year ICU sepsis survivors, the incidence rate ratio for a new cancer diagnosis ranged from 1.31 to 1.74 depending on sex, relative to the general population.[34] However, this association may be partly explained by residual confounding and surveillance bias and requires further confirmation.

Sepsis Survivors Suffer From Long-Term Health Impairments

Cognitive impairment

Sepsis survivors can experience substantial and persistent impact on cognitive function.[36] During acute illness, many patients develop septic-associated encephalopathy (SAE),[37] an umbrella term for sepsis-related acute brain dysfunction ranging from mild confusion to delirium and coma. SAE, particularly when complicated by delirium,[38] has been linked to adverse long-term cognitive outcomes such as attention, memory, and executive functioning.[24] An ICU-based, prospective cohort study found neuropsychological impairment in 34% of sepsis survivors 6 months after discharge.[39] Additionally, a prospective cohort study including all sepsis survivors showed an increase in moderate to severe cognitive impairment of 10.6% after sepsis, persisting for up to 8 years of follow-up even after accounting for baseline cognitive status.[11] Sepsis has also been associated with a faster decline in cognitive performance compared to pre-sepsis slopes.[40] Poorer cognitive performance was further associated with greater activities of daily living (ADL) dependence and reduced survival.[40]

Functional decline

A considerable proportion of sepsis survivors experience persistent limitations in daily activities. In a large longitudinal cohort study involving 1194 ICU and ward patients in the United States, severe sepsis was associated with the acquisition of approximately 1 to 2 new ADL or instrumental ADL limitations among patients without prior functional impairment.[11] While partial recovery of physical function is commonly observed during 6 to 12 months of follow-up, functional performance often remains below population norms and does not consistently return to pre-sepsis levels.[11] In line with these findings, sepsis survivors demonstrate reduced tolerance to physical exertion, reflecting impaired exercise capacity during recovery.[41,42] Furthermore, in a prospective survey study, sepsis survivors reported a significant increase in sensory, digestive, breathing, chest pain, and musculoskeletal problems.[43] Fatigue is a prominent feature of PSS and is reported by approximately 67.8% of sepsis survivors at 6 months after hospitalization.[44] Mental health problems are also frequent, as illustrated by a large population-based German cohort study that reported mental health impairment in 54.8% of patients within the first year following sepsis hospitalization.[28]

PROPOSED MECHANISMS

The pathogenesis of PSS remains poorly defined; however, proposed contributing mechanisms include chronic low-grade inflammation, persistent immunosuppression, mitochondrial dysregulation, endothelial dysfunction, and microbiome disruption (**Fig. 2**). Notably, many of these mechanisms are not unique to sepsis: they overlap substantially with etiopathogenesis proposed for post-acute infection syndromes (PAIS; **Box 1**).

Immune Dysregulation

Chronic low-grade inflammation

The most commonly proposed mechanism behind PSS is persistent immune dysregulation, characterized by ongoing inflammation alongside immunosuppression

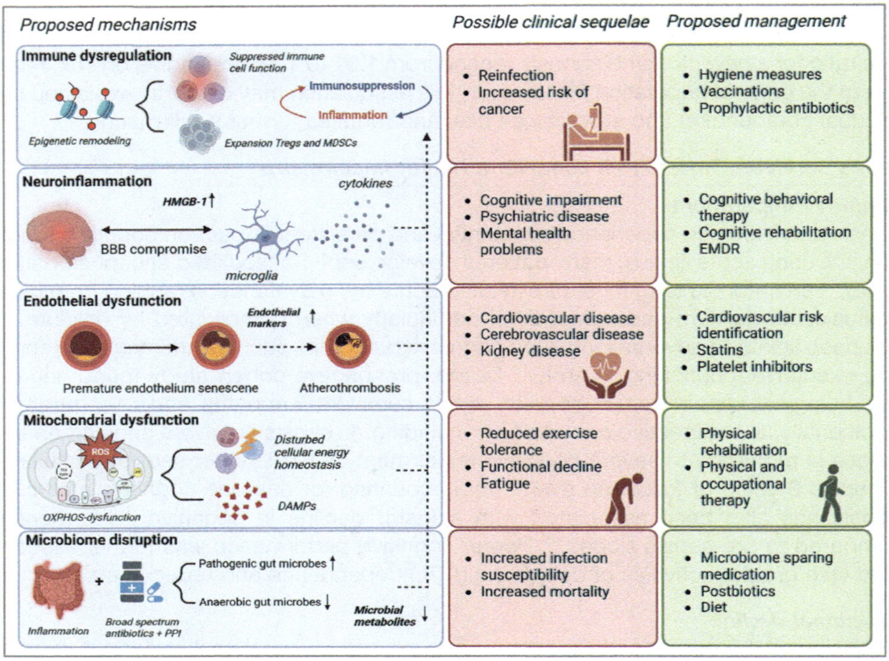

Fig. 2. Overview of proposed mechanisms of post-sepsis syndrome (PSS), the possible clinical sequalae, and proposed management strategies. Post-sepsis immune dysregulation may arise from epigenetic remodeling with impaired immune-cell function and expansion of regulatory T cells (Tregs) and myeloid-derived suppressor cells (MDSCs). Neuroinflammation, endothelial dysfunction, mitochondrial dysfunction, and microbiome disruption may contribute to this. Neuroinflammation may involve high-mobility group box 1 (HMGB1) and blood–brain barrier (BBB) disruption, promoting microglial activation and cytokine release. Endothelial senescence can contribute to endothelial dysfunction and downstream vascular complications, while mitochondrial abnormalities may perpetuate low-grade inflammation via damage-associated molecular patterns (DAMPs). Microbiome disruption due to inflammation and/ortherapy, may reduce beneficial microbes and impair immune regulation, increasing infection susceptibility. These interacting pathways may contribute to persistent symptoms after sepsis and highlight targets for mechanism-based therapies and follow-up care. (Created in BioRender. Appelman, B. (2026) https://BioRender.com/q4k3sf.)

following acute sepsis. Prospective cohort studies have identified persistent elevation of inflammatory markers, including interleukin (IL)-6, IL-10, and high-sensitivity C-reactive protein (CRP) at discharge and up to 1 year after sepsis in a subgroup of survivors.[47,48] Persistent elevation of proinflammatory cytokines is associated with long-term mortality and readmissions, particularly from cardiovascular disease and cancer.[47,48] Persistent inflammation after sepsis may also be mediated by damage-associated molecular patterns (DAMPs), particularly high-mobility group box 1 (HMGB1). Elevated plasma HMGB1 levels have been reported following sepsis and may contribute to sustained innate immune activation by acting as a potent DAMP, modulating neuroinflammatory signaling.[49] Persistently elevated HMGB1 levels were associated with memory impairment lasting up to 4 weeks after sepsis.[50]

Neuroinflammation may be amplified by blood–brain barrier (BBB) disruption after sepsis, as shown in MRI studies in patients with sepsis, potentially facilitating central

Box 1
Post-sepsis syndrome in the context of post-acute infection syndromes: from infection to impaired recovery

Post-acute infection syndromes (PAIS) have moved to the forefront since the COVID-19 pandemic, largely driven by recognition of post-COVID syndrome (long COVID). However, persistent post-infectious symptoms have been described across multiple pathogens well before COVID-19, including Epstein–Barr virus, *Coxiella burnetii*, and *Borrelia burgdorferi*. Across PAIS, symptom profiles are heterogeneous yet strikingly overlapping. Fatigue is the most frequently reported symptom. An important feature of post-COVID syndrome is post-exertional malaise: a delayed and disproportionate worsening of symptoms following physical or cognitive effort.[45] Cognitive dysfunction, myalgia, muscle weakness, and arthralgia are consistently reported in post-COVID syndrome, post-treatment Lyme disease syndrome, and Q-fever fatigue syndrome. Similar symptom clusters such as fatigue, reduced exercise tolerance, and cognitive impairment are also prominent in PSS.

Beyond clinical overlap, biological hypotheses suggest shared underlying mechanisms. Persistent immune activation, driven by residual pathogen components or sustained autoimmunity, has been proposed across PAIS. Neuroinflammation, as well as epigenetic and metabolic reprogramming, have been described after both sepsis and SARS-CoV-2 infection.[46] The overlap in symptoms and proposed mechanisms raises the question whether these conditions should be considered distinct entities, or instead represent the same spectrum after infection. If so, synergies from PSS and PAIS research should be increasingly utilized.

nervous system exposure to circulating inflammatory mediators.[51] Cerebral ischemia and systemic inflammation during sepsis can promote BBB permeability and microglial activation, leading to sustained cytokine production and further compromise of BBB integrity.[52,53] Together, these processes provide a potential mechanistic link between systemic immune dysregulation and long-term neurologic sequelae in PSS.

Immunosuppression

Immunosuppression is hypothesized as a key component of PSS and may contribute to the increased susceptibility to recurrent infections after sepsis.[15] Several mechanisms have been proposed to underlie sustained post-sepsis immunosuppression, including epigenetic reprogramming of both innate and adaptive immune cells.[54] Experimental data support the concept that epigenetic reprogramming affects innate immune cells after sepsis. In a murine cecal ligation and puncture (CLP) model, repressive epigenetic modifications at inflammatory gene promoters persisted after recovery up to 4 weeks after sepsis.[55] In addition, persistently reduced expression of monocytic human leukocyte antigen (mHLA)–DR, a key molecule for antigen presentation, has also been observed in sepsis survivors for up to 2 months after discharge and was independently associated with reinfection and mortality.[56]

Adaptive immune dysregulation further contributes to sustained immunosuppression after sepsis. In a prospective cohort study, low absolute lymphocyte counts 4 days after sepsis onset were independently associated with increased 28-day and 1-year mortality and a higher risk of secondary infections.[57] In parallel, regulatory T cells remain expanded for 5 to 10 months following sepsis hospitalization,[58] potentially shifting to an immunoregulatory milieu which may impair antitumor immune surveillance.[59] Myeloid-derived suppressor cells (MDSCs), which can inhibit T-cell activation and antigen-presenting cell function,[54] have also been reported to expand for at least 4 weeks following sepsis and are clinically associated with secondary infections.[60,61] Functional evidence, although limited, is consistent with these cellular changes. In a small translational study using ex vivo whole-blood stimulation months to years after sepsis, survivors showed reduced cytokine responses to immune challenges, including lower IL-6 and tumor necrosis factor (TNF) after zymosan stimulation and diminished IL-10 production following lipopolysaccharide (LPS) stimulation.[62] Taken together, these findings suggest impaired responsiveness to secondary immune challenges involving both innate and adaptive pathways in sepsis survivors. However, the extent to which these observations directly contribute to clinical outcomes such as secondary infections remains uncertain, with findings largely based on circulating markers that may not capture, among other factors, relevant immune processes at local sites of infection and damaged organs.

Mitochondrial Dysfunction

Mitochondrial dysfunction is hypothesized to play a central role in the metabolic alterations associated with PSS. Sepsis induces persistent mitochondrial abnormalities which can cause incomplete mitochondrial recovery and defective homeostatic mechanisms.[63] These alterations may sustain low-grade inflammation through DAMP release and compromise immune-cell bioenergetics, leading to reduced cytokine responsiveness.[64,65] Immunometabolic perturbations have further been linked to immunoregulatory phenotypes, including upregulation of programmed death-ligand 1 (PD-L1) and persistent metabolic impairment in circulating MDSCs months after sepsis.[66,67] The extent to which sepsis-induced mitochondrial damage is reversible remains uncertain. Experimental data indicate that mitochondrial DNA damage can persist for several days after resolution of acute sepsis and that impaired mitochondrial quality control may hinder full metabolic recovery.[63] In a translational two-stage longitudinal study, mitochondrial-related pathways were the only pathways consistently enriched at both 7 days and 6 months after ICU discharge.[68] Detailed functional analyses demonstrated that this was accompanied by impaired oxidative phosphorylation, accumulation of dysfunctional mitochondria, and defective mitophagy in skeletal muscle, collectively driving sustained post-sepsis muscle weakness.[68] Notably, complementary evidence from murine CLP models shows that mitochondrial-targeting synthetic tetrapeptide SS-31 prevented post-sepsis skeletal muscle weakness after inducing sepsis.[69] Mitochondrial dysregulation may therefore represent a common pathway linking immunometabolic imbalance to impaired recovery after sepsis.

Endothelial Dysfunction

Sepsis triggers cardiovascular complications through demand ischemia, endothelial injury, procoagulant states, and inflammatory plaque destabilization.[70] Inflammatory mediators released during sepsis have been shown to accelerate atherosclerosis through endothelial injury and activation.[71,72] Persistent vascular inflammation may destabilize pre-existing plaques and promotes atherothrombotic events well-beyond hospital discharge. Elevated inflammatory and endothelial activation markers have been linked to increased cardiovascular risk months to years after sepsis.[73] Although not focused on sepsis, a prospective study showed that elevated cardiac and endothelial biomarkers in patients hospitalized with community-acquired pneumonia were independently associated with both early and 30-day cardiovascular events after adjustment for pre-existing cardiovascular disease.[74]

A potential unifying mechanism is accelerated vascular aging, also referred to as premature endothelial senescence, occurring irrespective of age. This state is characterized by loss of endothelial regenerative capacity and sustained endothelial activation, leading to a proinflammatory and prothrombotic vascular state.[75,76] Experimental rat CLP models demonstrate sepsis-induced premature senescence in aortic tissue, peaking 3 months after the septic insult.[75] Comparable senescence-like endothelial responses have been described in humans following acute respiratory distress syndrome (ARDS) and AKI, conditions frequently associated with sepsis and linked to subsequent chronic organ dysfunction.[77,78]

Microbiome Disruption

The gut microbiome is increasingly recognized as an important contributing factor in sepsis, influencing susceptibility, disease onset, and recovery.[70] During hospitalization for sepsis, the gut microbiome is highly vulnerable to disruption due to both the underlying disease and treatments patients receive. In particular, antibiotic therapy frequently induces intestinal loss of commensal microbes causing impaired gut barrier integrity, facilitating translocation of microbial products and increasing susceptibility to secondary infections.[79] In addition, depletion of commensal microbes reduces colonization resistance, allowing overgrowth of pathobionts. Enterococcus domination, in particular, has been linked to higher infection risk and mortality in ICU patients,[80] and anti-anaerobic antibiotic exposure has been associated with increased mortality in sepsis.[81] Gut microbiome disruption after sepsis is not limited to bacteria, a prospective cohort study examined the mycobiome dysbiosis in ICU sepsis patients 2 to 3 weeks after discharge.[82] Compared to healthy controls, sepsis survivors had gut dysbiosis characterized by reduced diversity of the mycobiome, with an increase of pathogenic fungi such as *Candida* and loss of commensal fungi. Strategies to restore the gut microbiota after sepsis, such as prebiotics, probiotics, and synbiotics, are promising but require confirmation in well-designed clinical studies. The PAM-ICU trial is currently evaluating postdischarge supplementation with pasteurized *Akkermansia muciniphila* to support gut microbiota restoration and immune recovery in ICU sepsis survivors (ClinicalTrials.gov: NCT07295353).

MANAGEMENT OF POST-SEPSIS SYNDROME

Prevention of Post-Sepsis Syndrome During Hospitalization

Most current sepsis guidelines primarily focus on reducing short-term mortality, while providing limited guidance on preventing long-term morbidity and PSS. Fluid management appears particularly relevant for neurologic recovery: although conservative fluid strategies may shorten length of stay, they have been associated with worse late cognitive outcomes, potentially due to impaired cerebral perfusion.[83] Stress ulcer prophylaxis is commonly achieved with proton pump inhibitors (PPIs); however, PPIs may adversely affect the gut microbiome by increasing gastric pH and have been associated with higher rates of secondary infections.[5] Delirium during sepsis is strongly associated with subsequent cognitive impairment, and longer delirium duration is associated with poorer cognitive outcome.[38] Multicomponent delirium prevention bundles, which include avoidance or minimization of deliriogenic medications, have been associated with reduced incidence and duration of delirium in hospitalized patients.[84]

Post-discharge Rehabilitation

Evidence supporting post-discharge interventions is emerging but remains limited, especially high-quality studies including ward-treated sepsis remain scarce. A recent systematic review summarizing 14 post-acute intervention studies reports overall improvements in long-term outcomes after hospitalization for sepsis, particularly successful for programs emphasizing physical rehabilitation, mental health support, and care coordination.[85] Rehabilitation programs were associated with improved long-term survival up to 10 years after sepsis, while care coordination was linked to reductions in mortality and hospital readmissions.[85] Large observational data show improved long-term survival after rehabilitation for both ICU and non-ICU treated sepsis patients. A German retrospective cohort including 83,974 sepsis-associated hospitalizations showed significantly improved 5-year survival among sepsis patients discharged to rehabilitation facilities compared to matched sepsis patients discharged home or to self-care.[86] More recently, the Sepsis Transition and Recovery (STAR) trial randomized 3548 sepsis patients to a nurse-led transitional care program focused on medication review, identification of new disabilities, and surveillance of treatable conditions.[87] Although the intervention did not reduce 90 day readmissions compared with usual care, it was associated with lower 90-day mortality. In contrast, another RCT of a nurse navigator-led, multicomponent transition program in 691 sepsis survivors reported reductions in both 30-day mortality and readmission rates.[88]

The Role of Primary Care Postdischarge

The majority of PSS complaints do not lead to hospital readmission and are seen and managed in primary and outpatient care settings.[89] Approximately 40 to 42% causes of early readmission are potentially preventable, such as exacerbation of underlying chronic diseases (chronic obstructive pulmonary disease [COPD], asthma, heart failure), medication updates, and functional decline.[5] Even though there are large differences in primary care organization and delivery throughout the world,[90] the main focus is on the continuum from health promotion and disease prevention to treatment, rehabilitation, and palliative care, all of which should be accessible, continuous, and close to people's everyday environment.[91] In hierarchical primary care models, general practitioners (GPs) are the cornerstone of the health system and typically maintain long-standing relationships with patients and have detailed knowledge of local support services. This positions them in a central role to coordinate post-sepsis care and implement individualized prevention strategies. Several randomized trials have evaluated broader transitional care approaches for a longer time period.[85] A German RCT of 143 ICU sepsis survivors receiving structured primary care management showed no improvement in mental health–related quality of life at 6 or 24 months, but did demonstrate better physical functioning and ADL at 6 months.[92,93]

Primary care can already implement several pragmatic, risk-stratified strategies (**Box 2**, **Fig. 3**). As recurrent infections represent the leading cause of rehospitalization after sepsis, targeted prevention deserves particular attention. This includes optimization of vaccination status, hygiene counseling, nutritional support, and patient and

Box 2
Risk stratification in post-sepsis syndrome

Structured transitional care alone has not consistently reduced morbidity or mortality, suggesting that post-sepsis management likely requires individualized, risk-specific interventions rather than generic care coordination. One explanation may be the marked heterogeneity among sepsis survivors. A large retrospective observational study identified early survivorship phenotypes based on clinical characteristics at hospital discharge that were associated with differential risks of 30-day readmission and mortality.[96] Extending this concept to longer-term recovery trajectories, a large retrospective cohort study identified distinct post-sepsis subtypes using a parsimonious algorithm incorporating Charlson Comorbidity Index, length of stay, and discharge destination.[97] These subtypes predicted 3-month mortality, 6-month, and 12-month quality of life, and limitations in activities of daily living, though not readmission risk. This indicates that clinical phenotyping may help identify patients who require intensified follow-up, an approach that should be prospectively validated and implemented in future care pathways.

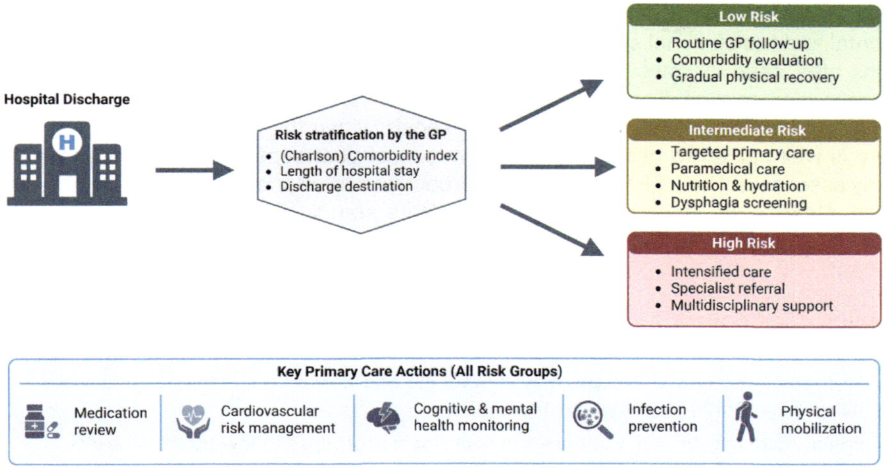

Fig. 3. Proposed follow-up pathway after sepsis hospitalization in primary care. After sepsis hospitalization, general practitioners (GPs) should risk-stratify survivors based on comorbidities, length of stay, and discharge destination. Follow-up intensity can then be tailored to risk level. Core actions across all risk groups include medication review, cardiovascular risk management, screening and monitoring for cognitive and mental health problems, infection prevention, and early mobilization/rehabilitation. (Created in BioRender. Appelman, B. (2026) https://BioRender.com/4hy7iak.)

caregiver education. Aspiration pneumonia is among the most frequent causes of readmission following severe sepsis.[6] Dysphagia is a well-recognized risk factor for aspiration-related pulmonary infection and is very common after sepsis.[15,94] Early swallow screening, dietary modification, and referral to speech and language therapy have reduced pneumonia risk in other high-risk populations,[95] suggesting a plausible opportunity for prevention in sepsis survivors as well.

Beyond infection prevention, primary care provides a natural setting for optimization of cardiovascular risk factors, monitoring of renal function, and referral for physical rehabilitation.[89] Given the elevated long-term risk, optimization of traditional cardiovascular risk factors through pharmacologic treatment and lifestyle interventions appears justified and could be incorporated into routine primary care follow-up of sepsis survivors. Importantly, GPs also play a key role in identifying cognitive impairment and mental health sequelae, providing continuity of care and validation of patient-reported symptoms. Many sepsis survivors experience fragmented follow-up across specialties, contributing to underrecognition of PSS.[98] As an example, post-COVID care pathways have demonstrated how centralized outpatient clinics can facilitate recognition, multidisciplinary assessment, and coordinated management of complex postinfectious sequelae. Improving awareness among clinicians and patients, alongside structured primary care follow-up, may therefore be essential to ensure timely recognition and management of PSS.

SUMMARY

PSS is an increasingly important challenge in the growing population of sepsis survivors. Survivors face high risks of early readmission and new disease, and many experience persistent physical, cognitive, and psychological sequelae that impair daily functioning and quality of life. Mechanistic understanding is still incomplete. Parallels with other PAIS, including long COVID, indicate shared etiopathogenesis. Experimental and translational studies suggest durable immune and inflammatory perturbations after sepsis. However, their persistence and clinical relevance require further investigation on the full spectrum of sepsis survivors. In addition to post critical illness follow-up services offered to survivors of sepsis within the hospital system, primary care is well placed to become the cornerstone of post-sepsis management through early assessment, risk stratification, and proactive surveillance for treatable complications. Greater recognition of PSS may facilitate standardized care transitions while improving clinical acknowledgment of survivors' persistent symptoms and their impact.

CLINICS CARE POINTS

- Persistent symptoms after sepsis may indicate PSS and warrant active follow-up to avoid delayed recognition and management.
- Primary care may be well positioned to coordinate post-sepsis follow-up for survivors, supporting continuity throughout recovery.
- Early assessment and risk stratification may help tailor care and focus intensified follow-up on those most likely to benefit.
- Proactive surveillance for treatable complications, particularly recurrent infection, cardiovascular, kidney, and psychiatric disease, could reduce early readmission.
- Evaluation and counseling regarding cognition, mental health, and physical functioning may improve quality of life.

DISCLOSURES

The authors have nothing to disclose.

REFERENCES

1. Singer M, Deutschman CS, Seymour CW, et al. The third international consensus definitions for sepsis and septic shock (Sepsis-3). JAMA 2016;315:801–10.
2. Gray AP, Chung E, Hsu RL, et al. Global, regional, and national sepsis incidence and mortality, 1990-2021: a systematic analysis. Lancet Global Health 2025;13: e2013–26.
3. Kaukonen KM, Bailey M, Suzuki S, et al. Mortality related to severe sepsis and septic shock among critically ill patients in Australia and New Zealand, 2000-2012. JAMA 2014;311:1308–16.
4. Kox M, Bauer M, Bos LDJ, et al. The immunology of sepsis: translating new insights into clinical practice. Nat Rev Nephrol 2025;22:30–49.
5. Prescott HC, Angus DC. Enhancing recovery from sepsis: a review. JAMA 2018; 319:62–75.
6. Prescott HC, Langa KM, Iwashyna TJ. Readmission diagnoses after hospitalization for severe sepsis and other acute medical conditions. JAMA 2015;313: 1055–7.
7. Inghammar M, Linder A, Lengquist M, et al. Long-term mortality and hospital readmissions among survivors of sepsis in Sweden: a population-based cohort study. Open Forum Infect Dis 2024;11:ofae331.
8. Prescott HC, Osterholzer JJ, Langa KM, et al. Late mortality after sepsis: propensity-matched cohort study. Br Med J 2016;353:i2375.

9. Shankar-Hari M, Saha R, Wilson J, et al. Rate and risk factors for rehospitalisation in sepsis survivors: systematic review and meta-analysis. Intensive Care Med 2020;46:619–36.
10. Pandolfi F, Brun-Buisson C, Guillemot D, et al. One-year hospital readmission for recurrent sepsis: associated risk factors and impact on 1-year mortality-a French nationwide study. Crit Care 2022;26:371.
11. Iwashyna TJ, Ely EW, Smith DM, et al. Long-term cognitive impairment and functional disability among survivors of severe sepsis. JAMA 2010;304:1787–94.
12. Jentzer JC, Lawler PR, Van Houten HK, et al. Cardiovascular events among survivors of sepsis hospitalization: a retrospective cohort analysis. J Am Heart Assoc 2023;12:e027813.
13. Fleischmann-Struzek C, Rose N, Freytag A, et al. Epidemiology and costs of postsepsis morbidity, nursing care dependency, and mortality in Germany, 2013 to 2017. JAMA Netw Open 2021;4:e2134290.
14. Mostel Z, Perl A, Marck M, et al. Post-sepsis syndrome—an evolving entity that afflicts survivors of sepsis. Mol Med 2019;26(1):6.
15. van der Slikke EC, An AY, Hancock REW, et al. Exploring the pathophysiology of post-sepsis syndrome to identify therapeutic opportunities. EBioMedicine 2020; 61:103044.
16. Wiersinga WJ, van der Poll T. Immunopathophysiology of human sepsis. EBioMedicine 2022;86:104363.
17. Prescott HC, Antonelli M, Alhazzani W, et al. Surviving sepsis campaign: international guidelines for management of sepsis and septic shock 2026. Critical Care Medicine 2026;54(4):725–812.
18. McPeake J, Oakes M, Graham C, et al. Top ten research priorities for sepsis research determined by patietns, carers and clinicians. Lancet Respir Med 2024;12:e68–9.
19. Demerle KM, Royer SC, Mikkelsen ME, et al. Readmissions for recurrent sepsis: new or relapsed infection? Crit Care Med 2017;45:1702.
20. Guirgis FW, Brakenridge S, Sutchu S, et al. The long-term burden of severe sepsis and septic shock: sepsis recidicism and organ dysfunction. J Trauma Acute Care Surg 2016;81:525–32.
21. Shen HN, Lu CL, Yang HH. Risk of recurrence after surviving severe sepsis. Crit Care Med 2016;44:1833–41.
22. Kosyakovsky LB, Angriman F, Katz E, et al. Association between sepsis survivorship and long-term cardiovascular outcomes in adults: a systematic review and meta-analysis. Intensive Care Med 2021;47:931–42.
23. Wu Z, Chen F, Xiao C, et al. Long-term cardiovascular outcomes in adult sepsis survivors: a systematic review and meta-analysis. World J Emerg Med 2025;16: 423–30.
24. Ackermann K, Lynch I, Aryal N, et al. Hospital readmission after surviving sepsis: a systematic review of readmission reasons and meta-analysis of readmission rates. J Crit Care 2025;85:154925.
25. Yende S, Linde-Zwirble W, Mayr F, et al. Risk of cardiovascular events in survivors of severe sepsis. Am J Respir Crit Care Med 2014;189:1065–74.
26. Ou SM, Chu H, Chao PW, et al. Long-term mortality and major adverse cardiovascular events in sepsis survivors. A nationwide population-based study. Am J Respir Crit Care Med 2016;194:209–17.
27. Li D, Zhang X, Lu Y, et al. Post-sepsis psychiatric disorder: pathophysiology, prevention, and treatment. Neurol Sci 2024;45:3093–105.

28. Sell S, Fleischmann-Struzek C, Spoden M, et al. Mental health in the first year after ICU-treated sepsis: analysis of administrative diagnoses in German health claims data. Gen Hosp Psychiatry 2025;93:109–15.
29. Calsavara AJ, Costa PA, Nobre V, et al. Prevalence and risk factors for post-traumatic stress, anxiety, and depression in sepsis survivors after ICU discharge. Braz J Psychiatry 2021;43:269–76.
30. Oh TK, Park HY, Song IA. Depression and long-term survival among South Korean sepsis survivors: a nationwide cohort study from 2011 to 2014. Crit Care Med 2021;49:1470–80.
31. Hatch R, Young D, Barber V, et al. Anxiety, Depression and Post Traumatic Stress Disorder after critical illness: a UK-wide prospective cohort study. Crit Care 2018;22:310.
32. Peerapornratana S, Manrique-Caballero CL, Gómez H, et al. Acute kidney injury from sepsis: current concepts, epidemiology, pathophysiology, prevention and treatment. Kidney Int 2019;96:1083–99.
33. Arshad A, Ayaz A, Rehman S, et al. Progression of acute kidney injury to chronic kidney disease in sepsis survivors: 1-year follow-up study. J Intensive Care Med 2021;36:1366–70.
34. Hästbacka J, But A, Strandberg G, et al. Risk of malignant disease in 1-year sepsis survivors, a registry-based nationwide follow-up study. Crit Care 2023;27:376.
35. Mirouse A, Vigneron C, Llitjos JF, et al. Sepsis and cancer: an interplay of friends and foes. Am J Respir Crit Care Med 2020;202:1625–35.
36. Basu S, Wei ZJ, Laor A, et al. Health-related quality of life among patients who have survived an episode of sepsis in the united states: a systematic review. Infect Dis Ther 2025;14:385–400.
37. Sonneville R, Benghanem S, Jeantin L, et al. The spectrum of sepsis-associated encephalopathy: a clinical perspective. Crit Care 2023;27:386.
38. Atterton B, Paulino MC, Povoa P, et al. Sepsis-associated delirium. Medicina 2020;56:240.
39. Jackson JC, Hart RP, Gordon SM, et al. Six-month neuropsychological outcome of medical intensive care unit patients. Crit Care Med 2003;31:1226–34.
40. Wang HE, Kabeto MM, Gray M, et al. Trajectory of cognitive decline after sepsis. Crit Care Med 2021;49:1083–94.
41. Mart MF, Gordon JI, González-Seguel F, et al. Muscle dysfunction and physical recovery after critical illness. J Intensive Care Med 2025;41(3):214–30.
42. Borges RC, Carvalho CRF, Colombo AS, et al. Physical activity, muscle strength, and exercise capacity 3 months after severe sepsis and septic shock. Intensive Care Med 2015;41:1433–44.
43. Huang CY, Daniels R, Lembo A, et al. Life after sepsis: an international survey of survivors to understand the post-sepsis syndrome. Int J Qual Health Care 2019;31:191–8.
44. Stallmach A, Kesselmeier M, Bauer M, et al. Comparison of fatigue, cognitive dysfunction and psychological disorders in post-COVID patients and patients after sepsis: is there a specific constellation? Infection 2022;50:661–9.
45. Appelman B, Charlton BT, Goulding RP, et al. Muscle abnormalities worsen after post-exertional malaise in long COVID. Nat Commun 2024;15:17.
46. Al-Aly Z, Davis H, McCorkell L, et al. Long COVID science, research and policy. Nat Med 2024;30:2148–64.

47. Yende S, Kellum JA, Talisa VB, et al. Long-term host immune response trajectories among hospitalized patients with sepsis. JAMA Netw Open 2019;2: e198686.
48. Yende S, D'Angelo G, Kellum JA, et al. Inflammatory markers at hospital discharge predict subsequent mortality after pneumonia and sepsis. Am J Respir Crit Care Med 2008;177:1242–7.
49. Gritte RB, Souza-Siqueira T, Curi R, et al. Why septic patients remain sick after discharge? Front Immunol 2021;11:605666.
50. Chavan SS, Huerta PT, Robbiati S, et al. HMGB1 mediates cognitive impairment in sepsis survivors. Mol Med 2012;18:930–7.
51. Sharshar T, Carlier R, Bernard F, et al. Brain lesions in septic shock: a magnetic resonance imaging study. Intensive Care Med 2007;33:798–806.
52. Barichello T, Sayana P, Giridharan VV, et al. Long-term cognitive outcomes after sepsis: a translational systematic review. Mol Neurobiol 2019;56:186–251.
53. Hoogland ICM, Houbolt C, van Westerloo DJ, et al. Systemic inflammation and microglial activation: systematic review of animal experiments. J Neuroinflammation 2015;12:114.
54. Torres LK, Pickkers P, van der Poll T. Sepsis-induced immunosuppression. Annu Rev Physiol 2022;84:157–81.
55. Davis FM, Schaller MA, Dendekker A, et al. Sepsis induces prolonged epigenetic modifications in bone marrow and peripheral macrophages impairing inflammation and wound healing. Arterioscler Thromb Vasc Biol 2019;39:2353–66.
56. Yin J, Mao W, Xiao X, et al. Immune dysfunction is associated with readmission in survivors of sepsis follwoing infected pancreatic necrosis. J Inflamm Res 2021; 14:5433–42.
57. Drewry A, Samra N, Skrupky L, et al. Persistent lymphopenia after sepsis predicts mortality. Shock 2014;42:383–91.
58. Cavassani KA, Carson WF, Moreira AP, et al. The post sepsis-induced expansion and enhanced function of regulatory T cells create an environment to potentiate tumor growth. Blood 2010;115:4403–11.
59. Torres JSS, Tamayo-Giraldo FJ, Bejarano-Zuleta A, et al. Sepsis and post-sepsis syndrome: a multisystem challenge requiring comprehensive care and management-a review. Front Med 2025;12:1560737.
60. Uhel F, Azzaoui I, Grégoire M, et al. Early expansion of circulating granulocytic myeloid-derived suppressor cells in septic shock. Am J Respir Crit Care Med 2017;196:315–27.
61. Mathias B, Delmas AL, Ozrazgat-Baslanti T, et al. Human myeloid-derived suppressor cells are associated with chronic immune suppression after severe sepsis/septic shock. Ann Surg 2017;265:827–34.
62. Arens C, Bajwa SA, Koch C, et al. Sepsis-induced long-term immune paralysis–results of a descriptive, explorative study. Crit Care 2016;20:93.
63. Rocheteau P, Chatre L, Briand D, et al. Sepsis induces long-term metabolic and mitochondrial muscle stem cell dysfunction amenable by mesenchymal stem cell therapyLong-term metabolic and mitochondrial dysfunction after sepsis. Nat Commun 2015;6:10145.
64. Hu D, Prabhakaran HS, Zhang YY, et al. Mitochondrial dysfunction in sepsis: mechanisms and therapeutic perspectives. Crit Care 2024;28:292.
65. Gorecki GP, Bodor A, Novac MB, et al. Rethinking post-sepsis syndrome: linking cellular dysfunction to the clinical picture. Crit Care 2025;29:418.
66. Zhang T, Li YJ, Ma T. Role of regulation of PD-1 and PD-L1 expression in sepsis. Front Immunol 2023;14:1029438.

67. Rodhouse C, Barrios EL, Zeumer-Spataro L, et al. Prolonged loss of oxidative phosphorylation and mitochondrial mass characterize CD66b^{+} leukocytes from patients with sepsism. bioRxiv [Preprint] 2025. https://doi.org/10.64898/2025.12.16.694726.
68. Pierre A, Favory R, Brassart B, et al. Sepsis induces long-term muscle and mitochondrial dysfunction dueo to autophagy disruption amenable by urolithin A. J Cachexia Sarcopenia Muscle 2025;16:e70041.
69. Kingren MS, Keeble AR, Galvan-Lara AM, et al. Post-sepsis chronic muscle weakness can be prevented by pharmacological protection of mitochondria. Mol Med 2024;30:221.
70. Wiersinga WJ, van der Poll T. Biological drivers of the host response in sepsis. Thorax 2025;2024–222012.
71. Kaynar AM, Yende S, Zhu L, et al. Effects of intra-abdominal sepsis on atherosclerosis in mice. Crit Care 2014;18:469.
72. Hansson GK, Robertson AKL, Söderberg-Nauclér C. Inflammation and atherosclerosis. Annu Rev Pathol 2006;1:297–329.
73. Yende S, D'Angelo G, Mayr F, et al. Elevated hemostasis markers after pneumonia increases one-year risk of all-cause and cardiovascular deaths. PLoS One 2011;6:e22847.
74. Menéndez R, Méndez R, Aldás I, et al. Community-acquired pneumonia patients at risk for early and long-term cardiovascular events are identified by cardiac biomarkers. Chest 2019;156:1080–91.
75. Merdji H, Kassem M, Chomel L, et al. Septic shock as a trigger of arterial stress-induced premature senescence: a new pathway involved in the post sepsis long-term cardiovascular complicationse. Vasc Pharmacol 2021;141:106922.
76. Martín-Vicente P, López-Martínez C, Rioseras B, et al. Activation of senescence in critically ill patients: mechanisms, consequences and therapeutic opportunities. Ann Intensive Care 2024;14:2.
77. Huidobro C, Martín-Vicente P, López-Martínez C, et al. Cellular and molecular features of senescence in acute lung injury. Mech Ageing Dev 2021;193:111410.
78. Li S, Livingston MJ, Ma Z, et al. Tubular cell senescence promotes maladaptive kidney repair and chronic kidney disease after cisplatin nephrotoxicity. JCI Insight 2023;8:e166643.
79. Sung J, Rajendraprasad SS, Philbrick KL, et al. The human gut microbiome in critical illness: disruptions, consequences, and therapeutic frontiers. J Crit Care 2024;79:154436.
80. Freedberg DE, Zhou MJ, Cohen ME, et al. Pathogen colonization of the gastrointestinal microbiome at intensive care unit admission and risk for subsequent death or infection. Intensive Care Med 2018;44:1203–11.
81. Baggs J, Jernigan JA, Halpin AL, et al. Risk of subsequent sepsis within 90 days after a hospital stay by type of antibiotic exposure. Clin Infect Dis 2018;66:1004.
82. Park G, Munley JA, Kelly LS, et al. Gut mycobiome dysbiosis after sepsis and trauma. Crit Care 2024;28:18.
83. Mikkelsen ME, Christie JD, Lanken PN, et al. The adult respiratory distress syndrome cognitive outcomes study: long-term neuropsychological function in survivors of acute lung injury. Am J Respir Crit Care Med 2012;185:1307–15.
84. Herling SF, Greve IE, Vasilevskis EE, et al. Interventions for preventing intensive care unit delirium in adults. Cochrane Database Syst Rev 2018;11(11):CD009783.

85. Bircak-Kuchtova B, Rose N, Geis C, et al. Effectiveness of targeted post-acute interventions and follow-up services for sepsis survivors: a systematic review. Crit Care 2025;29:351.
86. Rahmel T, Schmitz S, Nowak H, et al. Long-term mortality in hospital survivors of septic shock, sepsis, and severe infections: the importance of aftercare. PLoS One 2020;15:e0228952.
87. Taylor SP, Eaton T, Rios A, et al. Proactive telehealth-based sepsis transition and recovery support, hospital readmission, and mortality: a randomized clinical trial. JAMA Intern Med 2025;185:1238–46.
88. Taylor SP, Murphy S, Rios A, et al. Effect of a multicomponent sepsis transition and recovery program on mortality and readmissions after sepsis: the improving morbidity during post-acute care transitions for sepsis randomized clinical trial. Crit Care Med 2022;50:469–79.
89. Taylor R, Vollam S, McKechnie SR, et al. Improving outcomes in survivors of sepsis-the transition from secondary to primary care, and the role of primary care: a narrative review. J Clin Med 2025;14:2582.
90. Akman M, Ayhan Başer D, Usanma Koban B, et al. Organization of primary care. Prim Health Care Res Dev 2022;23:e49.
91. OECD. Realising the potential of primary health care. Paris: OECD Publishing; 2020.
92. Schmidt K, Worrack S, von Korff M, et al. Effect of a primary care management intervention on mental health-related quality of life among survivors of sepsis: a randomized clinical trial. JAMA 2016;315:2703–11.
93. Schmidt KF, Schwarzkopf D, Baldwin LM, et al. Long-term courses of sepsis survivors: effects of a primary care management intervention. Am J Med 2020;133:381–5.
94. Sasegbon A, O'Shea L, Hamdy S. Examining the relationship between sepsis and oropharyngeal dysphagia in hospitalised elderly patients: a retrospective cohort study. Frontline Gastroenterol 2018;9:256–61.
95. Palli C, Fandler S, Doppelhofer K, et al. Early dysphagia screening by trained nurses reduces pneumonia rate in stroke patients: a clinical intervention study. Stroke 2017;48:2583–5.
96. Taylor SP, Bray BC, Chou SH, et al. Clinical subtypes of sepsis survivors predict readmission and mortality after hospital discharge. Ann Am Thorac Soc 2022;19:1355–63.
97. Flick RJ, Kamphuis LA, Valley TS, et al. Sepsis survivor subtypes with long-term mortality and disability after discharge: a retrospective cohort study. Crit Care Med 2026;54:45–54.
98. Duda J. The walking wounded: sepsis survivors grapple with post-sepsis syndrome. Lancet Respir Med 2025;13:786–8.

Principles of Immunotherapeutic Drug Discovery for Severe Infections Using Extreme Phenotypes

Clark D. Russell, MBChB, PhD[a,*], Annette C. Westgeest, MD, PhD[b]

KEYWORDS

- Extreme phenotype • Host-directed therapy • Critical illness • HIV elite controller
- Interferon gamma • Hyper-virulent pathogen variants • Subphenotypes

KEY POINTS

- Extreme infection phenotypes are those at the very upper or lower end of the overall distribution, due to either host or pathogen traits.
- Host traits expressed as extreme phenotypes can be classified as resistance (related to pathogen clearance) or tolerance (related to immunopathology). Pathogen hypervirulence can present as invasive disease in otherwise healthy hosts.
- Extreme phenotypes can have a genetic basis (host or pathogen) or be the consequence of cumulative environmental exposures across the life course (the exposome).
- Characterizing host responses associated with extreme infection phenotypes can prioritize targets for host-directed therapies: augmenting protective responses or inhibiting deleterious responses.

INTRODUCTION

Host-Directed Immunotherapies for Severe Infections

Enabling patients to survive severe infection is a fundamental goal of critical care medicine, encompassing both infection as the primary insult leading to critical illness and secondary infections acquired after admission to a critical care unit. Aside from provision of organ support, in current clinical practice our ability to modify the pathogen-host interaction is mainly limited to the use of antimicrobials. While antimicrobial therapy represented a massive advance when first implemented at scale more than 80 years ago, and remains the cornerstone of managing most severe infections, the approach suffers from 3 main limitations.

[a] Centre for Inflammation Research, Institute for Regeneration and Repair, University of Edinburgh, Edinburgh, UK; [b] Leiden University Center for Infectious Diseases (LUCID), Leiden University Medical Center, Albinusdreef 2, Leiden, The Netherlands
* Corresponding author.
E-mail address: clark.russell@ed.ac.uk

Crit Care Clin 42 (2026) 763–775
https://doi.org/10.1016/j.ccc.2026.05.004 criticalcare.theclinics.com
0749-0704/26/

Abbreviations	
hvKp	hypermucoviscous *Klebsiella pneumoniae*
JAK	Janus kinase
PVL	Panton-Valentine leucocidin

1. Death and morbidity due to severe infection occurs despite receipt of antimicrobials with *in vitro* antimicrobial activity against the causative pathogen;
2. Antimicrobials have built-in redundancy: evolution of antimicrobial resistance is inevitable;
3. Antimicrobial therapy is associated with adverse ecological events for recipients, predisposing to colonization with resistant pathogens, *Clostridioides difficile* infection, and invasive *Candida* infections.

A conceptually attractive adjunctive or even alternative strategy is to therapeutically optimize the host immune response using immunotherapies.[1] Two main strands of evidence support this approach: Firstly, host defense against pathogens is usually extremely successful. Despite frequent exposure to and colonization with pathogenic microbes such as *Streptococcus pneumoniae* or *Staphylococcus aureus*, invasive disease is a very uncommon outcome.[2–5] Identifying and augmenting the components of normally successful host defense that fail during disease therefore represents an attractive therapeutic strategy, referred to here as "host-directed" anti-infective therapy. This also extends to suppressing immunopathologic inflammatory responses. Secondly, there is substantial variability between different individuals in the outcome of infection with the same pathogen: spanning life-threatening disease to asymptomatic infection. Broadly, survival from infection requires the correct balance of resistance (ability to control the pathogen load) and tolerance (ability to limit immunopathology in response to a given pathogen load).[6] Host-directed therapies have the potential to restore a resistant or tolerant phenotype on an otherwise susceptible or intolerant host (**Fig. 1**).

Challenge: Complexity of the Host Response

While conceptually attractive, there are limited examples of host-directed therapies in routine clinical usage. Existing approaches mainly relate to augmenting tolerance through use of anti-inflammatory drugs, for example, immunomodulatory treatment of Coronavirus disease 2019 (Covid-19) using steroids,[7] interleukin 6 receptor blockers,[8] and Janus kinase (JAK) inhibitors[9] (discussed later).

There is an unmet need to develop host-directed therapies for a broader range of indications, especially drugs to augment pathogen clearance (ie, resistance), which is especially important in the context of antimicrobial resistance. Achieving this is complicated by the difficulty in identifying therapeutic targets in severe infection. Host responses are multi-layered, incorporate redundancy, and are heterogeneous between individuals. We lack a granular understanding of which host responses deterministically contribute to successful defense against specific pathogens or cause harmful immunopathology. Innovative research strategies are required to overcome these challenges.

Solution: Biologically Informative Extreme Phenotypes

In this article, we will discuss how studying extreme infection phenotypes can provide a solution to this problem. In this context, an "extreme phenotype" broadly identifies the observable outcome of a pathogen:host interaction that is either at the very upper

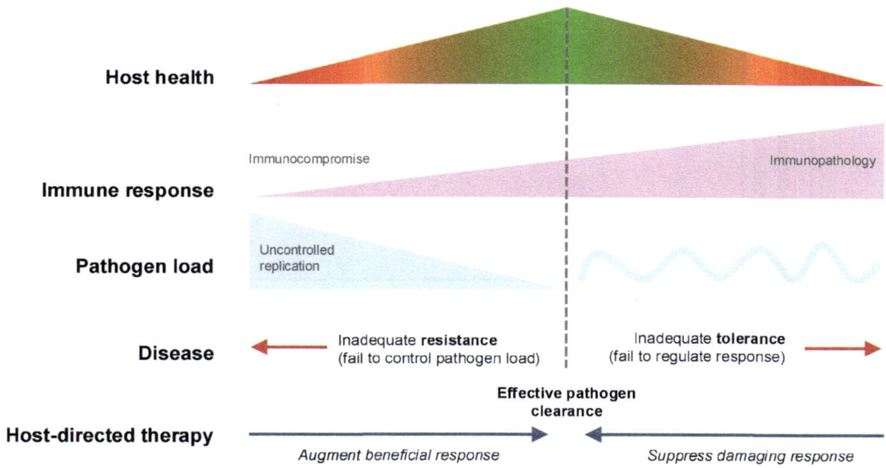

Fig. 1. Host-directed immunotherapies. Schematic of the role of resistance and tolerance in host defense against infection, and the role of host-directed therapies to re-calibrate these when they fail. For host health, red shading indicates clinically apparent disease, morbidity, or mortality, whereas green indicates recovery, survival, or asymptomatic infection. (*Created using* PowerPoint and GraphPad Prism.)

or lower end of the overall distribution, due to either host or pathogen traits (**Fig. 2**). Extreme host phenotypes include unusual disease severity (high or low), resistance to pathogen replication, or susceptibility to low virulence organisms. While the extreme phenotype concept originates in genetics, this can be extended to any extreme observable phenotype arising as a consequence of an individual's cumulative environmental exposures across the life course (the exposome), for example, comorbidities and age-related biological changes. Extreme pathogen phenotypes can also be informative, for example, pathogen variants with an unusually high capacity to cause severe disease in otherwise healthy people (ie, hyper-virulent).

Studying extreme infection phenotypes has the potential to amplify biological signal over noise, facilitating the identification of host responses mediating disease severity (eg, immunopathology) or protection (eg, pathogen clearance). Host responses identified in this way are rationale candidates for host-directed therapeutic targeting.

CURRENT EVIDENCE

Critical Illness in Covid-19

The concept of selectively studying extreme phenotypes is well established in the field of genetics, where extreme phenotype sampling is a method used to increase statistical power for identifying genetic associations compared with random sampling of all individuals with the phenotype.[10] This approach is the foundation of the GenOMICC study (https://genomicc.org/), which recruits individuals with critical illness caused by diseases of interest, rather than individuals with less severe manifestations. Infection with SARS-CoV-2 results in a wide range of outcomes, including asymptomatic infection, a mild respiratory tract infection, or viral pneumonitis. The latter, now largely restricted to unvaccinated or immunocompromised individuals, also presents as a spectrum, with a small proportion of individuals requiring critical care, thus representing an extreme phenotype of SARS-CoV-2 infection. GenOMICC performed several genome wide association studies (GWAS),[11–13] comparing critical Covid-19 to

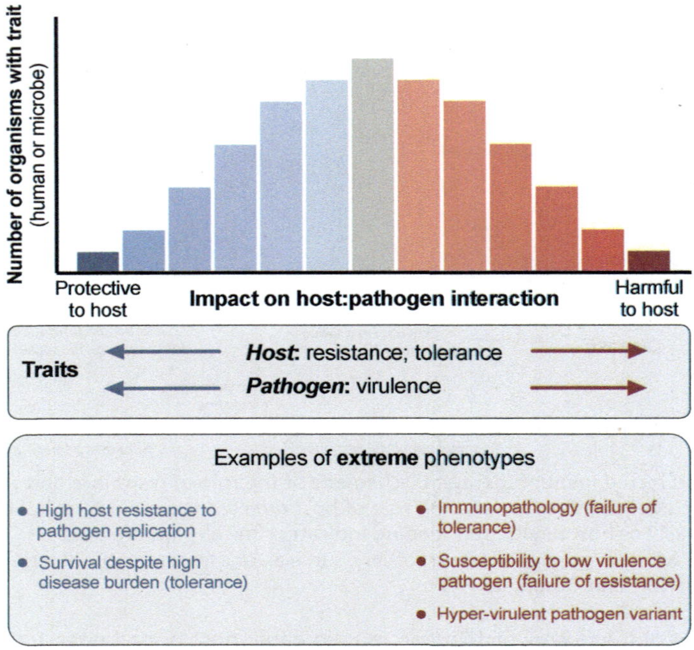

Fig. 2. Extreme infection phenotypes. Schematic representation of the concept of an "extreme phenotype": clinical features of infection that are either at the very upper or lower end of the overall distribution, and can be the result of host or pathogen traits. The *y*-axis indicates the number of organisms with the trait, either the host or the pathogen. The *x*-axis indicates the impact of the host or pathogen trait on the infection phenotype, representing a spectrum between most and least harm to the host. (*Created using* PowerPoint and GraphPad Prism.)

controls, and identifying an unprecedented number of genotype-phenotype associations for an infectious disease. These included variants in genes encoding effectors of the host anti-viral responses (eg, *IFNAR1*, *IFNAR2*) and regulators of myeloid cell inflammation (eg, *TYK2*, *JAK1*, *DPP9*). Orthogonal evidence from studies of bronchoalveolar lavage fluid,[14] circulating inflammatory mediators,[15,16] peripheral blood mononuclear cells,[17] and tissue immunopathology[16,18–22] concurrently identified a central role for macrophage-mediated inflammation in the pathogenesis of critical Covid-19. Specifically, expansion of pulmonary interstitial monocyte-derived macrophages was observed in critical Covid-19, occurring to a greater extent than in bacterial pneumonia or influenza virus infection.[21] Activation signals included M-CSF, GM-CSF, IL-6, and C5a, and recruitment axes included CCR2::MCP-3/MCP-1 and C5AR1::C5a. The finding that dexamethasone reduced mortality in individuals with Covid-19 associated with hypoxia[7] confirmed that suppressing the inflammatory response was beneficial. A humanized mouse model provided evidence this benefit was through augmenting tolerance by limiting the expansion of interstitial monocyte-derived macrophages identified in humans. In this model, dexamethasone reduced inflammatory macrophage recruitment and weight loss but increased the viral load.[23] Signaling through Janus kinase (JAK) family tyrosine kinases is a major pathway in pro-inflammatory macrophage activation, so the identification of the association of genetic variants in the JAK kinases *TYK2* and *JAK1* with critical Covid-19 supported the re-purposing of the JAK inhibitor baricitinib. In particular, genetic evidence identified that increased *TYK2* expression was associated with critical Covid-19. Baricitinib treatment was found to reduce 28-day mortality by 13% and remained beneficial even for individuals receiving corticosteroids or IL-6 receptor blockers.[9] This example provides important proof of principle that insights from studying extreme infection phenotypes can directly translate into therapeutically actionable information.

HIV Elite Controllers

The concept of HIV elite controllers provides another example of how studying extreme phenotypes may ultimately lead to therapeutic insights. Elite controllers are individuals able to suppress HIV-1 replication to undetectable or very low levels in plasma in the absence of anti-retroviral therapy, indicating unusually successful host defense. This phenotype is identified in less than 1% of people living with HIV.[24] This phenotype can be conferred to otherwise susceptible individuals, as demonstrated by lymphocyte transfer from an elite controller to a recipient with progressive HIV infection, which was associated with a transient reduction in viral load before clearance of the donor cells.[25]

Several facets of this extreme infection phenotype are informing development of lymphocyte-targeted immunotherapies for HIV-1 infection. Elite controllers are characterized by distinct CD8 T-cell effector phenotypes and resistance to exhaustion,[25–27] identifying immune checkpoint inhibitors as a candidate approach with pre-clinical data suggesting this could enhance vaccine-induced CD8 T-cell responses.[28] In addition, CD4 T cells from elite controllers exhibit up-regulation of the cyclin-dependent kinase inhibitor p21, which promotes resistance to viral replication, identifying CDK inhibitors as a therapeutic strategy.[29,30]

Inborn Errors of Interferon Gamma Immunity

Exposure to non-tuberculous mycobacteria (including the attenuated *Mycobacterium bovis* used in BCG vaccination), *Candida* spp., and non-typhoidal *Salmonella* spp. generally does not result in clinically significant disease among immunocompetent individuals. However, invasive, recurrent, or chronic infections with these organisms is an identifier of Mendelian susceptibility to mycobacterial disease (MSMD). MSMD represents an extreme infection susceptibility phenotype, caused by mutations in one of greater than 20 components of the interferon gamma response (including *IFNG*, *IFNGR1*, *IFNGR2*, *IL12 B*, *IL12RB1*, *IL12RB2*, *IL23R*), predominantly acquired through autosomal recessive inheritance.[31] As a result of impaired interferon gamma production or signaling (or both), affected individuals have a defect in macrophage intracellular killing of specific pathogens. In addition to the weakly virulent organisms already mentioned, this susceptibility appears to extend to additional intra-macrophagic organisms such as *Histoplasma* and *Leishmania*. Importantly, identifying that defective interferon gamma signaling is causal in the MSMD phenotype means that treatment with exogenous interferon gamma can be offered to patients with mutations resulting in impaired production. Although this strategy has not been evaluated in a clinical trial, in part due to the rarity of MSMD, cumulative evidence suggests there is clinical benefit.[32–35] Furthermore, by identifying interferon gamma as a key mediator of host resistance to mycobacterial disease, adjunctive interferon gamma has been evaluated as an adjunct to antimycobacterial treatment in patients without MSMD, with evidence from a small clinical trial indicating there may be clinical benefit.[36] This example highlights that defining the mechanistic basis of extreme susceptibility to specific pathogens can identify non-redundant elements of the host response against that pathogen that could be targeted using host-directed anti-infective therapies.

Hypervirulent Pathogen Variants

The immune system exerts demonstrable selective pressure on pathogen evolution, resulting in the emergence of immune-adaptive pathogen variants. For example, HIV-1 escape from CD8 T-cell recognition,[37] host-adaptation of *Mycobacterium abscessus* spp. and *S. aureus* during chronic endobronchial infection,[38,39] and differential *S aureus* toxin specificity in response to inter-species diversifying immune selective pressure.[40] Experimental passage of *Legionella pneumophila*[41] or *S aureus*[42] through macrophages in cell culture results in emergence of adaptive mutants with enhanced intra-macrophagic survival. Therefore, within the genetic heterogeneity naturally present in all bacterial species, certain adaptations will represent a footprint of immune selective pressure exerted by the host. Such variants will be resistant to specific host defense mechanisms (eg, cytotoxic T-cell recognition, macrophage intracellular killing) and be identifiable by their association with distinct clinical phenotypes during infection, for example, hyper-virulence (**Fig. 3**A), thus representing extreme pathogen phenotypes. While more challenging to identify than extreme host phenotypes, studying extreme pathogen phenotypes also has the potential to deliver therapeutic insights. Specifically, by asking the question "*which host responses has a hypervirulent pathogen variant evolved to escape*?" Immune-adaptive pathogen variants could be used as tools to identify elements of the host response as therapeutic targets.

Serotype 1 *S pneumoniae* are associated with disease that is clinically and epidemiologically distinct from pneumococcal disease due to other serotypes, representing putative adaptive variants. They exhibit a strong association with invasive pneumococcal disease (including extra-pulmonary) in young healthy hosts including empyema, peritonitis and salpingitis (**Fig. 3**B).[44–46] A further characteristic is their ability to cause disease outbreaks, often in conditions of close living such as prisons and schools, but also epidemics of meningitis in sub-Saharan Africa.[47–51] Overall, serotype 1 pneumococci represent an extreme pathogen phenotype, behaving as hypervirulent primary pathogens whereas most other pneumococci are opportunists. In a study providing proof of principle of this approach, clinical isolates of serotype 1 *S pneumoniae* were identified with an unusual resistance to macrophage intracellular killing.[52] This led to the identification of macrophage microbicidal responses these variants escaped from, which were confirmed to be key mediators of normally successful bacterial killing against *S pneumoniae* and related gram-positive organisms

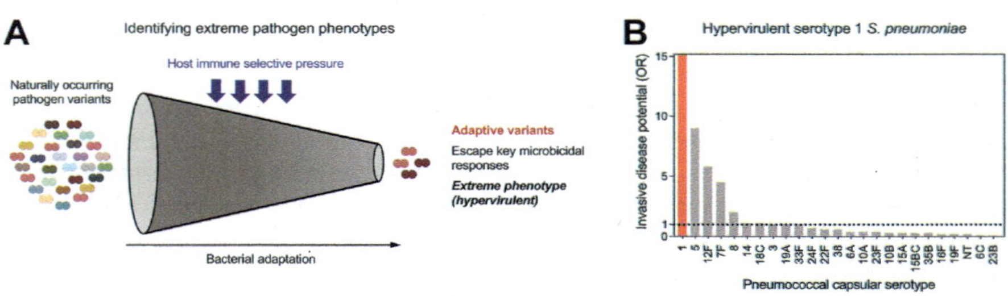

Fig. 3. Extreme pathogen phenotypes. (*A*) Identification of immune-adaptive pathogen variants. (*B*) Invasive disease potential of pneumococcal capsular serotypes. Data from reference.[43] The graph shows the OR of isolates recovered from invasive disease versus carriage, stratified by capsular serotype. An OR greater than 1 (*dotted line*) indicates a serotype is more likely to be associated with invasive disease than carriage, identifying the capacity of serotype 1 pneumococci to cause invasive disease as an extreme phenotype. OR, odds ratio. (Created in BioRender. Russell, C. (2026) https://BioRender.com/9xxegiv.)

(*S agalactiae*, *S pyogenes*, and *Enterococcus faecium*). Specifically, P2RX7 signaling was identified as a host defense factor that could be augmented in mouse and zebrafish larvae models by re-purposing of the anti-histamine clemastine. Treatment with clemastine led to pathogen clearance without the requirement for conventional antimicrobials. This example shows that extreme pathogen phenotypes, characterized by hyper-virulence, can be used to pinpoint elements of host defense that normally control the pathogen and can be therapeutically targeted. While the genetic basis for serotype 1 *S pneumoniae* hypervirulence has not been established, distinct gene expression profiles have been described compared with less virulent isolates.[53] Several other examples of extreme pathogen phenotypes exist and could be leveraged to define host defense mechanisms, for example,.

- *S aureus* USA300 North American epidemic clone, associated with necrotizing pneumonia, severe skin and soft tissue infections, and metastatic complications during bacteraemia.[54–56]
- Hypermucoviscous *Klebsiella pneumoniae* (hvKp), associated with hematogenous liver abscesses and endogenous endophthalmitis.[57]

While the genetic basis for these extreme pathogen phenotypes remains to be confirmed (and may be context specific), candidate genes exist for both examples: the Panton-Valentine leucocidin (PVL) toxin, enterotoxin variants, and the arginine catabolic mobile element for USA300,[58] and the regulator of mucoid phenotype genes (eg, *rmpA*) for hvKp. More definitively, a bacterial GWAS has established the role of PVL in tropical pyomyositis caused by *S aureus*.[59]

Patient Stratification

The examples considered so far rely on clinical, epidemiological, and microbiological observation to identify extreme phenotypes to study. Approaches for patient stratification also offer opportunities to identify extreme infection phenotypes and may be particularly well suited to infections or syndromes with a high degree of clinical heterogeneity. For example, critical illness in COVID-19 is a clearly identifiable, homogenous subgroup. In contrast, identifying an extreme phenotype within a more heterogeneous syndrome is more challenging and well exemplified by the difficulties identifying therapeutically-relevant sub-groups within sepsis (comprehensively reviewed in[60]). Important proof of principle comes from the similarly heterogeneous syndrome of acute respiratory distress syndrome, where two disease subphenotypes (hyper-inflammatory and hypo-inflammatory) can be reproducibly identified in different cohorts, using routinely available clinical variables, associated with differences in outcome and also response to ventilation strategy and simvastatin.[61,62] An inevitable tension exists in efforts to classify patients into subphenotypes: clinical applicability of the approach (ie, can the relevant classifying measurements be made in routine clinical practice) versus the depth of biological insight (using deep phenotyping methods not routinely available). While decades of sepsis immunobiology have established that some patients suffer organ dysfunction due to excessive inflammation (loss of tolerance), whereas others exhibit immune exhaustion and susceptibility to secondary infections (loss of resistance), until recently this had not led to successful drug discovery. However, a recently reported approach for patient stratification in sepsis has succeeded in identifying a clinically applicable and therapeutically relevant approach, using measurement of circulating ferritin and HLA-DR expression on CD45/CD14 monocytes. Patients with ferritin greater than 4420 ng/mL were classified as having a hyper-inflammatory macrophage-activation like syndrome subphenotype, and patients with ferritin less than or equal to 4420 ng/mL and monocyte HLA-DR expression less than 5000/cell were classified as having sepsis-induced immunoparalysis subphenotype.[63,64] These represent extreme phenotypes within sepsis, and patients with ferritin less than or equal to 4420 ng/mL but HLA-DR expression greater than or equal to 5000/cell were considered unclassifiable and not belonging to one of these extremes. The macrophage-activation like phenotype was treated with the interleukin-1 receptor antagonist anakinra and the sepsis-induced immunoparalysis phenotype was treated with recombinant interferon-gamma. In a randomized, placebo-controlled trial of this approach, personalized host-directed immunotherapy was associated with an improvement in day 9 Sequential Organ Failure Assessment score.[64] This is a particularly noteworthy finding considering the large number of negative trials investigating immunotherapy in sepsis. This example highlights the role of biomarker-based patient stratification in defining extreme phenotypes that would otherwise not be observable.

DISCUSSION

Immunotherapeutic drug discovery for severe infections remains a major challenge, evidenced by our ongoing reliance on conventional antimicrobials, despite their intrinsic limitations. The complexity of the host immune response underpins this difficulty and innovative solutions are required to overcome this. The examples discussed earlier illustrate that identifying host responses associated with extreme infection phenotypes provides a method to prioritize therapeutic targets, and has several strengths.

- Comparison of individuals at the extreme end of a trait distribution can improve the signal:noise ratio, filtering potential targets to facilitate identification of those with causal relevance;
- Statistical power is increased in GWAS since extreme phenotypes are likely to be enriched for causal genetic variants (eg, critical COVID-19). Objective evidence for this is provided by the increased discovery power of GenOMICC compared with other COVID-19 GWAS[13];
- Extreme phenotypes with a monogenic basis are readily interpretable from a mechanistic perspective (eg, mutations in the interferon gamma response in MSMD).

As with any research method there are potential limitations to this approach:

- The generalizability of findings is not guaranteed, particularly as translating pathways identified in extreme phenotypes into effective host-directed therapies may be limited by disease heterogeneity, timing, and patient selection. For example, despite the association of type 1 interferon genetic variants with critical COVID-19 (eg, reduced *IFNAR2* expression in individuals with the risk allele for critical illness),[11] trials of exogenous interferon in unselected patients were generally negative;
- Not all extreme phenotypes will have a genetic basis, thus deep phenotyping and consideration of the exposome will be required to identify mechanisms that can be therapeutically modified;
- Extreme phenotypes are by definition uncommon, which can lead to recruitment difficulties. This is somewhat context dependent since critical Covid-19 was unfortunately common during the pandemic. In contrast HIV elite controllers and individuals with MSMD are rare within the population.

GOALS AND FUTURE CONSIDERATIONS

1. *Research capacity within critical care.* As exemplified by the GenOMICC critical COVID-19 GWAS, critical illness caused by a pathogen, especially if a homogenous

Table 1
How to identify extreme infection phenotypes

Extreme Phenotype	Clinical Identifiers	Example
Resistance (high)	Control of pathogen load without antimicrobials	HIV elite controllers[24]
Resistance (low)	Invasive, recurrent, or chronic infection with low virulence organisms	MSMD[31] Sepsis-induced immunoparalysis[63]
Tolerance (high)	High pathogen load without severe disease	Sickle hemoglobin and malaria[65,66]
Tolerance (low)	Immunopathology causing morbidity/ mortality	Critical Covid-19[11] Macrophage-activation like syndrome in sepsis[63]
Hypervirulent pathogen	Invasive disease in healthy hosts	Serotype 1 *S pneumoniae*[67]

disease manifestation (eg, hypoxemic respiratory failure caused by respiratory viruses; toxic shock syndrome caused by *S pyogenes*), represents a tractable extreme phenotype to study. The capacity to recruit such patients to research studies and obtain relevant biological samples should be embedded within critical care units where possible.
2. *Identification of rare inborn errors of immunity.* Monogenic disorders such as MSMD can be highly informative, but are rare, can have variable clinical presentations, and can have a diverse genetic basis to a single syndrome. Improved access to whole genome sequencing in clinical settings to investigate suspected cases will lead to additional insights and should be considered when patients unexpectedly present with invasive, recurrent, or chronic infections with low virulence organisms.
3. *Identification of immune-adaptive pathogen variants.* Identification of potentially informative variants requires integration of clinical observations, epidemiologic investigation, and microbiologic characterization.
4. *Patient stratification.* Defining subphenotypes with distinct disease outcomes has the potential to identify extreme phenotypes for further mechanistic investigation.

SUMMARY

We propose the following identifiers of extreme phenotypes for application in clinical and research practice (**Table 1**).

DISCLOSURES

C.D. Russell was supported by the Chief Scientist Office (CSO) Scotland (PCL/25/21).

REFERENCES

1. Watson K, Russell CD, Baillie JK, et al. Developing novel host-based therapies targeting microbicidal responses in macrophages and neutrophils to combat bacterial antimicrobial resistance. Front Immunol 2020;11:786.

2. Smith EL, Wheeler I, Adler H, et al. Upper airways colonisation of Streptococcus pneumoniae in adults aged 60 years and older: a systematic review of prevalence and individual participant data meta-analysis of risk factors. J Infect 2020;81(4):540–8.
3. Sakr A, Brégeon F, Mège JL, et al. Staphylococcus aureus nasal colonization: an update on mechanisms, epidemiology, risk factors, and subsequent infections. Front Microbiol 2018;9:2419.
4. Lexau CA, Lynfield R, Danila R, et al. Changing epidemiology of invasive pneumococcal disease among older adults in the era of pediatric pneumococcal conjugate vaccine. JAMA 2005;294(16):2043–51.
5. Laupland KB, Lyytikäinen O, Søgaard M, et al. The changing epidemiology of Staphylococcus aureus bloodstream infection: a multinational population-based surveillance study. Clin Microbiol Infection 2013;19(5):465–71.
6. Medzhitov R, Schneider DS, Soares MP. Disease tolerance as a defense strategy. Science 2012;335(6071):936–41.
7. Horby P, Lim WS, Emberson JR, et al. Dexamethasone in hospitalized patients with Covid-19. N Engl J Med 2021;384(8):693–704.
8. Abani O, Abbas A, Abbas F, et al. Tocilizumab in patients admitted to hospital with COVID-19 (RECOVERY): a randomised, controlled, open-label, platform trial. Lancet 2021;397(10285):1637–45.
9. RECOVERY Collaborative Group. Baricitinib in patients admitted to hospital with COVID-19 (RECOVERY): a randomised, controlled, open-label, platform trial and updated meta-analysis. Lancet 2022;400(10349):359–68.
10.. Amanat S, Requena T, Lopez-Escamez JA. A systematic review of extreme phenotype strategies to search for rare variants in genetic studies of complex disorders. Genes 2020;11(9):987.
11. Pairo-Castineira E, Clohisey S, Klaric L, et al. Genetic mechanisms of critical illness in COVID-19. Nature 2021;591(7848):92–8.
12. Kousathanas A, Pairo-Castineira E, Rawlik K, et al. Whole-genome sequencing reveals host factors underlying critical COVID-19. Nature 2022;607(7917):97–103.
13. Pairo-Castineira E, Rawlik K, Bretherick AD, et al. GWAS and meta-analysis identifies 49 genetic variants underlying critical COVID-19. Nature 2023;617(7962):764–8.
14. Liao M, Liu Y, Yuan J, et al. Single-cell landscape of bronchoalveolar immune cells in patients with COVID-19. Nat Med 2020;26(6):842–4.
15.. Thwaites RS, Sanchez Sevilla Uruchurtu A, Siggins MK, et al. Inflammatory profiles across the spectrum of disease reveal a distinct role for GM-CSF in severe COVID-19. Sci Immunol 2021;6(57):eabg9873.
16. Carvelli J, Demaria O, Vély F, et al. Association of COVID-19 inflammation with activation of the C5a-C5aR1 axis. Nature 2020;588(7836):146–50.
17. Stephenson E, Reynolds G, Botting RA, et al. Single-cell multi-omics analysis of the immune response in COVID-19. Nat Med 2021;27(5):904–16.
18. Dorward DA, Russell CD, Um IH, et al. Tissue-specific immunopathology in fatal COVID-19. Am J Respir Crit Care Med 2021;203(2):192–201.
19. Russell CD, Valanciute A, Gachanja NN, et al. Tissue proteomic analysis identifies mechanisms and stages of immunopathology in fatal COVID-19. Am J Respir Cell Mol Biol 2022;66(2):196–205.
20.. Hönzke K, Obermayer B, Mache C, et al. Human lungs show limited permissiveness for SARS-CoV-2 due to scarce ACE2 levels but virus-induced expansion of inflammatory macrophages. Eur Respir J 2022;60(6):2102725.

21. Rendeiro AF, Ravichandran H, Bram Y, et al. The spatial landscape of lung pathology during COVID-19 progression. Nature 2021;593(7860):564–9.
22. Melms JC, Biermann J, Huang H, et al. A molecular single-cell lung atlas of lethal COVID-19. Nature 2021;595(7865):114–9.
23. Sefik E, Israelow B, Mirza H, et al. A humanized mouse model of chronic COVID-19. Nat Biotechnol 2022;40(6):906–20.
24. Okulicz JF, Lambotte O. Epidemiology and clinical characteristics of elite controllers. Curr Opin HIV AIDS 2011;6(3):163–8.
25.. Migueles SA, Chairez C, Lin S, et al. Adoptive lymphocyte transfer to an HIV-infected progressor from an elite controller. JCI Insight 2019;4(18):e130664.
26. Jones AD, Capriotti Z, Santos E, et al. HIV-1 controllers possess a unique CD8+ T cell activation phenotype and loss of control is associated with increased expression of exhaustion markers. PLoS One 2025;20(8):e0328706.
27. Migueles SA, Osborne CM, Royce C, et al. Lytic granule loading of CD8+ T cells is required for HIV-infected cell elimination associated with immune control. Immunity 2008;29(6):1009–21.
28. Marin M, Ruiz A, Ouchi D, et al. PD-1 blockade enhances functional vaccine-induced HIV-1 CD8(+) T-cell responses in PWH receiving early ART. EBioMedicine 2026;123:106070.
29. Horvath RM, Brumme ZL, Sadowski I. CDK8 inhibitors antagonize HIV-1 reactivation and promote provirus latency in T cells. J Virol 2023;97(9):e0092323.
30. Chen H, Li C, Huang J, et al. CD4+ T cells from elite controllers resist HIV-1 infection by selective upregulation of p21. J Clin Investig 2011;121(4):1549–60.
31. Casanova JL, MacMicking JD, Nathan CF. Interferon-γ and infectious diseases: lessons and prospects. Science 2024;384(6693):eadl2016.
32. Ulrichs T, Fieschi C, Nevicka E, et al. Variable outcome of experimental interferon-gamma therapy of disseminated Bacillus Calmette-Guerin infection in two unrelated interleukin-12Rbeta1-deficient Slovakian children. Eur J Pediatr 2005; 164(3):166–72.
33. Rosenzweig SD, Yancoski J, Bernasconi A, et al. Thirteen years of culture-positive M. bovis-BCG infection in an IL-12Rbeta1 deficient patient: treatment and outcome. J Infect 2006;52(3):e69–72.
34. Errami A, Baghdadi JE, Ailal F, et al. Mendelian susceptibility to mycobacterial disease (msmd): clinical, immunological, and genetic features of 22 patients from 15 moroccan kindreds. J Clin Immunol 2023;43(4):728–40.
35. Khavandegar A, Mahdaviani SA, Zaki-Dizaji M, et al. Genetic, immunologic, and clinical features of 830 patients with Mendelian susceptibility to mycobacterial diseases (MSMD): a systematic review. J Allergy Clin Immunol 2024;153(5): 1432–44.
36. Milanés-Virelles MT, García-García I, Santos-Herrera Y, et al. Adjuvant interferon gamma in patients with pulmonary atypical Mycobacteriosis: a randomized, double-blind, placebo-controlled study. BMC Infect Dis 2008;8:17.
37. Leslie A, Kavanagh D, Honeyborne I, et al. Transmission and accumulation of CTL escape variants drive negative associations between HIV polymorphisms and HLA. J Exp Med 2005;201(6):891–902.
38. Kreutzfeldt KM, McAdam PR, Claxton P, et al. Molecular longitudinal tracking of Mycobacterium abscessus spp. during chronic infection of the human lung. PLoS One 2013;8(5):e63237.
39. McAdam PR, Holmes A, Templeton KE, et al. Adaptive evolution of Staphylococcus aureus during chronic endobronchial infection of a cystic fibrosis patient. PLoS One 2011;6(9):e24301.

40. Wilson GJ, Seo KS, Cartwright RA, et al. A novel core genome-encoded superantigen contributes to lethality of community-associated MRSA necrotizing pneumonia. PLoS Pathog 2011;7(10):e1002271.
41. Ensminger AW, Yassin Y, Miron A, et al. Experimental evolution of legionella pneumophila in mouse macrophages leads to strains with altered determinants of environmental survival. PLoS Pathog 2012;8(5):e1002731.
42. Alves J, Vrieling M, Ring N, et al. Experimental evolution of Staphylococcus aureus in macrophages: dissection of a conditional adaptive trait promoting intracellular survival. mBio 2024;15(6):e0034624.
43. Balsells E, Dagan R, Yildirim I, et al. The relative invasive disease potential of Streptococcus pneumoniae among children after PCV introduction: a systematic review and meta-analysis. J Infect 2018;77(5):368–78.
44. Sirotnak AP, Eppes SC, Klein JD. Tuboovarian abscess and peritonitis caused by Streptococcus pneumoniae serotype 1 in young girls. Clin Infect Dis 1996;22(6):993–6.
45. Harboe ZB, Thomsen RW, Riis A, et al. Pneumococcal serotypes and mortality following invasive pneumococcal disease: a population-based cohort study. PLoS Med 2009;6(5):e1000081.
46. Brueggemann AB, Spratt BG. Geographic distribution and clonal diversity of Streptococcus pneumoniae serotype 1 isolates. J Clin Microbiol 2003;41(11):4966–70.
47. Mehiri-Zghal E, Decousser JW, Mahjoubi W, et al. Molecular epidemiology of a Streptococcus pneumoniae serotype 1 outbreak in a Tunisian jail. Diagn Microbiol Infect Dis 2010;66(2):225–7.
48. Mercat A, Nguyen J, Dautzenberg B. An outbreak of pneumococcal pneumonia in two men's shelters. Chest 1991;99(1):147–51.
49. Dagan R, Gradstein S, Belmaker I, et al. An outbreak of Streptococcus pneumoniae serotype 1 in a closed community in southern Israel. Clin Infect Dis 2000;30(2):319–21.
50. Gupta A, Khaw FM, Stokle EL, et al. Outbreak of Streptococcus pneumoniae serotype 1 pneumonia in a United Kingdom school. Br Med J 2008;337:a2964.
51. Leimkugel J, Adams Forgor A, Gagneux S, et al. An outbreak of serotype 1 Streptococcus pneumoniae meningitis in northern Ghana with features that are characteristic of Neisseria meningitidis meningitis epidemics. J Infect Dis 2005;192(2):192–9.
52. Russell CD, Marshall J, McHugh BJ, et al. Immune-adaptive pathogen variation reveals targetable mediators of gram-positive bacterial killing in macrophages. Sci Adv 2026;12(9):eaea0375.
53.. Pongchaikul P, Hokamp K, Kjos M, et al. Transcriptomic analysis of Streptococcus pneumoniae serotype 1 reveals serotype-specific gene regulation. Microb Genom 2025;11(12):001582.
54. Miller LG, Perdreau-Remington F, Rieg G, et al. Necrotizing fasciitis caused by community-associated methicillin-resistant Staphylococcus aureus in Los Angeles. N Engl J Med 2005;352(14):1445–53.
55. Francis JS, Doherty MC, Lopatin U, et al. Severe community-onset pneumonia in healthy adults caused by methicillin-resistant Staphylococcus aureus carrying the Panton-Valentine leukocidin genes. Clin Infect Dis 2005;40(1):100–7.
56. Souli M, Ruffin F, Choi SH, et al. Changing characteristics of staphylococcus aureus bacteremia: results from a 21-year, prospective, longitudinal study. Clin Infect Dis 2019;69(11):1868–77.

57. Fang CT, Chuang YP, Shun CT, et al. A novel virulence gene in Klebsiella pneumoniae strains causing primary liver abscess and septic metastatic complications. J Exp Med 2004;199(5):697–705.
58. Diep BA, Gill SR, Chang RF, et al. Complete genome sequence of USA300, an epidemic clone of community-acquired meticillin-resistant Staphylococcus aureus. Lancet 2006;367(9512):731–9.
59. Young BC, Earle SG, Soeng S, et al. Panton–Valentine leucocidin is the key determinant of Staphylococcus aureus pyomyositis in a bacterial GWAS. eLife 2019;8: e42486.
60. Shankar-Hari M, Calandra T, Soares MP, et al. Reframing sepsis immunobiology for translation: towards informative subtyping and targeted immunomodulatory therapies. Lancet Respir Med 2024;12(4):323–36.
61. Calfee CS, Delucchi K, Parsons PE, et al, NHLBI ARDS Network. Subphenotypes in acute respiratory distress syndrome: latent class analysis of data from two randomised controlled trials. Lancet Respir Med 2014;2(8):611–20.
62. Calfee CS, Delucchi KL, Sinha P, et al. Acute respiratory distress syndrome subphenotypes and differential response to simvastatin: secondary analysis of a randomised controlled trial. Lancet Respir Med 2018;6(9):691–8.
63. Leventogiannis K, Kyriazopoulou E, Antonakos N, et al. Toward personalized immunotherapy in sepsis: the PROVIDE randomized clinical trial. Cell Rep Med 2022;3(11):100817.
64.. Giamarellos-Bourboulis EJ, Kotsaki A, Kotsamidi I, et al. Precision immunotherapy to improve sepsis outcomes: the immunosep randomized clinical trial. JAMA 2026;335(9):775–86.
65. Williams TN. Human red blood cell polymorphisms and malaria. Curr Opin Microbiol 2006;9(4):388–94.
66. Ferreira A, Marguti I, Bechmann I, et al. Sickle hemoglobin confers tolerance to Plasmodium infection. Cell 2011;145(3):398–409.
67. Chaguza C, Yang M, Jacques LC, et al. Serotype 1 pneumococcus: epidemiology, genomics, and disease mechanisms. Trends Microbiol 2022;30(6):581–92.

The Nonimmune Aspects of Sepsis

Nicole P. Juffermans, MD, PhD[a,*], Lies Langouche, MSc, PhD[b],
Nathan D. Nielsen, MD, MSc[c]

KEYWORDS

• Sepsis • Hemodynamics • Hemostasis • Neuroendocrine • Maladaptive

KEY POINTS

- Vascular, hemostatic and neuroendocrine processes during sepsis can become maladaptive.
- These are driven by inflammation.
- They determine whether the host maintains homeostasis or progresses to multiorgan failure.

INTRODUCTION

Sepsis is defined by a dysregulated immune response to infection, causing organ dysfunction. However, there are many pathophysiological processes in sepsis that are not directly mediated by immune cells, yet they determine patient outcome. These encompass vascular, hemostatic, metabolic and neuroendocrine changes that collectively determine whether the host maintains homeostasis or progresses to multiorgan failure. While adaptations of all of these pathways are essential for mounting an adequate host response to pathogens, dysregulation contributes to progression into the sepsis syndrome, with adverse outcome. This article describes the adaptive and maladaptive nonimmune responses during sepsis, with the aim to provide a more comprehensive approach to diagnosis, risk stratification, and potential therapeutic targeting of sepsis that reaches beyond immunomodulation alone.

[a] Department of Intensive Care, The Emergency, Perioperative and Intensive Care Laboratory (EPIC Lab), Erasmus Medial Center, Rotterdam, the Netherlands; [b] Clinical Division and Laboratory of Intensive Care Medicine, Department of Cellular and Molecular Medicine, KU Leuven, Leuven, Belgium; [c] Division of Pulmonary, Critical Care and Sleep Medicine, Section of Transfusion Medicine and Therapeutic Pathology, University of New Mexico School of Medicine, Albuquerque, NM, USA

* Corresponding author. Department of Intensive Care, The Emergency, Perioperative and Intensive Care Laboratory (EPIC Lab), Erasmus Medial Center, Dr Molewaterplein 40, 3015 GD Rotterdam, the Netherlands.

E-mail address: n.juffermans@erasmusmc.nl

Crit Care Clin 42 (2026) 777–793
https://doi.org/10.1016/j.ccc.2026.05.005 criticalcare.theclinics.com
0749-0704/26/

Abbreviations	
DAMPs	damage-associated molecular patterns
DIC	disseminated intravascular coagulation
EC	endothelial cell
NET	neutrophil extracellular trap
PAMPs	pathogen-associated molecular patterns
TF	tissue factor
TSH	thyroid-stimulating hormone

PERFUSION ALTERATIONS TO SEPSIS

Adaptive Hemodynamic Responses

Macro hemodynamic adaptations to sepsis

These include changes in the systemic circulation that initially serve to maintain organ perfusion but can become maladaptive as sepsis progresses. These are summarized in **Table 1**. The primary macrocirculatory adaptation in sepsis is arterial vasodilation, resulting in decreased systemic vascular resistance and hypotension. This vasodilation is driven by cytokine-mediated upregulation of inducible nitric oxide synthase and increased nitric oxide production, as well as activation of adenosine triphosphate (ATP)-sensitive potassium channels in vascular smooth muscle, which impairs vasoconstrictor responses to endogenous catecholamines and angiotensin II.[1]

Table 1
Hemodynamic alterations in sepsis

System	Adaptive Responses in Early Sepsis	Maladaptive Responses in Late Sepsis
Arterial vasodilation	• Increased NO production • K^+ channel activation causing vasodilation	• Increased NO and ATP-sensitive K^+ channels activation • Cytokines downregulate adrenergic and AT receptors
Sympathetic nervous system	• Activated by baroreceptor unloading due to hypotension • Increased catecholamine release	• Reduced response to catecholamines • Diminished vascular constriction despite high levels of catecholamines
Cardiac function	• Increased heart rate and contractility from adrenergic stimulation	• Myocardial dysfunction due to continued catecholamine stimulation
Renin–angiotensin–aldosterone system	• Renin release leads to increased AT II production, inducing vasoconstriction and Na^+ retention	• Diminished response to AT and adrenergic stimulation • Vasodilation and reduced preload
Vasopressin release	• Vasopressin release promotes vasoconstriction	• Relative vasopressin deficiency occurs, contributing to vasodilation
Microcirculation	• Capillary recruitment • Redistribution of blood flow to hypoxic areas	• Uncoupling of O2 sensing from blood flow • Capillary clogging • Microcirculatory heterogeneity

To compensate for arterial underfilling, the sympathetic nervous system is activated, leading to increased release of catecholamines, which stimulate β-adrenergic receptors in the heart, resulting in positive chronotropy and inotropy.[2] This sympathetic drive is triggered by baroreceptor unloading due to hypotension and is further amplified by inflammatory mediators and prostaglandins.[3] Low circulating blood volume also activates the renin–angiotensin–aldosterone axis.[4] Renin release leads to increased angiotensin II, which acts as a systemic vasoconstrictor and also stimulates aldosterone secretion. Angiotensin II increases venous return, thereby increasing preload, through vasoconstriction and sodium retention. In addition, arterial underfilling induces baroreceptor-mediated stimulation of the hypothalamus and posterior pituitary, resulting in vasopressin release. Vasopressin causes vasoconstriction through binding to V1 receptors on vascular smooth muscle, thereby increasing vascular tone and arterial blood pressure.[5]

Microhemodynamic adaptations to sepsis

The microcirculatory compartment adapts early in the course of sepsis, by autoregulatory attempts to preserve capillary flow. These include vasodilation of local capillaries and low-frequency oscillations in vessel diameter that help redistribute blood flow to hypoxic tissues.[6] This response is partially mediated by increased nitric oxide production, which promotes vasodilation and enhances flow to areas of relative hypoxia. In addition, there is recruitment of reserve capillaries to maximize the surface area for oxygen diffusion. These hemodynamic alterations early in the course of sepsis collectively support cardiac output at the macro circulatory level and tissue perfusion at the microcirculatory level.

Maladaptive Hemodynamic Responses in Sepsis

Maladaptive macrocirculatory alterations

During the trajectory of sepsis, proinflammatory cytokines and nitric oxide induce downregulation and desensitization of adrenergic and angiotensin II type 1 receptors, leading to diminished vascular contractile responses to norepinephrine and angiotensin II, even at high doses.[7] Also, as septic shock persists, vasopressin levels decline to inappropriately low concentrations relative to the degree of hypotension. This phenomenon is termed relative vasopressin deficiency, which can occur in up to one-third of patients with septic shock.[5] Vasopressin deficiency is thought to result from depletion of neuro hypophyseal stores after sustained baroreceptor stimulation. Clinically, this manifests as a requirement for escalating doses of catecholamines to maintain target mean arterial pressure, with reduced efficacy and increased risk of adverse effects such as arrhythmias and tissue ischemia. High levels of nitric oxide and inflammatory cytokines further blunt vascular responsiveness to vasopressors, exacerbating shock and tissue hypoperfusion.[1]

Maladaptive microcirculatory alterations

Microcirculatory maladaptations include excessive microvascular vasoconstriction due to neurohumoral activation, which can impair organ perfusion and precipitate organ injury, despite systemic vasodilation. Other maladaptive alterations in microcirculatory function are characterized by a loss of microvascular autoregulation, with delayed capillary response to hypoxia and reduced erythrocyte ATP efflux, resulting in uncoupling of local oxygen sensing from flow regulation. Microvascular flow heterogeneity is the hallmark of maladaptation. Some capillaries have high flow, resulting in a transit time too short to exchange oxygen, while others are clogged by microthrombi.[8] Capillary density is decreased, included occluded capillaries, even after resuscitation, further impairing oxygen delivery to tissues. Importantly, these microcirculatory changes can occur, despite normal or restored arterial blood pressure and cardiac output, a situation referred to as *uncoupling*. Ultimately, these maladaptive responses are associated with multiorgan dysfunction and increased mortality in septic shock.[8,9]

Applying Knowledge of Hemodynamic Alterations in Sepsis to Bedside Care

Norepinephrine is recommended as the first-line vasopressor to restore perfusion pressure,[10] but receptor saturation and downregulation may limit its effectiveness at higher doses. Vasopressin and angiotensin II can be used as adjuncts to reduce catecholamine requirements. Addition of vasopressin is further associated with a lower risk of atrial fibrillation,[11] likely due to reduction in catecholamine exposure and limitation of adrenergic toxicity. However, these strategies do not overcome receptor downregulation or vascular hyporesponsiveness. A simulation study with a machine learning model suggested that earlier start of vasopressin as an adjunctive to norepinephrine in sepsis patients was associated with reduced mortality,[12] but clinical trials are lacking s.

Identification of patient subgroups most likely to benefit is a therapeutic goal. However, there currently is no validated bedside biomarker for vasopressin deficiency. From a pathophysiological standpoint, patients with elevated serum renin or a high angiotensin I/II ratio may derive the greatest benefit of early start of vasopressin, as these markers indicate impaired endogenous angiotensin II production and are associated with vasopressor responsiveness.[13]

At the microcirculatory level, knowledge of uncoupling of the microcirculation from the macrocirculation has put emphasis on the assessment of efficacy of therapies improving microcirculatory perfusion. Microcirculatory-guided therapy with capillary refill time as compared to standard care in septic patients led to faster organ dysfunction recovery and less fluid administration, but no impact on mortality.[14] Inodilators such as levosimendan, has shown improvement in microvascular flow in some studies, though outcome benefit is unproven.[15] Vasodilators such as prostacyclin and nitric oxide donors recruit microcirculatory vessels, but with inconsistent outcome data.[16]

Taken together, hemodynamic alterations in sepsis profoundly impact patient outcome. Improved knowledge on these alterations is highly likely to improve care of sepsis patients.

ENDOTHELIAL ALTERATIONS TO SEPSIS

Adaptation of the Endothelium to Sepsis

The vascular endothelium acts as an adaptive *gatekeeper* that orchestrates local containment processes to prevent the spread of a pathogen beyond the primary site.[17] During infection, endothelial cells (ECs) actively coordinate the immune response to trap and eliminate pathogens, reviewed in detail elsewhere.[18] Nonimmune mechanisms, or more accurately, indirect immune mechanisms include a range of physiologic pathways.

Walling off pathogens via coagulation

To restrict the endovascular spread of pathogens, endothelial activity shifts from antithrombotic to a prothrombotic state. This induces local thrombin generation and fibrin formation, effectively *walling off* the infection within the local microvasculature, in concert with local vasoconstrictive effects also mediated by ECs.[19]

Targeted leukocyte recruitment

At baseline, ECs express adhesion molecules such as intercellular adhesion molecule 1 and vascular cell-adhesion molecule 1. During infection, ECs universally upregulate the expression of adhesion molecules, which act as *traps* to ensnare circulating leukocytes and facilitate leukocyte recruitment to the tissue endothelial beds to kill pathogens.[20]

Controlled permeability

A transient and controlled increase in endothelial permeability via intercellular gap formation allows leukocyte transit from the bloodstream into the affected tissues, as well as the passage of antibodies and other immunomodulatory molecules into the interstitial spaces. The permeability in a controlled infectious response is balanced such that useful mediators can pass to the affected site without causing tissue edema.[21]

Maladaptation of the Endothelium to Sepsis

While infection-induced endothelial changes are needed for leukocyte recruitment and transition into the site of infection to promote bacterial elimination, uncontrolled or persistent endothelial changes may contribute to organ failure (**Fig. 1**). An overwhelming or persistent infection can lead to systemic endothelial activation and a shift toward a proapoptotic, proinflammatory, proadhesive, and procoagulant phenotype, a key factor in the progression from sepsis to organ failure and sepsis-mediated death.[17]

Glycocalyx shedding

The glycocalyx is a heparan sulfate–rich layer of glycosaminoglycans and proteoglycans that coats the inner wall of vascular endothelia, forming a dense gel-like surface layer ranging from 0.5 to greater than 10 mm thick. It is critically involved in vascular integrity and leukocyte trafficking.[22]

The glycocalyx can be degraded by inflammatory processes. Its destruction exposes the procoagulant surface of the endothelium, increases the permeability of the endothelium to macromolecules and increases leukocyte adhesion in the microcirculation.[23] Furthermore, loss of heparan sulfate glycosaminoglycans results in impaired nitric oxide (NO) production, which affects the ability of the endothelium to vasodilate in response to shear stress.[22] The summation of these deleterious processes contributes to alterations in microvascular rheology, affecting capillary blood flow, and ultimately decreasing tissue perfusion.[24]

Direct measurements of the glycocalyx thickness can only be done in experimental settings. Indirect biomarkers are levels of glycocalyx components that are shed into the plasma, such as syndecan-1 and hyaluronan. The levels of these markers are consistently correlated with disease severity in septic patients.[25,26]

After the acute septic insult, it can take up to 5 to 7 days for the glycocalyx to be restored structurally, and even longer to fully recover hydrodynamic regulatory

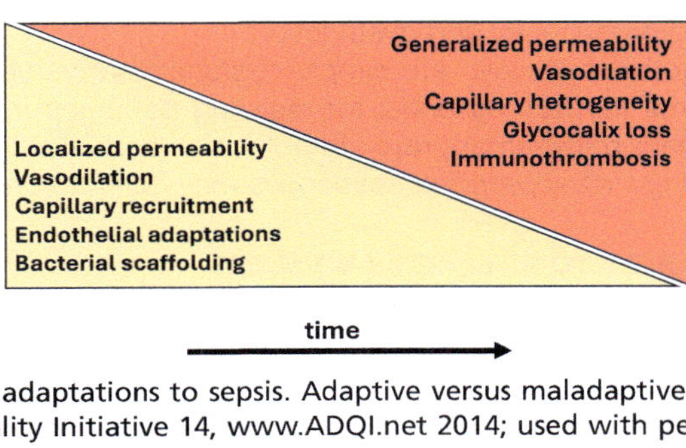

Fig. 1. Endothelial adaptations to sepsis. Adaptive versus maladaptive responses to sepsis. (Acute Dialysis Quality Initiative 14, www.ADQI.net 2014; used with permission.[51])

function.[27] The delay in functional glycocalyx recovery explains, at least in part, persistent microcirculatory dysfunction in septic shock despite the normalization of the macrocirculation.[28,29]

Uncontrolled vascular permeability and edema

For some time, it was held that vascular leakage is a necessary step for leukocyte transit from the blood into the tissue, and that modulating leakage may also alter the local immune response. However, recent studies have found that leukocyte trafficking and vascular permeability are regulated through distinct pathways,[30] suggesting that the maladaptive sepsis-related capillary leakage could be modulated without adversely affecting leukocyte recruitment.[31,32] In response to damage- (DAMPs) or pathogen-associated molecular patterns (PAMPs), there is glycocalyx breakdown, EC death and junction protein dysregulation. Endothelial intercellular permeability is regulated by adherens junctions (cadherin–cadherin) and tight junctions (claudin/occludin). During acute inflammation, phosphorylation of the vascular endothelial–cadherin intracellular domain leads to its deconstruction and endocytosis.[16] Claudin proteins, the primary regulators of tight junction permeability[32] are elevated in sepsis, which lead to the disassembly of endothelial tight junctions, contributing to capillary leak.[20] The heightened expression of angiopoietin-2 and lower expression of angiopoietin-1, results in inhibiting of Tie-2 activation and signaling, leading to endothelial permeability and other dysregulations of vascular homeostasis through multiple signaling pathways.[17] The net result of these synergistic maladaptations is the *capillary leak syndrome*, where plasma and proteins can pass freely into the interstitium, contributing to edema and injury.

Regulated endothelial cell death

ECs can undergo acceleration of programmed cell death following pathogen invasion.[33] PAMPs and DAMPs, in concert with oxidative stress from reactive oxygen species bursts, can trigger programmed cell death pathways in ECs.[16] Such pathways include apoptosis (vesicle formation and DNA/protein fragmentation), necroptosis (cell membrane rupture), pyroptosis (membrane pore formation), and ferroptosis (cell death by iron overload). The loss of cells resulting from these programmed cell death pathways leads to gaps in vessel walls, further contributing to edema-causing processes. Also, the subsequent release of proinflammatory mediators and cellular debris from dead and dying ECs further amplifies the septic process.[34]

In summary, during infection, exogenous PAMPs and endogenous DAMPs can trigger an array of pathophysiological pathways involving the endothelium that can impair its structure and/or function and even result in the death of its constituent cells. The damage to the glycocalyx, loss of vascular patency and EC apoptosis lead to an increase in permeability to proteins and fluids, causing interstitial leakage, tissue edema and resulting organ injury and dysfunction.

As these maladaptive pathways are simply dysfunctional versions of protective, adaptive mechanisms that are essential for resisting pathogen invasion, it is challenging to discriminate between appropriate activation and endothelial dysfunction, especially considering that *appropriate* responses may differ among organs.[35,36]

COAGULATION CHANGES TO INFECTION AND SEPSIS

Beneficial Adaptation of the Coagulation System to Sepsis

In the early stages of an infection, coagulation acts as a crucial element of the innate immune defense. A blood clot is a highly effective bactericidal device. Immunothrombi can limit pathogen spreading, augment bacterial killing, and provide physical anchors for immune cell localization and activation. When confined to the site of pathogen invasion, coagulation and coagulation-linked defense pathways can be highly effective contributors to a successful and controlled immune response. Key elements of a beneficial immunothrombotic response are pathogen/toxin containment, neutrophil extracellular traps (NETs) formation, and immune scaffold construction.[37]

Pathogen/toxin containment

On sensing PAMPs and/or DAMPs, myeloid cells become activated and induce fibrin formation. The resulting fibrin lattices facilitate the detection, containment and elimination of pathogens,[38] acting as a mechanical *trap* by immobilizing and killing the micro-organisms and preventing their spread into the systemic circulation. The entrapment of pathogens is mediated by the cross-linking of bacteria to fibrin fibers by the action of coagulation factor XIII.[39] Mechanical pressure from clot contracture may tear bacterial capsules and walls, causing the squeezing out of bacterial contents and cell death.[40] The fibrin lattices can also capture significant quantities of lipopolysaccharide, mitigating potential damage from gram negative bacilli.[41]

Neutrophil extracellular traps formation

NETs are complexes of neutrophil DNA and histones causing a multitude of immunothrombotic sequelae resulting from pathogen-induced activation of neutrophils in a process referred to as NETosis. These released *webs* of DNA, histones, enzymes, and antimicrobial proteins trap bacteria, induce both core coagulation pathways (resulting in additional fibrin formation), and provide a surface around the invading pathogens for further coagulation and immune activities.[38]

Immune scaffolding

Developing blood clots, particularly the fibrin and NET components, can act as *immune scaffolding*, recruiting immune cells (primarily neutrophils and macrophages) to the sites of infection. Such activity reflects the merging of coagulation and innate immunity pathways to restrict pathogen dissemination by focusing immune antimicrobial activity to the invaded tissue.[42]

Maladaptation of the Coagulation System to Sepsis

When coagulation localization is lost, microthrombus and macrothrombus formation can contribute to morbidity and mortality.[37] A fine balance between a protective immunothrombosis[43] and uncontrolled pathologic thrombosis is required.[44] The widespread, reciprocal and self-amplifying activation of blood coagulation and innate immune mechanisms is known as disseminated intravascular coagulation (DIC), which carries a high morbidity and mortality.[38] Mechanisms of DIC have been well addressed elsewhere.[37] Here, major elements of sepsis-induced coagulation maladaptation that lead to DIC are discussed.

Widespread tissue factor activity and thrombin generation

In sepsis-associated DIC, inflammatory cytokines are the key mediators of the *first phase* systemic procoagulable process[45] The extralocal cytokine burst triggers a massive upregulation, expression and release of tissue factor (TF) from circulating and anchored monocytes and monocyte-derived microparticles,[46] which in combination with increased TF exposure at endothelial surfaces that have lost their protective glycocalyx layer,[37] results in a major shift toward a procoagulant state in the normally coagulation-balanced microcirculatory environment. The major increase in TF activity results in the amplified generation of thrombin followed by the conversion of fibrinogen to fibrin, with resulting uncontrolled clot formation at sites far distant from the initial infection site – the *sine qua non* of DIC.

Failure of natural anticoagulants

During sepsis-induced maladaptive coagulation, the function of all 3 physiologic endogenous anticoagulant pathways (the *brakes*) are impaired. First, antithrombin (which complexes with and inhibits thrombin and factor Xa) levels are markedly reduced via a combination of processes, including reduced synthesis, increased clearance from the formation of protease–antithrombin complexes, extravascular loss due to increased vascular permeability and direct degradation by neutrophil elastases.[37] Second, the activity of Protein C (a potent inhibitor of factors Va and VIIIa and downregulator of thrombin) is similarly reduced due to a combination of decreased synthesis, reduced substrate affinity, increased consumption, and inhibited activation.[47] The third major anticoagulant system, based on the action of TF pathway inhibitor inhibiting the procoagulant effects of TF VIIa complexes, is also disrupted in sepsis, due at least in part due to cleavage from enzymes released by NETs.[48] These NET enzymes also degrade thrombomodulin, further removing a *brake* on unchecked thrombin formation.[49]

Fibrinolysis inhibition

At the peak of sepsis-induced accelerated thrombus formation and anticoagulation pathway inhibition, endogenous fibrinolysis is almost completely shut down,[50] further cementing microthrombi in place. The initial fibrinolytic reaction to inflammatory mediators is an increase in tissue-type plasminogen activator and urokinase-type plasminogen activator release from the endothelium[51] with the resulting generation of high levels of plasmin, favoring net clot lysis. This is followed by an even greater, and persistent, increase in the levels of plasminogen activator inhibitor 1. The latter results in a sustained suppression of endogenous fibrinolysis, further adding to uncontrolled disseminated thrombus propagation.

In summary, while coagulation pathways form a critical element of innate immunity contributing to pathogen containment, when these pathways become unchecked, they can become major contributors to endothelial damage, microvascular flow compromise, tissue ischemia, and resulting organ damage.

NEUROENDOCRINE REPROGRAMMING IN SEPSIS—A BIPHASIC PATTERN

The endocrine and metabolic reactions seen in sepsis—initiated by PAMPs—closely resemble those observed in other forms of critical illness driven by DAMPs. Nevertheless, because sepsis typically induces a more intense hyperinflammatory state, its associated metabolic and hormonal disturbances tend to be more marked than those triggered by major surgery or trauma.[52] Combined, the neuroendocrine response follows a biphasic pattern: an early, acute phase that is mostly adaptive and oriented toward survival, and a later, protracted phase that may become maladaptive as critical illness persists (**Fig. 2**).

The Adrenal Axis

Activation of the adrenal axis is a first crucial neuroendocrine response to sepsis. In the acute phase, cytokines and neuronal stress signals stimulate hypothalamic corticotropin-releasing hormone (CRH) and arginine vasopressin (AVP) release, activating the pituitary to secrete adrenocorticotropic hormone (ACTH) which concomitantly stimulates the adrenal cortex to produce and release cortisol. Although cortisol levels remain high during sepsis, ACTH concentrations are only very acutely elevated and are

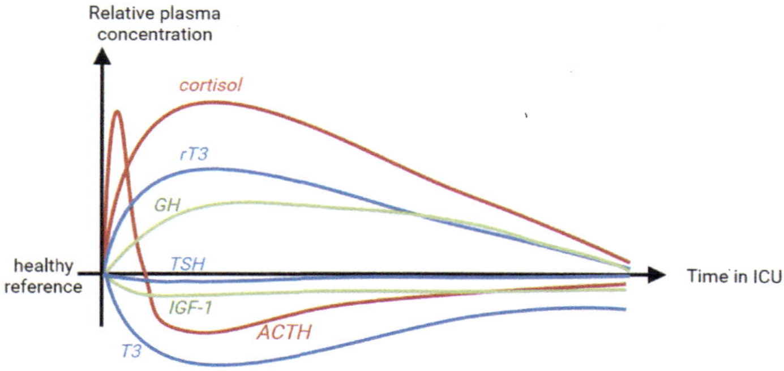

Fig. 2. Schematic representation of the adrenal, thyroid and growth hormone axis during acute and prolonged sepsis. (Created in BioRender. Langouche, L. (2026) https://BioRender.com/nfth3pf.)

often already low to normal when patients enter the intensive care unit (ICU).[53] Other non–ACTH-driven mechanisms increase the availability of free cortisol during sepsis, with decreased cortisol breakdown and reduced levels of cortisol-binding proteins being the most important, rather than an ongoing increased production.[54] The sustained elevated cortisol levels provide negative feedback at the pituitary level, impairing the processing of pro-opiomelanocortin into ACTH, thereby reducing ACTH in the circulation.[55] In the acute phase of sepsis, these changes can be interpreted as adaptive and beneficial for the host as this energy-efficient increase in plasma cortisol—reducing breakdown rather than increasing production—may support hemodynamic stability, enhance vascular responsiveness to catecholamines, maintain fluid balance and limit excessive inflammation. Tissue-specific alterations in expression of metabolizing enzymes and of the glucocorticoid nuclear receptor GRα further titrate cortisol actions in vital organs, whereas immune-suppressive off-target effects are prevented by reduced GRα actions in neutrophils.[56] Where these alterations might be beneficial in the short term, sustained hypercortisolemia with suppressed ACTH levels in patients who remain critically ill for several weeks may create a form of central adrenal insufficiency.[57,58] Furthermore, persistently elevated cortisol may contribute to hyperglycemia, muscle wasting and infection susceptibility. Current guidelines recommend the use of glucocorticoids only in patients with refractory septic shock resistant to fluids and vasopressors, with stress doses (200 mg/day) of hydrocortisone.[10] The vasopressor-reducing effect of this treatment is pharmacologic and should not be administered on the assumption of insufficient cortisol availability or general glucocorticoid resistance, also taking into account possible off-target effects.[59] Indeed, the tissue-specific GRα actions do not support a general glucocorticoid resistance in septic shock and normal incremental ACTH responses to a CRH stimulation test were reported in the acute phase of sepsis.

The Thyroid Axis

Sepsis also causes rapid and profound alterations in the thyroid axis. Immediately after onset, triiodothyronine (T3) levels fall, rT3 rises, while thyroid-stimulating hormone (TSH) remains normal to elevated.[60] This shift is due to an upregulated peripheral deiodination of T4 to the inactive rT3 instead of to the active T3 due to tissue specific changes in expression and activity of deiodinasing enzymes D1 and D3.[61,62] This *low T3 syndrome* or *nonthyroidal illness* is considered adaptive in the acute phase, reducing energy expenditure and protein catabolism.[63] Both inflammation and a reduced nutritional intake or major contributors to this constellation.[64,65] In prolonged critical illness, both central and peripheral regulation of the axis become suppressed, with now also a suppression of thyrotropin-releasing hormone (TRH) and TSH and a further decline in both T3 and T4.[60] While statistical modeling suggest that these chronic changes may be maladaptive,[64] clinical trials using T3 or T4 replacement have not shown benefit, likely because peripheral hormone administration bypasses normal feedback.[60] Infusion of TRH in prolonged ICU patients restored physiologic patterns of TSH and thyroid hormone secretion,[66] but its effect on clinical outcomes remains unknown.

The Growth Hormone Axis

Acute sepsis increases GH pulse amplitude and frequency, but also nonpulsatile growth hormone (GH) secretion.[67] The high abundance of proinflammatory ctyokines simultaneously induce peripheral GH resistance, reflected in lowered levels of low insulin-like growth factor 1 (IGF-I), and binding proteins IGFBP-3 and ALS.[68] This acute response supports the catabolic effects of GH with increased lipolysis, as such providing substrates for energy, but suppresses the anabolic IGF-1 regulated effects of GH.[69] In chronic critical illness, both GH secretion and its downstream anabolic mediators remain severely depressed, likely contributing to the muscle wasting seen in prolonged sepsis.[70] An attempt to treat prolonged ICU patients with high-dose GH worsened mortality,[71] whereas more physiologic approaches using GHRH and GH secretagogues, combined with TRH, have shown promising metabolic responses, but clinical outcome data are lacking.[72]

The Lactotrophic Axis

Prolactin initially rises as part of the stress response of sepsis, but later becomes suppressed, potentially contributing to immune dysfunction.[73,74] In men, a cytokine-induced increased aromatization lowers testosterone availability, while luteinizing hormone (LH) remains normal or elevated.[75] The increase in estradiol and simultaneous decrease in testosterone continues into the prolonged phase of sepsis, whereas also LH levels drop, deepening hypogonadism.[76,77] Pulsatile gonadotropin-releasing hormone (GnRH) administration, in combination with other hypothalamic releasing factors, is able to transiently restore the gonadal axis.[78]

Metabolic Reprogramming—from Stress Hyperglycemia to Anabolic Resistance

Stress hyperglycemia

The above described endocrine changes in the acute phase of sepsis, with hypercortisolemia, elevated GH but low IGF-1 and low testosterone adds up to the high circulating cytokine levels and catecholamines. This cocktail of inflammatory regulators and catabolic hormones creates a hypercatabolic response leading to hyperglycemia and insulin resistance. Historically this hyperglycemia was regarded as an adaptive response to the septic insult, to provide energy to vital tissues and immune cells that do not need insulin for glucose uptake.[79] The degree of hyperglycemia strongly correlates with worse outcomes and several randomized controlled trial (RCTs) have made clear that lowering hyperglycemia with insulin improves outcome.[80,81] Mechanistic studies indicate that glycemic control with insulin protects cells from glucose toxicity, thereby reducing organ failure. However, the large NICE-SUGAR RCT reported increased mortality with tight glycemic control, which was attributed to a 14-fold increase in hypoglycemia.[82] The earlier RCT's showing benefit, were mainly conducted in a context of early parenteral nutrition, which likely exacerbated hyperglycemia to more harmful levels.[83] The most recent large RCT on this topic showed that during late parenteral nutrition, tight glycemic control did not influence mortality, but reduced severity of acute kidney injury and cholestatic liver dysfunction.[84] Current evidence supports avoiding iatrogenic contributors to hyperglycemia such as early parenteral nutrition or liberal corticosteroid administration, but tight glycemic control requires highly accurate monitoring tools and protocols before it can be endorsed.

Hypercatabolism

Inflammatory cytokines together with high cortisol and GH, combined with low IGF-1 and low testosterone and insulin resistance fuels not only hyperglycemia, but also protein breakdown in liver and muscle tissue together with reduced protein synthesis.[85,86] The catabolic cocktail together with insulin resistance promotes adipose tissue lipolysis and blunts lipogenesis.[87] Overall, this acute hypercatabolic state combined with anabolic resistance might initially be adaption, prioritizing survival over growth and anabolism. In response to sepsis, patients usually develop anorexia and can develop feeding intolerance.[88] The orexigenic hormone ghrelin[89] and the satiety hormone leptin[90]—both of which also exert immunomodulatory effects—along with the metabolic regulators fibroblast growth factor 21[91] and growth differentiation factor-15,[92] may contribute to this illness-induced anorexia. Moreover, several of acute alterations in circulating neuroendocrine hormones seen with sepsis, especially low T3, high cortisol, and low IGF-1, largely resemble those observed in healthy individuals following a period of fasting.[93] From an evolutionary perspective, fasting naturally accompanies severe physical injury, and the hormonal responses triggered by both fasting and inflammation are therefore likely adaptive, helping the organism withstand and recover from a major physiologic insult. Ongoing hypercatabolism however will further promote the development of ICU acquired muscle weakness, which delays recovery and increases mortality.

SUMMARY

Maladaptive pathways are dysfunctional versions of protective, adaptive mechanisms that are essential for resisting pathogen invasion. Discriminating between appropriate activation and unchecked and overactivated processes, is likely to contribute to novel discoveries that aim to improve the management of sepsis.

CLINICS CARE POINTS

- Adaptive responses in sepsis aim to preserve homeostasis by improving capillary flow to organs, by orchestrating a coordinated host response to pathogens while ensuring efficient use of energy.
- A dysregulated inflammatory response drives maladaptive processes, including systemic vasodilation while the microcirculation is vasoconstricted, hampering oxygen extraction.
- Uncontrolled inflammation leads to loss of coagulation localization with systemic microthrombi formation. A hypercatabolic response with blunted lipogenesis promote muscle weakness and delayed recovery.

DISCLOSURE

N.P. Juffermans receives funding from the Landsteiner Foundation to investigate mechanisms of anemia in sepsis and serves on the advisory board for Bayer, for investigator-driven research on shock-induced vascular permeability from

Octapharma, and for research materials from Werfen. N.D. Nielson serves on advisory boards for 4Teen4, Aurobac, Bayer, and Grand Medical. The remaining author discloses no conflicts.

REFERENCES

1. Landry DW, Oliver JA. The pathogenesis of vasodilatory shock. N Engl J Med 2001;345:588–95.
2. Ramchandra R, Wan L, Hood SG, et al. Septic shock induces distinct changes in sympathetic nerve activity to the heart and kidney in conscious sheep. Am J Physiol Regul Integr Comp Physiol 2009;297(5):R1247–53.
3. Booth LC, Ramchandra R, Calzavacca P, et al. Role of prostaglandins in determining the increased cardiac sympathetic nerve activity in ovine sepsis. Am J Physiol Regul Integr Comp Physiol 2014;307(1):R75–81.
4. Legrand M, Khanna AK, Ostermann M, et al. The renin–angiotensin–aldosterone-system in sepsis and its clinical modulation with exogenous angiotensin II. Crit Care 2024;28(1):389.
5. Landry DW, Levin HR, Gallant EM, et al. Vasopressin deficiency contributes to the vasodilation of septic shock. Circulation 1997;95(5):1122–5.
6. Bateman RM, Sharpe MD, Jagger JE, et al. Sepsis impairs microvascular autoregulation and delays capillary response within hypoxic capillaries. Crit Care 2015;19:389.
7. Bucher M, Frieder K, Taeger K, et al. Cytokines down-regulate α_1-adrenergic receptor expression during endotoxemia. Crit Care Med 2003;31(2):566–71.
8. Kanoore EV, Enrico C, Laviolle B, et al. Quantitative assessment of the microcirculation in healthy volunteers and in patients with septic shock. Crit Care Med 2012;40(5):1443–8.
9. De Backer D, Ricottilli F, Ospina-Tascón G. Septic shock: a microcirculation disease. Curr Opin Anaesthesiol 2021 1;34(2):85–9.
10. Evans L, Rhodes A, Alhazzani W, et al. Surviving sepsis campaign: international guidelines for management of sepsis and septic shock 2021. Intensive Care Med 2021;47:1181–247.
11. McIntyre WF, Um KJ, Alhazzani W, et al. Association of vasopressin plus catecholamine vasopressors vs CatecholaminesAlone with atrial fibrillation in patients with distributive shock. A systematic review and meta-analysis. JAMA 2018;319-(18):1889–900.
12. Kalimouttou A, Kennedy JA, Feng J, et al. Optimal vasopressin initiation in septic ShockThe OVISS reinforcement learning Study. JAMA 2025;333(19):1688–98.
13. Senatorea F, Balakumarb P, Jagadeeshc G. Dysregulation of the renin-angiotensin system in septic shock: mechanistic insights and application of angiotensin II in clinical management. Pharmacol Res 2021;174:105916.
14. The ANDROMEDA-SHOCK-2 Investigators for the ANDROMEDA Research Network, Spanish Society of Anesthesiology, Reanimation and PainTherapy (SEDAR), and Latin American Intensive Care Network (LIVEN), Hernandez G, Ospina-Tascón GA, Kattan E, et al. Personalized hemodynamic resuscitation targeting capillary refill time in early septic shock. The ANDROMEDA-SHOCK-2 randomized clinical trial. JAMA 2025;334(22):1988–99.
15. Morelli A, Donati A, Ertmer C, et al. Levosimendan for resuscitating the microcirculation in patients with septic shock: a randomized controlled study. Crit Care 2010;14(6):R232.

16. Sathianathan S, Sachar S, Berro J, et al. Vasoactive medications and the microcirculation in septic shock: a scoping review. Crit Care Med 2026;13. https://doi.org/10.1097/CCM.0000000000007016.
17. Joffre J, Hellman J, Ince C, et al. Endothelial responses in sepsis. Am J Respir Crit Care Med 2020;202(3):361–70.
18. Amersfoort J, Eelen G, Carmeliet P. Immunomodulation by endothelial cells — partnering up with the immune system? Nat Rev Immunol 2022;22:576–88.
19. Dolmatova EV, Wang K, Mandavilli R, et al. The effects of sepsis on endothelium and clinical implications. Cardiovasc Res 2021;117(1):60–73.
20. Ma Z, Pierce RW, Lucas CL, et al. Roles of endothelial cells during infection. Curr Opin Immunol 2025;97:102648.
21. Vermette D, Hu P, Canarie MF, et al. Tight junction structure, function, and assessment in the critically ill: a systematic review. ICM Experimental 2018;6:37.
22. Reitsma S, Slaaf DW, Vink H, et al. The endothelial glycocalyx: composition, functions, and visualization. Pflugers Arch 2007;454:345–59.
23. Kataoka H, Ushiyama A, Akimoto Y, et al. Structural behavior of the endothelial glycocalyx is associated with pathophysiologic status in septic mice: an integrated approach to analyzing the behavior and function of the glycocalyx using both electron and fluorescence intravital microscopy. Anesth Analg 2017;125: 874–83.
24. Lipowsky HH, Gao L, Lescanic A. Shedding of the endothelial glycocalyx in arterioles, capillaries, and venules and its effect on capillary hemodynamics during inflammation. Am J Physiol Heart Circ Physiol 2011;301:H2235–45.
25. Ostrowski SR, Haase N, Müller RB, et al. Association between biomarkers of endothelial injury and hypocoagulability in patients with severe sepsis: a prospective study. Crit Care 2015;19:191.
26. Smart L, Macdonald SPJ, Burrows S, et al. Endothelial glycocalyx biomarkers increase in patients with infection during emergency department treatment. J Crit Care 2017;42:304–9.
27. Potter DR, Jiang J, Damiano ER. The recovery time course of the endothelial cell glycocalyx *in vivo* and its implications *in vitro*. Circ Res 2009;104:1318–25.
28. Verdant CL, De Backer D, Bruhn A, et al. Evaluation of sublingual and gut mucosal microcirculation in sepsis: a quantitative analysis. Crit Care Med 2009; 37:2875–81.
29. Sakr Y, Dubois MJ, De Backer D, et al. Persistent microcirculatory alterations are associated with organ failure and death in patients with septic shock. Crit Care Med 2004;32:1825–31.
30. Filewod NC, Lee WL. Inflammation without vascular leakage: science fiction no longer? Am J Respir Crit Care Med 2019;200:1472–6.
31. Goldenberg NM, Steinberg BE, Slutsky AS, et al. Broken barriers: a new take on sepsis pathogenesis. Sci Transl Med 2011;3:88ps25.
32. Gunzel D, Yu AS. Claudins and the modulation of tight junction permeability. Physiol Rev 2013;93:525–69.
33. Bao Y, Yang X, Zhao P, et al. Research advances on the role of programmed endothelial cell death in sepsis. Cell Death Discov 2025;11:426.
34. Lin X, Ouyang S, Zhi C, et al. Focus on ferroptosis, pyroptosis, apoptosis and autophagy of vascular endothelial cells to the strategic targets for the treatment of atherosclerosis. Arch Biochem Biophys 2022;715:109098.
35. Aird WC. Endothelial cell heterogeneity. Cold Spring Harb Perspect Med 2012;2: a006429.

36. Aird WC. Phenotypic heterogeneity of the endothelium: II. Representative vascular beds. Circ Res 2007;100:174–90.
37. Gando S, Levi M, Toh CH. Disseminated intravascular coagulation. Nat Rev Dis Primers 2016;2:16037.
38. Schulz C, Engelmann B, Massberg S. Crossroads of coagulation and innate immunity: the case of deep vein thrombosis. J Thromb Haemostasis 2013;11: 233–41.
39. Schroeder V, Kohler HP. New developments in the area of factor XIII. J Thromb Haemost 2013;11(2):234–44.
40. Si F, Li B, Margolin W, et al. Bacterial growth and form under mechanical compression. Sci Rep 2015;5:11367.
41. Minasyan H, Flachsbart F. Blood coagulation: a powerful bactericidal mechanism of human innate immunity. Int Rev Immunol 2019;38(1):3–17.
42. Antoniak S. The coagulation system in host defense. Research and Practice in Thrombosis and Haemostasis 2018;2(3):549–57.
43. Esmon CT, Xu J, Lupu F. Innate immunity and coagulation. J Thromb Haemostasis 2011;9:182–8.
44. Clark SR, Ma AC, Tavener SA, et al. Platelet TLR4 activates neutrophil extracellular traps to ensnare bacteria in septic blood. Nat Med 2007;13(4):463–9.
45. Girardis M, David S, Ferrer R, et al. Understanding, assessing and treating immune, endothelial and haemostasis dysfunctions in bacterial sepsis. Intensive Care Med 2024;50(10):1580–92.
46. Laursen MA, Larsen JB, Hvas AM. Platelet function in disseminated intravascular coagulation: a systematic review. Platelets 2018;29(3):238–48.
47. Coloretti I, Corcione A, De Pascale G, et al. Protein C in adult patients with sepsis: from pathophysiology to monitoring and supplementation. J Anesth Analg Crit Care 2025;5(1):21.
48. Keragala CB, Draxler DF, McQuilten ZK, et al. Haemostasis and innate immunity–a complementary relationship: a review of the intricate relationship between coagulation and complement pathways. Br J Haematol 2018;180(6):782–98.
49. Levi M, van der Poll TA. Short contemporary history of disseminated intravascular coagulation. Semin Thromb Hemost 2014;40:874–80.
50. Biemond BJ, Levi M, Ten Cate H, et al. Plasminogen activator and plasminogen activator inhibitor I release during experimental endotoxaemia in chimpanzees: effect of interventions in the cytokine and coagulation cascades. Clin Sci 1995; 88(5):587–94.
51. Ince C, Mayeux PR, Nguyen T, et al, ADQI XIV Workgroup. The endothelium in sepsis. Shock 2016;45(3):259–70.
52. Haug VF, Tapking C, Panayi AC, et al. Long-term sequelae of critical illness in sepsis, trauma and burns: a systematic review and meta-analysis. J Trauma Acute Care Surg 2021;91(4):736–47.
53. Langouche L, Teblick A, Gunst J, et al. The hypothalamus-pituitary-adrenocortical response to critical illness: a concept in need of revision. Endocr Rev 2023;44(6):1096–106.
54. Boonen E, Vervenne H, Meersseman P, et al. Reduced cortisol metabolism during critical illness. N Engl J Med 2013;368(16):1477–88.
55. Teblick A, Vander Perre S, Pauwels L, et al. The role of pro-opiomelanocortin in the ACTH-cortisol dissociation of sepsis. Crit Care 2021;25(1):65.
56. Teblick A, Van Dyck L, Van Aerde N, et al. Impact of duration of critical illness and level of systemic glucocorticoid availability on tissue-specific glucocorticoid

receptor expression and actions: a prospective, observational, cross-sectional human and two translational mouse studies. EBioMedicine 2022;80:104057.
57. Peeters B, Meersseman P, Vander Perre S, et al. Adrenocortical function during prolonged critical illness and beyond: a prospective observational study. Intensive Care Med 2018;44(10):1720–9.
58. Peeters B, Meersseman P, Vander Perre S, et al. ACTH and cortisol responses to CRH in acute, subacute, and prolonged critical illness: a randomized, double-blind, placebo-controlled, crossover cohort study. Intensive Care Med 2018;44-(12):2048–58.
59. Teblick A, Gunst J, Van den Berghe G. Critical illness-induced corticosteroid insufficiency: what it is not and what it could be. J Clin Endocrinol Metab 2022; 107(7):2057–64.
60. Fliers E, Bianco AC, Langouche L, et al. Thyroid function in critically ill patients. Lancet Diabetes Endocrinol 2015;3(10):816–25.
61. Peeters RP, Wouters PJ, Kaptein E, et al. Reduced activation and increased inactivation of thyroid hormone in tissues of critically ill patients. J Clin Endocrinol Metab 2003;88(7):3202–11.
62. Boelen A, Boorsma J, Kwakkel J, et al. Type 3 deiodinase is highly expressed in infiltrating neutrophilic granulocytes in response to acute bacterial infection. Thyroid 2008;18(10):1095–103.
63. Van den Berghe G. On the neuroendocrinopathy of critical illness. Perspectives for feeding and novel treatments. Am J Respir Crit Care Med 2016;194(11): 1337–48.
64. Langouche L, Vander Perre S, Marques M, et al. Impact of early nutrient restriction during critical illness on the nonthyroidal illness syndrome and its relation with outcome: a randomized, controlled clinical study. J Clin Endocrinol Metab 2013; 98(3):1006–13.
65. Boelen A, Kwakkel J, Fliers E. Beyond low plasma T3: local thyroid hormone metabolism during inflammation and infection. Endocr Rev 2011;32(5):670–93.
66. Van den Berghe G, de Zegher F, Bowers CY, et al. Pituitary responsiveness to GH-releasing hormone, GH-releasing peptide-2 and thyrotrophin-releasing hormone in critical illness. Clin Endocrinol (Oxf) 1996;45(3):341–51.
67. Van den Berghe G, de Zegher F, Bouillon R. Clinical review 95: acute and prolonged critical illness as different neuroendocrine paradigms. J Clin Endocrinol Metab 1998;83(6):1827–34.
68. Timmins AC, Cotterill AM, Hughes SCC, et al. Critical illness is associated with low circulating concentrations of insulin-like growth factors-I and -II, alterations in insulin-like growth factor binding proteins, and induction of an insulin-like growth factor binding protein 3 protease. Crit Care Med 1996;24(9):1460–6.
69. Bentham J, Rodriguez-Arnao J, Ross RJ. Acquired growth hormone resistance in patients with hypercatabolism. Horm Res 1993;40(1–3):87–91.
70. Yildizdas D, Onenli-Mungan N, Yapicioglu H, et al. Thyroid hormone levels and their relationship to survival in children with bacterial sepsis and septic shock. J Pediatr Endocrinol Metab 2004;17(10):1435–42.
71. Takala J, Ruokonen E, Webster NR, et al. Increased mortality associated with growth hormone treatment in critically ill adults. N Engl J Med 1999;341(11): 785–92.
72. Van den Berghe G, Wouters P, Weekers F, et al. Reactivation of pituitary hormone release and metabolic improvement by infusion of growth hormone-releasing peptide and thyrotropin-releasing hormone in patients with protracted critical illness. J Clin Endocrinol Metab 1999;84(4):1311–23.

73. Van den Berghe G, Wouters P, Bowers CY, et al. Growth hormone-releasing peptide-2 infusion synchronizes growth hormone, thyrotrophin and prolactin release in prolonged critical illness. Eur J Endocrinol 1999;140(1):17–22.
74. Van den Berghe G, de Zegher F, Veldhuis JD, et al. Thyrotrophin and prolactin release in prolonged critical illness: dynamics of spontaneous secretion and effects of growth hormone-secretagogues. Clin Endocrinol (Oxf) 1997;47(5):599–612.
75. Noel GL, Suh HK, Stone JG, et al. Human prolactin and growth hormone release during surgery and other conditions of stress. J Clin Endocrinol Metab 1972; 35(6):840–51.
76. Christeff N, Benassayag C, Carli-Vielle C, et al. Elevated oestrogen and reduced testosterone levels in the serum of male septic shock patients. J Steroid Biochem 1988;29(4):435–40.
77. Van den Berghe G, Weekers F, Baxter RC, et al. Five-day pulsatile gonadotropin-releasing hormone administration unveils combined hypothalamic-pituitary-gonadal defects underlying profound hypoandrogenism in men with prolonged critical illness. J Clin Endocrinol Metab 2001;86(7):3217–26.
78. Van den Berghe G, Baxter RC, Weekers F, et al. The combined administration of GH-releasing peptide-2 (GHRP-2), TRH and GnRH to men with prolonged critical illness evokes superior endocrine and metabolic effects compared to treatment with GHRP-2 alone. Clin Endocrinol (Oxf) 2002;56(5):655–69.
79. Gunst J, De Bruyn A, Van den Berghe G. Glucose control in the ICU. Curr Opin Anaesthesiol 2019;32(2):156–62.
80. Van den Berghe G, Wouters P, Weekers F, et al. Intensive insulin therapy in critically ill patients. N Engl J Med 2001;345(19):1359–67.
81. Vlasselaers D, Milants I, Desmet L, et al. Intensive insulin therapy for patients in paediatric intensive care: a prospective, randomised controlled study. Lancet 2009;373(9663):547–56.
82. Investigators N-S, Finfer S, Chittock DR, et al. Intensive versus conventional glucose control in critically ill patients. N Engl J Med 2009;360(13):1283–97.
83. Van den Berghe G, Vanhorebeek I, Langouche L, et al. Our scientific journey through the ups and downs of blood glucose control in the ICU. Am J Respir Crit Care Med 2024;209(5):497–506.
84. Gunst J, Debaveye Y, Guiza F, et al, TGC-Fast Collaborators. Tight blood-glucose control without early parenteral nutrition in the ICU. N Engl J Med 2023;389(13): 1180–90.
85. Preiser JC, Ichai C, Orban JC, et al. Metabolic response to the stress of critical illness. Br J Anaesth 2014;113(6):945–54.
86. Friedrich O, Reid MB, Van den Berghe G, et al. The sick and the weak: neuropathies/myopathies in the critically ill. Physiol Rev 2015;95(3):1025–109.
87. Wasyluk W, Zwolak A. Metabolic alterations in sepsis. J Clin Med 2021;10(11).
88. Reintam Blaser A, Preiser JC, Fruhwald S, et al, Working Group on Gastrointestinal Function within the Section of Metabolism, Endocrinology and Nutrition MEN Section of ESICM. Gastrointestinal dysfunction in the critically ill: a systematic scoping review and research agenda proposed by the Section of Metabolism, Endocrinology and Nutrition of the European Society of Intensive Care Medicine. Crit Care 2020;24(1):224.
89. Nikitopoulou I, Kampisiouli E, Jahaj E, et al. Ghrelin alterations during experimental and human sepsis. Cytokine 2020;127:154937.
90. Langouche L, Vander Perre S, Frystyk J, et al. Adiponectin, retinol-binding protein 4, and leptin in protracted critical illness of pulmonary origin. Crit Care 2009; 13(4):R112.

91. Thiessen SE, Vanhorebeek I, Derese I, et al. FGF21 response to critical illness: effect of blood glucose control and relation with cellular stress and survival. J Clin Endocrinol Metab 2015;100(10):E1319–27.
92. Van Dyck L, Gunst J, Casaer MP, et al. The clinical potential of GDF15 as a "ready-to-feed indicator" for critically ill adults. Crit Care 2020;24(1):557.
93. Boelen A, Wiersinga WM, Fliers E. Fasting-induced changes in the hypothalamus-pituitary-thyroid axis. Thyroid 2008;18(2):123–9.

Antimicrobial Resistance in Patients with Sepsis

Alexandre P. Zavascki, MD, PhD[a,b], Ana C. Gales, MD, PhD[c], Paulo Mergulhao, MD[d], Andre C. Kalil, MD, MPH[e,*]

KEYWORDS

- Sepsis • Antimicrobial resistance • Antibiotics • Intensive care unit

KEY POINTS

- Sepsis diagnosis is often non-specific, so about one-third of "sepsis syndrome" cases may not have an infectious cause, and only approximately 60% to –70% of true infectious cases yield positive bacterial cultures, increasing risk of inappropriate empirical antibiotics.
- Antimicrobial resistance (AMR) burden in sepsis is global and increasing, with approximately 49 million sepsis cases (2017) and approximately 11 million deaths (~22.5%), disproportionately affecting low-income and middle-income countries; WHO AMR surveillance reports greater than 17% of infections due to AMR bacteria.
- Transmission within intensive care units (ICUs) drives much AMR, so the highest-impact prevention is infection prevention and control (IPC)—especially hand hygiene, environmental cleaning, and device-associated infection bundles—to reduce health care-associated resistant infections.
- AMR prevention also requires stewardship + communication, where antimicrobial stewardship improves appropriateness and protects host microbiota/colonization resistance, while multidisciplinary ICU communication (rounds, antibiotic "time-outs," audit/feedback) is the mechanism to implement IPC/antibiotic stewardship (AS) decisions consistently.
- Diagnostics and optimized treatment reduce harm and resistance selection: rapid diagnostics shorten time to targeted therapy, and optimal AMR treatment relies on mechanism-specific antibiotics (eg, newer beta-lactam/beta-lactamase inhibitors for carbapenem-resistant *Enterobacterales*) plus pharmacokinetic/pharmacodynamic-informed dosing (eg, loading doses, prolonged/continuous beta-lactam infusions, and TDM when needed).

[a] Department of Internal Medicine, Universidade Federal do Rio Grande do Sul, Porto Alegre; [b] Infectious Diseases Service, Hospital de Clinicas de Porto Alegre, Infectious Diseases and Infection Control Service, Hospital Moinhos de Vento, Porto Alegre, Brazil; [c] Division of Infectious Diseases, Department of Internal Medicine, Universidade Federal de São Paulo, Antimicrobial Resistance Institute of São Paulo, São Paulo, São Paulo, Brazil; [d] Intensive Care Department, Hospital Lusíadas Porto, Grupo de Infeção e Desenvolvimento em Sepsis, Faculdade de Medicina da Universidade do Porto, Porto, Portugal; [e] Division of Infectious Diseases, Department of Internal Medicine, University of Nebraska Medical Center, Omaha, NE, USA
* Corresponding author.
E-mail address: akalil@unmc.edu

Crit Care Clin 42 (2026) 795–820
https://doi.org/10.1016/j.ccc.2026.05.006 **criticalcare.theclinics.com**

Abbreviations	
AMR	antimicrobial resistance
ASP	antimicrobial stewardship program
AST	antimicrobial susceptibility testing
BCID	Blood Culture Identification
BSI	bloodstream infection
CI	cardiac index
CRAB	carbapenem-resistant *Acinetobacter baumannii*
CRE	carbapenem-resistant *Enterobacterales*
CRPA	carbapenem-resistant *Pseudomonas aeruginosa*
ESBL	extended-spectrum β-lactamase
ICU	intensive care unit
IPC	infection prevention and control
LMICs	low-income and middle-income countries
MALDI-TOF MS	matrix-assisted laser desorption/ionization time-of-flight mass spectrometry
MIC	minimum inhibitory concentration
mNGS	metagenomic next-generation sequencing
MRSA	methicillin-resistant Staphylococcus aureus
NAAT	nucleic acid amplification test
PCR	polymerase chain reaction
PK/PD	pharmacokinetic/pharmacodynamic
TAT	turnaround time
VRE	vancomycin-resistant enterococci

INTRODUCTION

Antimicrobial resistance (AMR) in patients with sepsis is a growing problem worldwide.[1,2] However, the more subjective the sepsis clinical syndrome is, the less specific the actual sepsis diagnosis. Sepsis illustrates this dilemma, that is, about one-third of the cases defined by the sepsis clinical syndrome do not have an infectious etiology.[3] To make matters more complex, out of the patients who actually have an infectious etiology for sepsis, only 60% to 70% have a positive bacterial culture from any site, which makes the selection of antibiotics more prone to errors due to the lack of susceptibility patterns.[1] In addition, the vast majority of IV antibiotics are administrated in intensive care units (ICUs) around the world.[4] The combination of these 3 factors is the inevitable over utilization of inappropriate antibiotics, which may lead to individual harm due to the direct drug side effects in patients already critically ill, as well as to major shifts in the ICU microbial population, which may lead to more critically ill patients being exposed to multi-drug resistant infections.

This article will describe the most current world scenario of AMR in patients with sepsis, from epidemiology to diagnostics to therapeutics, in order to provide a comprehensive understanding of today's challenges and the potential solutions for the future.

WHAT IS THE EXTENT OF ANTIMICROBIAL RESISTANCE IN PATIENTS WITH SEPSIS WORLDWIDE?

Sepsis and AMR represent significant, growing, and intertwined threats to global health. Sepsis remains a major challenge in all settings, but one that disproportionately impacts lower income countries, regarding both incidence and mortality. Even in more affluent settings it remains a public health concern that is not likely to diminish any time soon due to the aging of the population and growing incidence of comorbid conditions.[5]

The growing awareness about the challenge of sepsis led the World Health Organization to publish their first global report on sepsis epidemiology.[6] According to data from the Global Burden of Disease study,[7] the number of sepsis cases, worldwide, in 2017 was estimated to be close to 49 million with approximately 11 million (~22.5%) sepsis-related fatalities reported. Of these, more than 80% of cases and deaths occurred in countries with low to middle socio-demographic indexes, highlighting the unequal burden that low-income and middle-income countries (LMICs) face.

The usual clinical requirement to initiate appropriate (ie, active in vitro against the causative organism) antimicrobials as soon as possible in septic shock and, to a lesser extent, in sepsis, often leads to the use of empirical broad spectrum antimicrobials. This strategy is particularly relevant in settings of widespread AMR and increases the risk of further development of resistant strains, thus potentially creating a vicious cycle.

In the recently published WHO global AMR surveillance report,[8,9] the percentage of infections caused by AMR bacteria is over 17% (meaning 1 out of every 6 infections regardless of setting). There is significant geographic heterogeneity but, even in the lower incidence areas of Europe and the western pacific, the percentage is around 10%.

The issue of resistance is particularly worrying in gram-negative bacteria where resistance to quinolones and 3rd generation cephalosporins has become endemic in several regions and resistance to carbapenems is showing an alarming growth.[10]

Of course, the impact of AMR is greatest in the critically ill as illustrated in the prospective Eurobact II cohort[11] where, among 2042 ICU patients with ICU-acquired bloodstream infection (BSI), those with DTR gram-negatives had significantly increased 28 day mortality when compared with those infected by susceptible strains (19.2 vs 10.1%; OR 1.71; $P<.001$). This scenario is clearly worse in LMICs, as demonstrated in a multicenter study in Brazil, where 50.5% of BSI among ICU patients were caused by an antimicrobial resistant bacteria from the WHO priority list, and reported carbapenem resistance rates in 45.5% and 94.4% of *Enterobacterales* and *Acinetobacter baumannii*, respectively.[12]

Another large study from the United States, also focusing on BSI analyzed the impact of "discordant" therapy (meaning that none of the empirically used antibiotics was active *in vitro* against the causative MO) in 26,036 patients.[13] Of these, 83% (n = 21,608; 42.2% with sepsis and 14.2% with septic shock) received antibiotics on the same day that blood cultures were collected, which was used as a surrogate marker for severe infection. Infection by an antimicrobial-resistant strain was associated with a markedly increased risk of receiving discordant therapy (aOR = 9.09 [95% CI 7.68–10.76]; $P<.001$). Discordant empirical therapy independently increased mortality by 37% (aOR = 1·37 [95%CI 1.24–1.51]; $P\leq.001$). Thus, sepsis represents an ongoing public health threat and the rising incidence of AMR increases the mortality risk by decreasing the proportion of patients receiving appropriate empirical antibiotics.

PREVENTION STRATEGIES TO MITIGATE ANTIMICROBIAL RESISTANCE IN PATIENTS WITH SEPSIS

This section focuses on prevention strategies aimed at mitigating AMR in patients with sepsis, with particular emphasis on interventions that reduce the incidence and transmission of infections at ICUs. The following strategies are framed within a preventive hierarchy, in which infection prevention and control (IPC) measures constitute the cornerstone strategy, antimicrobial stewardship provides complementary protection at the patient level and potentially to reduce overall AMR rates, and effective communication within ICU teams enables sustained implementation.

Infection Prevention and Control

IPC interventions represent the most robust and consistently effective measures to mitigate AMR in patients with sepsis. Almost the totality of infections caused by pathogens presenting the WHO-priority antimicrobial-resistant phenotypes, for example, carbapenem-resistant *Enterobacterales* (CRE), carbapenem-resistant *Acinetobacter baumannii* (CRAB), and carbapenemase-producing *Pseudomonas aeruginosa*, third-generation CRE (class A extend-spectrum beta-lactamase-producing isolates), methicillin-resistant *Staphylococcus aureus* (MRSA) and vancomycin-resistant *Enterococcus faecium*,[14] result from horizontal transmission within health care settings rather than from *de novo* emergence under antibiotic pressure in individual patients.[15–20] Consequently, measures that prevent health care-associated infections and interrupt transmission pathways directly reduce both the need for antimicrobial exposure and the dissemination of resistant pathogens.[21]

Hand hygiene remains the single most effective IPC intervention[22–24] Multimodal hand hygiene strategies, including alcohol-based hand rub availability, education, monitoring, and feedback, have been repeatedly associated with reductions in health care-associated infections and antimicrobial-resistant pathogens transmission across diverse health care systems.[22–24] Contemporary IPC compendia emphasize hand hygiene as a foundational measure, particularly in high-acuity settings such as ICUs, where care intensity and patient vulnerability amplify transmission risk.[23]

Environmental hygiene also plays a critical role in preventing antimicrobial-resistant pathogens.[25] High-touch surfaces and shared equipment may serve as reservoirs for resistant organisms, contributing to sustained environmental contamination and patient colonization. Enhanced environmental cleaning protocols, appropriate disinfectant use, and monitoring of cleaning performance have been associated with reduced environmental bioburden and downstream infection risk.[25]

In addition, evidence-based bundles for the prevention of device-associated infections, including central line-associated BSIs, ventilator-associated pneumonia, and catheter-associated urinary tract infections, constitute a central component of modern IPC programs.[26] Recent guidelines highlight that consistent bundle implementation leads to substantial and sustained reductions in HAIs.[27–29] By preventing infections altogether, these interventions indirectly but powerfully mitigate AMR by reducing antibiotic initiation, duration, and selection pressure.

IPC has been formally recognized as a core strategy for addressing AMR. The WHO Global Action Plan and Monitoring Framework on IPC (2024–2030) explicitly links the strengthening of IPC programs to reductions in HAI incidence and AMR burden, emphasizing governance, workforce training, surveillance, and sustained implementation as essential elements.[30] Importantly, this framework underscores the relevance of IPC in LMICs, where infrastructure gaps and overcrowding further amplify transmission dynamics.[21]

Taken together, IPC interventions address the dominant drivers of AMR by preventing infections and interrupting horizontal transmission, thereby exerting the greatest population-level impact on AMR.

Antimicrobial Stewardship

Antimicrobial stewardship programs (ASPs) remain an essential component of AMR prevention in sepsis, although their primary impact differs from that of IPC interventions. ASP initiatives consistently improve antimicrobial appropriateness, reduce unnecessary exposure, and decrease drug-related adverse events.[31] However, evidence demonstrating a direct and sustained reduction in AMR rates attributable solely to stewardship interventions is heterogeneous and context-dependent.[31] This limitation reflects the complex ecology of AMR in ICUs, where clonal dissemination and cross-transmission often predominate.[15–18,20] In such settings, stewardship interventions that focus exclusively on prescribing behavior may have limited impact on resistance epidemiology if not accompanied by robust IPC measures.[21,31,32]

Nevertheless, ASP exerts a biologically important preventive effect through preservation of the host microbiota.[33–35] Antibiotic exposure disrupts commensal microbial communities and compromises colonization resistance, facilitating intestinal overgrowth and subsequent infection or transmission of antimicrobial-resistant organisms.[35,36] Experimental and clinical studies have demonstrated that loss of microbiota-mediated colonization resistance increases susceptibility to infections caused by resistant organisms, particularly in critically ill patients.[36,37]

Through minimizing unnecessary antibiotic exposure, narrowing spectrum when clinically appropriate, and limiting treatment duration, ASP interventions help preserve microbiota integrity and maintain what is called "colonization resistance."[33,34] From this perspective, the main preventive value of antimicrobial stewardship in sepsis lies less in directly reducing institutional resistance rates and more in reducing individual patient vulnerability to colonization and infection by resistant pathogens. Thus, ASP complements IPC by mitigating antimicrobial-related ecological disruption at the patient-level, reinforcing prevention through preservation of colonization resistance rather than serving as a standalone solution to AMR.

Communication and Multidisciplinary Collaboration in the Intensive Care Unit

Effective communication within the ICU team is a critical enabler of both IPC and ASP strategies. Multidisciplinary collaboration involving intensivists, infectious diseases specialists, microbiologists, pharmacists, nurses, and infection prevention personnel facilitates adherence to prevention bundles, timely reassessment of antimicrobial therapy, and consistent application of IPC measures.[32,38,39]

Structured ICU rounds, antibiotic time-outs, and prospective audit and feedback embedded within multidisciplinary workflows have been associated with improved antimicrobial use and process outcomes in ICU settings.[38,39] Although direct evidence linking communication strategies alone to reductions in AMR is limited, these approaches support sustained implementation of prevention strategies by aligning clinical priorities and reinforcing shared accountability.

From an operational perspective, communication should be viewed not as an independent AMR intervention, but as the mechanism through which IPC and ASP are translated into routine ICU practice. In this context, effective communication strengthens prevention efforts by integrating IPC and adequate antimicrobial use principles into daily decision-making within the ICU team.

DIAGNOSTIC STEWARDSHIP IN SEPSIS

Early recognition of septic patients and the prompt initiation of appropriate antimicrobial therapy are associated with reduced mortality in septic shock patients.[40,41] In this context, the clinical microbiology laboratory plays a critical role in identifying infectious agents and determining their antimicrobial susceptibility profiles. Diagnostic stewardship is a systematic approach to optimizing test selection, execution, and result reporting to ensure that appropriate diagnostics are applied to the appropriate patient at the appropriate time, thereby generating accurate and clinically actionable information that guides therapeutic decision-making, promotes appropriate antimicrobial use, mitigates AMR, improve resource utilization, and ultimately enhance patient outcomes.[42,43]

Traditional culture-based methods are largely employed for pathogen identification and antimicrobial susceptibility testing, AST[44–46]]. Blood cultures processed through continuous monitored automated systems (eg, Bactec FX, VersaTREK, BacT/ALERT Virtuo) usually requires time to allow the growth of such pathogens and can be affected by numerous factors including skin antisepsis, blood volume collected, incubation delay of blood culture bottles, and previous administration of antibiotics.[45–50] Traditional diagnostic tests may require up to 96 hours to yield results, which limits their usefulness for timely antimicrobial decision-making. During this interval, patients typically remain on empirical therapy that may be ineffective or unnecessarily broad-spectrum, contributing to AMR, drug-related toxicity, and increased health care costs.[44,46–48,50,51]

The incorporation of matrix-assisted laser desorption/ionization time-of-flight mass spectrometry (MALDI-TOF MS) has revolutionized diagnostic speed by substantially reducing the time required for pathogen identification.[44,52] However, this methodology still depends on blood culture positivity that typically requires approximately 12 to 24 hours. Despite MALDI-TOF MS limitation such as reduced performance in polymicrobial infections, difficulty distinguishing closely related species, and inability to routinely detect resistance genes, it provides more accurate pathogen identification than conventional staining methods performed after blood culture positivity, thereby supporting more appropriate antimicrobial prescribing.[53] A meta-analysis of 21 studies including 14,515 patients demonstrated that MALDI-TOF MS significantly reduced the time to pathogen identification by 22.86 hours and the time to effective antibiotic therapy by 5.07 hours compared with conventional phenotypic methods. Earlier initiation of effective therapy was associated with a 23% reduction in in-hospital mortality among patients with BSIs, with greater benefit observed when MALDI-TOF MS was implemented alongside ASPs (35% mortality reduction).[54] In addition, implementation of MALDI-TOF MS was associated with a 0.73-day reduction in hospital length of stay and an average cost saving of US$ 4140.18 per hospitalization, despite the high upfront cost of the technology.[54] However, all analyzed studies were focused on patients with BSIs, which limits the ability to estimate its true impact on outcomes among patients with sepsis or septic shock. A single study evaluating septic patients found that a modified workflow using MALDI-TOF MS and rapid susceptibility testing for positive blood cultures reduced time to pathogen identification from 28.3 to approximately 10 hours and time to optimal antimicrobial therapy from 36.1 to 17.9 to 21.6 hours, accelerating targeted treatment and potentially improving outcomes.[55]

Similarly, to accelerate pathogen identification in septic patients, molecular assays, most based on multiplex real-time polymerase chain reaction (PCR), have been developed.[56] Assays like BioFire Blood Culture Identification (BCID and BCID 2; bioMérieux, Inc., Hazelwood, MO), Unyvero BCU Application (Curetis GmbH, Germany), and Verigene (Nanosphere, Northbrook, IL), can provide results between 1-6h, and when combined with knowledge of local epidemiology, may support antimicrobial optimization and de-escalation.[56–61] The operational advantages of multiplex PCR panels are as follows: (i) the ability to rapidly identify pathogens and resistance genes, including in polymicrobial infections; (ii) operational simplicity with reduced dependence on specialized expertise; and (iii) availability for continuous (24 hour) processing features that are particularly valuable during off-hours, when trained personnel may not be available.[52,56] However, key limitations include the requirement for positive blood cultures, incomplete coverage of less frequent bacterial/fungal species or resistance genes, and potential misidentification of closely related organisms.[44,52,56] Rapid diagnostic testing for BSIs was systematically evaluated by an expert panel convened by American Society for Microbiology in collaboration with Centers for Disease Control and Prevention and Battelle consultants using a GRADE-based approach across 51 studies.[62] Most available evidence on the clinical impact of rapid diagnostic testing derives from retrospective observational studies and is therefore of limited strength, with insufficient data to compare specific technologies (eg, molecular assays vs MALDI-TOF MS). Despite these limitations, expert consensus strongly supports implementing rapid diagnostics in combination with structured, active communication of actionable results, as this integrated approach consistently reduces time to targeted therapy and hospital length of stay, whereas rapid tests used in isolation are not recommended. Evidence for reductions in ICU length of stay remains limited. Rapid diagnostics with active communication may also contribute to lower nonspecific, in-hospital, and infection-related mortality; however, supporting evidence is low quality and recommendations are weak due to heterogeneity and uncertainty across studies.[62]

Detection of a resistance gene does not necessarily predict phenotypic resistance; therefore, AST remains essential to confirm susceptibility and guide therapeutic optimization. AST results are critical for adjusting antimicrobial regimen, particularly in septic patients, in whom determination of the minimum inhibitory concentration (MIC) of the causative pathogen enables dose optimization to maximize the probability of achieving pharmacokinetic/pharmacodynamic (PK/PD) targets.[63] To reduce AST turnaround time (TAT), both EUCAST and CLSI recommend the rapid antimicrobial susceptibility testing approach, which uses 150 μL of blood from a positive blood culture bottle to inoculate antimicrobial plates[64,65] Although this technique can shorten AST TAT, it increases laboratory workload because plates must be read at multiple time points. Another limitation is that interpretive breakpoints are standardized only for selected bacterial species.[64,65] To further reduce AST TAT, rapid antimicrobial susceptibility platforms have been developed. These systems rely on different technological principles as shown in **Table 1**.[66–71] To date, the clinical impact of novel rapid AST methodologies has been evaluated for the Accelerate PhenoTest BC Kit (AXDX). In the largest multicenter study, including 854 patients with BSIs, implementation of this platform significantly reduced the median time to optimal antimicrobial therapy from 40.9 to 23.7 hours (17.2 hour reduction; $P<.0001$), the time to first antimicrobial modification from 24.2 to 13.9 hours ($P<.0001$), and the time to antimicrobial de-escalation from 36.0 to 27.2 hours ($P = .0004$). Among patients with Gram-positive bacteremia, the system shortened the time to optimal therapy from 36.3 to 20.4 hours ($P = .01$) and reduced the duration of unnecessary MRSA coverage from 58.4 to 29.7 hours ($P = .04$). No differences in the mortality (8.7% vs 6.0%), length of stay (7.0 vs 6.5 days), and adverse drug events were noticed after employing AXDX[72] AST interpretations and PK/PD targets associated with clinical response are derived from breakpoints established using standardized reference methods that determine MICs with defined inocula.[63–65,72,73] Machine-learning approaches that infer antimicrobial susceptibility from genomic data show promise, particularly for pathogen–drug combinations in which resistance is predominantly driven by chromosomal mutations in well-characterized genes (eg, *Salmonella* spp. and fluoroquinolones)[74] However, predictive performance will be challenging for agents such as carbapenems and β-lactam/β-lactamase inhibitor combinations, in which mechanisms of resistance are complex and MIC values can be influenced by inoculum effect.[75,76]

Table 1
Rapid whole-blood diagnostic platforms for bloodstream pathogen detection

Technology (Manufacturer, Country)	Methodological Principle	Targets Detected	Resistance Gene Detection	TAT	Reported Identification Sensitivity/Specificity[a]
LightCycler® SeptiFast (Roche Molecular Diagnostics, Switzerland) - *Discontinued*	Multiplex real-time PCR targeting pathogen DNA directly from whole blood	Bacteria and fungi (25 pathogens)	Limited (eg, *mecA*)	6 h	65%–86%[77]
Magicplex™ Sepsis Test (Seegene, South Korea)	Multiplex real-time PCR with pathogen-specific primers	Bacteria and fungi (90 pathogens)	Yes (selected Gram-positive targets: *mecA, vanA, vanB*)	3–6 h	29%–47%/ 66%–95%[171,172]
VYOO® (Analytik Jena, Germany)—*Discontinued*	Broad-range PCR with pathogen DNA enrichment	Bacteria and fungi (40 pathogens)	Yes (*mecA, vanA, vanB,* bla_{SHV}, bla_{CTX-M})	~7 h	60%/75%[173]
SepsiTest® (Molzym, Germany)	Broad-range PCR followed by sequencing-based identification	Bacteria and fungi (385 pathogens)	No	~8 h	48%/86%[77]
IRIDICA™ BAC BSI (Abbott Molecular, United States)—*Discontinued*	PCR amplification coupled with electrospray ionization mass spectrometry (PCR–ESI-MS)	Bacteria and fungi (600 pathogens)	Yes	6–8 h	81%/84%[77]
T2Bacteria® Panel (T2MR) (T2 Biosystems, United States)—*Discontinued*	Mechanical lysis → PCR amplification → magnetic resonance detection via nanoparticle agglomeration	Bacteria (targeted panel—6 pathogens)	13 resistance genes including bla_{KPC} bla_{OXA-48}, bla_{NDM}, bla_{VIM}, bla_{IMP}	3–5 h 3.6–7.7 h	83.3%–90.0%/ 90.0%–97.6%[174,175]
InfectID-BSI	Real-time quantitative PCR assay	Bacteria and fungi (26 pathogens)	No	<3 h	Not reported[78] NPV: 99.7%

Abbreviations: ESI-MS, electrospray ionization mass spectrometry; MR, magnetic resonance; NPV, negative predictive value; PCR, polymerase chain reaction; TAT, turnaround time for final results.

[a] Sensitivity and specificity values derive from meta-analyses or representative clinical studies and may vary by population, comparator, and pathogen spectrum.

Roche Molecular Diagnostics introduced LightCycler SeptiFast as the first commercially available nucleic acid amplification test (NAAT) for the rapid identification of pathogens directly from whole blood, followed by the development of additional NAAT-based platforms. **Table 1** summarizes these NAAT technologies designed for the direct detection of microorganisms and selected resistance genes without the need for prior blood culture positivity.[52,77] Despite their rapid turnaround time, these assays have demonstrated heterogeneous diagnostic performance, including reports of suboptimal sensitivity, which are partly attributable to PCR inhibitors present in whole blood, as well as limitations in specificity coupled with the extensively MALDI-TOF MS use[52] Although these technologies enabled earlier pathogen identification, several platforms, including LightCycler SeptiFast, T2Bacteria, and IRIDICA BAC BSI, have been withdrawn from the market. InfectID-BSI (Microbio Ltd., Australia) is a recently developed molecular assay that uses 0.4 mL of whole blood to identify the 20 most common bacterial pathogens and 6 Candida species associated with sepsis within approximately 3 hours. In a 2 center study conducted in Australia, InfectID-BSI demonstrated superior detection compared with conventional blood cultures for both Gram-positive bacteria (56 vs 19 detections) and Gram-negative bacteria (46 vs 35 detections), while maintaining a very high negative predictive value (>99.0%). However, the current version of the assay does not include detection of AMR genes.[78] A new NAAT, UIICORE BSI, currently under development by deepull, is designed to identify pathogens (bacterial and fungal pathogens) and selected resistance markers directly from 8 mL of whole blood from patients with suspected infection or sepsis in under 1 hour.

Metagenomic next-generation sequencing (mNGS) has emerged as a rapid, culture-independent approach for pathogen detection in sepsis, demonstrating substantially higher detection rates than conventional blood cultures and enabling identification of a broad spectrum of organisms, including bacteria, viruses, fungi, and atypical pathogens. This technology is particularly valuable for detecting organisms difficult to culture, including viruses, *Mycobacterium tuberculosis*, atypical pathogens, and polymicrobial infections as it is less affected by antimicrobial use.,[79–81] Prospective studies report pathogen detection in approximately 67% to 92% of septic patients with mNGS, compared with 19% to 48% using blood cultures.[80–86] Turnaround times range from ~1.4 to 12 hours[83,87] Both plasma cell-free DNA and blood cell mNGS can be performed, with combined plasma and blood cell mNGS achieving 85.25% sensitivity, which is significantly higher than plasma alone (67.21%) or blood cultures (36.09%).[85] Plasma mNGS is particularly effective for detecting viruses and cell-free bacterial DNA, while blood cell mNGS better identifies viable intracellular bacteria.[85,88] However, the high analytical sensitivity of mNGS increases the likelihood of detecting contaminant DNA. Consequently, interpretation requires careful clinical correlation and expert judgment due to challenges distinguishing true pathogens from colonizers or contaminants, and the lack of unified diagnostic criteria.[80,89] Clinical impact studies show promising but mixed results on mortality. A retrospective study found routine blood culture combined with mNGS reduced 28-day mortality from 62.2% to 47.3% (P = .043), and early mNGS testing (<1 day) was associated with shorter hospital and ICU stays.[83] A large multicenter prospective study demonstrated that mNGS halved 7-day mortality (hazard ratio 0.44, P = .004) but showed no significant difference in 28-day mortality. [86] mNGS prompted antibiotic modifications in 29% to 60% of patients, including de-escalation in approximately 20% of cases.[82] To definitively assess whether combining mNGS-based diagnostics with standard culture-based methods improves clinical outcomes in patients with sepsis and septic shock, DigiSep-Trial a randomized, controlled, interventional, open-label, multicenter trial is ongoing.[90]

Without structured and timely communication, even the most advanced microbiological results will fail to translate into better patient outcomes. Effective implementation of diagnostic stewardship requires close alignment with antimicrobial stewardship and IPC practices, supported by timely and structured communication among these teams.[42,91] Active communication can be accomplished by phone calls, paging systems, or secure electronic messaging to enable efficient exchange of microbiological and clinical information, facilitating rapid interpretation of results and prompt therapeutic and infection control decisions.[62] This coordinated approach promotes appropriate antimicrobial use, reduces unnecessary exposure, and contributes to improved patient outcomes and more efficient utilization of health care resources. Ultimately, maximizing clinical success while minimizing the emergence of AMR depends on the integrated application of diagnostic stewardship, antimicrobial stewardship, and IPC strategies.[42,62,91]

WHAT ARE THE OPTIMAL TREATMENT CHOICES FOR PATIENTS WITH SEPSIS DUE TO ANTIMICROBIAL RESISTANCE INFECTIONS?

The optimal antimicrobial therapy in patients with sepsis caused by antimicrobial-resistant bacteria represents one of the greatest challenges in critical care. Although resistant pathogens encompass a broad range of organisms, both Gram-positive and Gram-negative bacteria, and both community-acquired and health care-associated infections, the burden of AMR severe infections is predominantly driven by Gram-negative bacteria causing health care-associated infections,[8,10] particularly those recognized by WHO as critical and high-priority antimicrobial-resistant bacteria, that is, CRE, CRAB, and carbapenem-resistant *Pseudomonas aeruginosa* (CRPA).[14] Multicenter studies confirm that these pathogens account for a large proportion of resistant BSI and have been associated with high mortality rates worldwide.[12,57,92–94] Third-generation CRE, either driven by extended-spectrum β-lactamase (ESBL) or AmpC enzymes also represent a common threat to hospitalized patients.[10,14]

The therapy for these antimicrobial-resistant Gram-negative bacteria has changed over the last decade due to the launching of many novel beta-lactamase-inhibitors combined with beta-lactams, new cephalosporins, such as ceftolozane and the siderophore cephalosporin, cefiderocol. These new antimicrobials now constitute the first-line therapy for carbapenem-resistant, gram-negative bacteria, as addressed in recent guidelines.[95,96] However, the access to these new drugs is very limited in low and middle-income countries, where the combination of old and less active agents, such as polymyxins and tigecycline, are still the cornerstone therapies for most of these infections.[97]

Although less frequent than antimicrobial-resistant gram-negative bacteria, gram-positive isolates, particularly, MRSA continues to cause severe infections with substantial mortality.[10,12,98] Globally, MRSA has shown the largest increases in resistance-associated mortality over recent decades.[10]

We will present an overview of the optimal antimicrobial therapy for the treatment of patients with sepsis caused by major resistant gram-negative bacteria, including carbapenem-resistant isolates, extended-spectrum β-lactamase-producing and AmpC-producing *Enterobacterales*, as well as MRSA and vancomycin-resistant enterococci (VRE), which together represent the pathogens of greatest therapeutic concern in severe health care-associated infections.

The antimicrobial therapy for CRE, of which *Klebsiella pneumoniae* isolates are by far the most common species, depends largely on the underlying resistance mechanism. KPC-producing isolates are typically susceptible to newer β-lactam/β-lactamase inhibitor combinations such as ceftazidime–avibactam, imipenem-relebactam or meropenem–vaborbactam, which are considered preferred agents for severe infections by these pathogens. Although only two small clinical trials comparing these agents against the best available therapy have been conducted,[99,100] several observational studies have reported lower mortality and toxicity rates with newer β-lactam/β-lactamase inhibitor, especially with ceftazidime-avibactam versus other older antimicrobials.[79,101] Comparative effectiveness of these antimicrobials is scarce and limited ceftazidime-avibactam versus meropenem–vaborbactam, which showed no difference in clinical effectiveness,[102] but ceftazidime-avibactam may be preferred for its narrow spectrum.[97] However, although still very uncommon, resistance to these agents may be drug-specific and the appropriate choice requires an antimicrobial susceptibility test.[103,104] No benefit has been shown with the combination of other drugs to ceftazidime-avibactam.[105]

Metallo-β-lactamase-producing CRE isolates, of which NDM-type is the most common, are resistant to these agents, and treatment often relies on aztreonam-based strategies combined with avibactam-containing regimens.[95–97] Combinations of aztreonam with either vaborbactam or relebactam have been shown to present inferior in vitro activity against metallo-β-lactamase isolates compared with avibactam.[106,107] Hence, either aztreonam combined to ceftazidime-avibactam or the recently launched aztreonam-avibactam[108] are the therapy of choice for patients with sepsis by metallo-β-lactamase-producing CRE isolates.

CRAB is particularly difficult to treat and is associated with some of the highest mortality rates among resistant pathogens.[10,12,57] The development of sulbactam–durlobactam represents an important advance, as this combination restores activity against many CRAB isolates by inhibiting class D carbapenemases,[109] the major mechanism of carbapenem resistance in *A baumannii*[15] In the seminal clinical trial, sulbactam–durlobactam administered with imipenem demonstrated improved outcomes compared with colistin plus imipenem-based therapy and is increasingly viewed as a preferred option when available.[109] Nevertheless, access remains limited in many regions, and alternative regimens, including high-dose sulbactam-containing combinations, polymyxins, or tigecycline derivatives, are still commonly employed.[97]

Pseudomonas aeruginosa poses additional therapeutic challenges because resistance mechanisms are multifactorial, involving β-lactamases, efflux pumps, porin loss, and target modifications, and even new antimicrobial agents may be commonly affected.[110] Ceftolozane–tazobactam has been the main therapeutic option against non-carbapenemase-producing CRPA and other difficult-to-treat *P aeruginosa* isolates,[95–97] which improved clinical effectiveness compared with polymyxins and aminoglycosides.[111] Ceftazidime–avibactam has been shown to present similar clinical effectiveness and is also an adequate option, which may also be active against class A (majorly KPC-type)-carbapenemase-producing isolates.[111] Imipenem-relebactam is also an option for CRPA, but comparative studies with other options are lacking. These agents may allow effective monotherapy when susceptibility is documented. Metallo-β-lactamases are the most common type of carbapenemase in *P aeruginosa*, but differently to CRE, the activity of aztreonam-avibactam may be affected by other non-enzymatic resistance mechanisms.[110] Although with a promising role in metallo-β-lactamase-producing *P aeruginosa*, currently there is no susceptibility breakpoint and reported clinical experience is still limited.[112] Polymyxins-based regimes combined with other antimicrobial agents have been used against carbapenemase-producing isolates or where these new drugs are not available.[95–97]

Cefiderocol, a siderophore cephalosporin with broad activity against carbapenem-resistant gram-negative organisms, offers an additional option for infections caused by DTR *P aeruginosa* and CRAB,[95,96] despite the fact that this is a newer drug that is not recommended as a first-line therapy in severe infections by carbapenem-resistant gram-negative bacteria. In fact, results of clinical trials have raised concerns regarding outcomes against CRAB[113] and other gram-negative bacteria.[114] However, cefiderocol remains an alternative, particularly when other active agents are unavailable or in combination schemes, with overall similar or superior results compared with best available therapy for CRAB infections in observational studies.[115,116] It may also be useful as part of combination schemes against CRE and CRPA, when first-line agents are not available.[95,96]

ESBL-producing and *Enterobacterales* with inducible or derepressed AmpC β-lactamases are among the most frequently encountered resistant pathogens, particularly in BSIs originating from urinary or intra-abdominal sources. Although both mechanisms confer resistance to third-generation cephalosporins, their therapeutic implications differ. For ESBL-producing *Enterobacterales*, carbapenems remain as first choice therapy in severe infections,[95–97] mostly relying on the results of the MERINO trial.[117] In addition, some concerns regarding ESBL inhibitory activity of tazobactam[95] and antimicrobial susceptibility tests in third-generation CRE[118] have also supported the recommendation for avoiding piperacillin-tazobactam in patients with sepsis by ESBL-producing *Enterobacterales*, despite some favorable results in some observational studies.[119,120] Cefepime-enmetazobactam is a newly approved combination with promising activity against ESBL-producing *Enterobacterales*[109]; however, its role as a carbapenem-sparing strategy in severe infections still needs to be determined.

AmpC-producing *Enterobacterales* present a distinct challenge because resistance may emerge during therapy through derepression of chromosomal AmpC enzymes. Cefepime is generally favored over third-generation cephalosporins and piperacillin-tazobactam due to greater stability against AmpC hydrolysis and lower risk of selecting resistant subpopulations. Carbapenems remain highly active and are commonly used in critically ill patients,[95–97] and has been the preferred agent particularly if the isolate is non-susceptible to one or more third-generation cephalosporins.[97] However, cefepime is a reliable option for infections by these pathogens, with effectiveness compared with meropenem in observational studies.[121]

Although multiple agents demonstrate *vitro* efficacy against MRSA and VRE, treating invasive infections due to these organisms continues to be challenging.[122,123] Optimal management of MRSA infections requires both appropriate antimicrobial therapy and effective source control. MRSA is resistant to most β-lactams, except ceftaroline and ceftobiprole, primarily due to alterations in penicillin-binding protein 2 encoded by *mec* genes.[124] Several newer agents demonstrate in vitro activity against MRSA, including daptomycin, linezolid, tetracycline derivatives (eg, tigecycline and eravacycline), and long acting lipoglycopeptides. However, only vancomycin, daptomycin, and ceftobiprole are approved by the FDA/EMA for treatment of MRSA BSI.[123,125]

Vancomycin remains widely used as first-line therapy because of its availability, large clinical experience, and relatively low cost, although its use is limited by the need for therapeutic drug monitoring and risk of toxicity.[123,125] Daptomycin is an effective alternative for bacteremia, and higher doses (8–10 mg/kg/day) are associated with improved clinical success in complicated MRSA BSIs[126] In the ERADICATE trial, ceftobiprole was noninferior to daptomycin for complicated MRSA bacteremia, with comparable microbiological outcomes and no significant difference in treatment success. Drug-related adverse events were more frequent with ceftobiprole, whereas serious adverse events were slightly more common with daptomycin[127]

Routine combination therapy for *S aureus* bacteremia is not supported by current evidence but may be considered in persistent bacteremia despite adequate therapy and source control[123] Observational studies suggest that combinations such as daptomycin plus ceftaroline may accelerate microbiological clearance and reduce clinical failure[128–130] Additional salvage strategies include adding cefazolin, fosfomycin, or ceftobiprole to vancomycin or daptomycin.[123,131,132]

Among long-acting lipoglycopeptides, dalbavancin has the strongest supporting clinical evidence, with studies suggesting a role as step-down therapy in selected patients after bloodstream clearance.[133–135] Oritavancin also demonstrates potent in vitro activity and offers simplified dosing due to its prolonged half-life, although clinical experience in invasive infections remains limited[136,137] Both agents may be considered as consolidation therapy when prolonged intravenous access is undesirable, but neither is recommended for initial treatment of MRSA bacteremia.

Despite not being approved by FDA/EMA for treatment of VRE infections, daptomycin has been recommended for treatment of infections caused by *Enterococcus* spp. resistant ampicillin and vancomycin, and along with linezolid constitute the main therapeutic options for treatment of VRE BSI.[122] Enterococci exhibit higher daptomycin MICs and intrinsic tolerance,[138] and inoculum effects may further reduce efficacy,[139] necessitating higher daptomycin doses to achieve PK/PD targets.[140] Clinical evidence supports a dose–response relationship, with standard dosing (6 mg/kg/day) associated with worse outcomes and higher doses ($\geq$9–12 mg/kg/day) linked to improved survival and microbiological response.[140–142] Outcomes worsen with increasing MIC, and optimal exposure may remain difficult when MICs are greater than or equal to 2 μg/mL.[140,142] Linezolid provides established clinical efficacy with advantages including reliable oral bioavailability and lower cost.[143] Comparative studies of linezolid and daptomycin show mixed results[144,145] outcomes appear similar when adequate daptomycin exposure is achieved, with excess mortality being associated with PK/PD target failure.[146,147] Tedizolid demonstrates potent in vitro activity, but it is not recommended for VRE bacteremia due to bacteriostatic activity, suboptimal pharmacodynamic exposure, and limited clinical evidence.[122,148]

Teicoplanin may retain activity against *vanB* VRE, but resistance emergence and inconsistent clinical outcomes limit its therapeutic role.[122,149] Among lipoglycopeptides, only oritavancin demonstrates activity against *vanA*-mediated and *vanB*-mediated VRE, with limited clinical evidence from case reports of successful use in complex hematologic patients.[150–152]

HOW TO BEST OPTIMIZE THE UTILIZATION OF NEW ANTIBIOTICS TO COMBAT ANTIMICROBIAL RESISTANCE INFECTIONS IN THE INTENSIVE CARE UNIT?

Among useful strategies to combat the threat posed by AMR in septic patients, the development of new drugs is paramount. Alas it is quite slow and, despite regulatory and financial incentives for drug companies, the availability of these newer compounds is not as fast as necessary.[153]

In a setting of widespread AMR prevalence, the empirical use of newer, broad spectrum antibiotics is often necessary to reduce the risk of initially inappropriate therapy that has long been associated with increased mortality in several different syndromes.[13,154–158] Effective communication with the microbiology laboratory is paramount.[159] Also, the judicious use of novel diagnostic techniques to minimize the time until appropriate therapy and for early de-escalation seems relevant. For example, the use of rapid molecular testing in BSI is associated with decreased mortality only when used within the context of an ASP.[160] Thus, optimal use of these limited resource is critical, both for maximizing their effectiveness and to reduce antibiotic pressure and, consequently, diminish the emergence of resistant strains as evidence suggests that, at a population level, AM use seems to have thresholds below which the emergence of resistance happens.[161]

As for effectiveness, the first consideration needs to be the diagnosis of the source of infection. This will allow for the selection of drugs with adequate penetration and activity and to assess the need for source control procedures. We should strive to obtain a microbiological diagnosis whenever possible, which has been shown to correlate with mortality.[162]

The optimal use of antimicrobials in critically ill patients should aim for ideal Pk/Pd parameters with adequate loading doses (regardless of ongoing organ dysfunction) and dosing intervals that are consistent with the Pd profile of the drug being used. The concept of "dose modulation" in critically ill patients as originally proposed in 2013[163] encompasses these ideas. This is well established for drugs with a narrow therapeutic window like aminoglycosides[164] or vancomycin[165,166] for which serum level monitoring is widely available.

Beta-lactam ABs are time-dependent drugs, commonly used as first-line options for severe infections, and data regarding the use of prolonged or continuous infusions to optimize their efficacy continue growing.[167] The recent Bling III trial,[168] focused specifically on this issue and added significant evidence in favor of these strategies.

In this open-label RCT, ICU patients receiving meropenem or piperacillin/tazobactam were randomized to either continuous (CI; n = 3498) or intermittent (II; n = 3533) AM infusions. The primary end-point of 90 day all-cause mortality was met in 24.9% of patients in the CI group versus 26.8% in the II group (OR 0.91 [95%CI 0.81–1.01]) and the secondary goal of clinical cure of the infection was significantly more frequent in the CI group (55.7 vs 50.0% OR 1.26 [95%CI 1.15–1.38];P<.001). The incidence of adverse events was low (0.3 vs 0.2% in the CI and II groups).This raises the issue of the variability of serum levels of antimicrobials in critically ill patients that can be at risk of underdosing and treatment failure[169] but also of toxicity. Interestingly, in the Eurobact II cohort,[11] the availability of TDM (for aminoglycosides and vancomycin) or of a clinical pharmacist were associated with decreased mortality. Thus, as is accepted standard of care for drugs such as voriconazole, the way forward is the use of TDM to allow for maximal, safe dosing of antibiotics in patients with sepsis.[170]

SUMMARY

Current evidence shows that the solution to reduce the growing rate of AMR in patients with sepsis requires an approach that expands from optimizing the individual bedside ICU care to a multi-disciplinary approach that encompasses the cohesive work of intensivists, infectious disease clinicians, nurses, pharmacists, microbiologists, infection prevention and antibiotic stewardship teams.

We propose that the combination of improved bedside microbiological diagnostics, more efficient PK/PD utilization of therapeutics by simultaneously reducing the utilization of unnecessary antibiotics and increasing patients' colonization resistance, in combination with effective and sustainable communication among the ICU and multidisciplinary teams is the most efficient strategy to prevent the further dissemination of AMR infections in patients with sepsis.

CLINICS CARE POINTS

- Optimize bedside microbiological diagnostics.
- Maximize the efficiecy of antibiotics by utilizing pharmacokinetic and pharmacodynamic principles.

- Mantain an antibiotic stewardship program.
- Aim to have a consistent multidisciplinary communication with the Intensive Care Unit team.
- The simultaneous action of the four factors above is essential to reduce the prevalence of AMR infections in patients with sepsis.

DISCLOSURES

The authors have no financial disclosures or conflicts of interest to disclose.

REFERENCES

1. Singer M, Angus DC, Annane D, et al. Sepsis. Lancet 2026;407(10535):1276–88.
2. La Via L, Ferlito S, Di Modica MS, et al. The global impact of sepsis: epidemiology, recognition, management, and health system challenges. Epidemiologia (Basel) 2026;7(1).
3. Rhee C, Kadri SS, Danner RL, et al. Diagnosing sepsis is subjective and highly variable: a survey of intensivists using case vignettes. Crit Care 2016;20:89.
4. Kalil AC. Sepsis and septic shock. Semin Respir Crit Care Med 2021;42(5): 639–40.
5. Walkey AJ, Lagu T, Lindenauer PK. Trends in sepsis and infection sources in the United States. A population-based study. Ann Am Thorac Soc 2015;12(2): 216–20.
6. Global report on the epidemiology and burden of sepsis Internet. Available at: https://www.who.int/news-room/fact-sheets/detail/sepsis (Accessed 26 April 2026), 2020.
7. Rudd KE, Johnson SC, Agesa KM, et al. Global, regional, and national sepsis incidence and mortality, 1990-2017: analysis for the global burden of disease study. Lancet 2020;395(10219):200–11.
8. Collaborators GBDGS. Global, regional, and national sepsis incidence and mortality, 1990-2021: a systematic analysis. Lancet Glob Health 2025;13(12): e2013–26.
9. Global antibiotic resistance surveillance report 2025 Internet. 2025. Available at: https://globalsepsisalliance.org/news/2025/11/4/new-global-estimates-from-the-lancet-166-million-sepsis-cases-and-21-million-deaths (Accessed 26 April 2026).
10. Collaborators GBDAR. Global burden of bacterial antimicrobial resistance 1990-2021: a systematic analysis with forecasts to 2050. Lancet 2024;404(10459): 1199–226.
11. Tabah A, Buetti N, Staiquly Q, et al, EUROBACT-2 Study Group, ESICM, ESCMID ESGCIP and the OUTCOMEREA Network. Epidemiology and outcomes of hospital-acquired bloodstream infections in intensive care unit patients: the EUROBACT-2 international cohort study. Intensive Care Med 2023;49(2):178–90.
12. Antochevis LC, Wilhelm CM, Arns B, et al, ASCENSION Study Group. World health Organization priority antimicrobial resistance in Enterobacterales, Acinetobacter baumannii, Pseudomonas aeruginosa, Staphylococcus aureus and Enterococcus faecium healthcare-associated bloodstream infections in Brazil (ASCENSION): a prospective, multicentre, observational study. Lancet Reg Health, Am 2025;43:101004.
13. Kadri SS, Lai YL, Warner S, et al, forming the National Insititutes of Health Antimicrobial Resistance Outcomes Research Initiative NIH-ARORI. Inappropriate

empirical antibiotic therapy for bloodstream infections based on discordant in-vitro susceptibilities: a retrospective cohort analysis of prevalence, predictors, and mortality risk in US hospitals. Lancet Infect Dis 2021;21(2):241–51.
14. Sati H, Carrara E, Savoldi A, et al, WHO Bacterial Priority Pathogens List Advisory Group. The WHO bacterial priority pathogens list 2024: a prioritisation study to guide research, development, and public health strategies against antimicrobial resistance. Lancet Infect Dis 2025;25(9):1033–43.
15. Castanheira M, Mendes RE, Gales AC. Global epidemiology and mechanisms of resistance of acinetobacter baumannii-calcoaceticus complex. Clin Infect Dis 2023;76(Suppl 2):S166–78.
16. Luterbach CL, Chen L, Komarow L, et al, Multi-Drug Resistant Organism Network Investigators Network Investigators and the Antibacterial Resistance Leadership Group. Transmission of carbapenem-resistant Klebsiella pneumoniae in US hospitals. Clin Infect Dis 2023;76(2):229–37.
17. Popovich KJ, Green SJ, Okamoto K, et al. MRSA transmission in intensive care units: genomic analysis of patients, their environments, and healthcare workers. Clin Infect Dis 2021;72(11):1879–87.
18. Blanco N, O'Hara LM, Harris AD. Transmission pathways of multidrug-resistant organisms in the hospital setting: a scoping review. Infect Control Hosp Epidemiol 2019;40(4):447–56.
19. The Lancet Regional H-E. Addressing sexually transmitted infections in Europe: challenges and strategies. Lancet Reg Health Eur 2023;34:100766.
20. Zhou X, Willems RJL, Friedrich AW, et al. Enterococcus faecium: from microbiological insights to practical recommendations for infection control and diagnostics. Antimicrob Resist Infect Control 2020;9(1):130.
21. Lewnard JA, Charani E, Gleason A, et al. Burden of bacterial antimicrobial resistance in low-income and middle-income countries avertible by existing interventions: an evidence review and modelling analysis. Lancet 2024;403(10442):2439–54.
22. Vermeil T, Peters A, Kilpatrick C, et al. Hand hygiene in hospitals: anatomy of a revolution. J Hosp Infect 2019;101(4):383–92.
23. Glowicz JB, Landon E, Sickbert-Bennett EE, et al. SHEA/IDSA/APIC practice recommendation: strategies to prevent healthcare-associated infections through hand hygiene: 2022 update. Infect Control Hosp Epidemiol 2023;44(3):355–76.
24. Pittet D, Hugonnet S, Harbarth S, et al. Effectiveness of a hospital-wide programme to improve compliance with hand hygiene. Infection control programme. Lancet 2000;356(9238):1307–12.
25. Dancer SJ. Controlling hospital-acquired infection: focus on the role of the environment and new technologies for decontamination. Clin Microbiol Rev 2014;27(4):665–90.
26. Yokoe DS, Advani SD, Anderson DJ, et al. Executive summary: a compendium of strategies to prevent healthcare-associated infections in acute-care hospitals: 2022 updates. Infect Control Hosp Epidemiol 2023;44(10):1540–54.
27. Buetti N, Marschall J, Drees M, et al. Strategies to prevent central line-associated bloodstream infections in acute-care hospitals: 2022 update. Infect Control Hosp Epidemiol 2022;43(5):553–69.
28. Klompas M, Branson R, Cawcutt K, et al. Strategies to prevent ventilator-associated pneumonia, ventilator-associated events, and nonventilator hospital-acquired pneumonia in acute-care hospitals: 2022 update. Infect Control Hosp Epidemiol 2022;43(6):687–713.

29. Patel PK, Advani SD, Kofman AD, et al. Strategies to prevent catheter-associated urinary tract infections in acute-care hospitals: 2022 update. Infect Control Hosp Epidemiol 2023;44(8):1209–31.
30. Global action plan and monitoring framework on infection prevention and control (IPC), 2024–2030. (Internet). 2024. Available at: https://globalsepsisalliance.org/news/2025/11/4/new-global-estimates-from-the-lancet-166-million-sepsis-cases-and-21-million-deaths (Accessed 26 April 2026).
31. Baur D, Gladstone BP, Burkert F, et al. Effect of antibiotic stewardship on the incidence of infection and colonisation with antibiotic-resistant bacteria and Clostridium difficile infection: a systematic review and meta-analysis. Lancet Infect Dis 2017;17(9):990–1001.
32. Gentry EM, Kester S, Fischer K, et al. Bugs and drugs: collaboration between infection prevention and antibiotic stewardship. Infect Dis Clin North Am 2020; 34(1):17–30.
33. Rosa R, Donskey CJ, Munoz-Price LS. The intersection between colonization resistance, antimicrobial stewardship, and Clostridium difficile. Curr Infect Dis Rep 2018;20(8):27.
34. Woerther PL, Lepeule R, Burdet C, et al. Carbapenems and alternative beta-lactams for the treatment of infections due to extended-spectrum beta-lactamase-producing enterobacteriaceae: what impact on intestinal colonisation resistance? Int J Antimicrob Agents 2018;52(6):762–70.
35. de Nies L, Kobras CM, Stracy M. Antibiotic-induced collateral damage to the microbiota and associated infections. Nat Rev Microbiol 2023;21(12):789–804.
36. Caballero-Flores G, Pickard JM, Nunez G. Microbiota-mediated colonization resistance: mechanisms and regulation. Nat Rev Microbiol 2023;21(6):347–60.
37. Ducarmon QR, Zwittink RD, Hornung BVH, et al. Gut microbiota and colonization resistance against bacterial enteric infection. Microbiol Mol Biol Rev 2019;83(3).
38. Mishima Y, Nawa N, Asada M, et al. Impact of antibiotic time-outs in multidisciplinary ICU rounds for antimicrobial stewardship program on patient survival: a controlled before-and-after study. Crit Care Explor 2023;5(1):e0837.
39. Seidelman JL, Turner NA, Wrenn RH, et al. Impact of antibiotic stewardship rounds in the intensive care setting: a prospective cluster-randomized crossover study. Clin Infect Dis 2022;74(11):1986–92.
40. Kumar A, Roberts D, Wood KE, et al. Duration of hypotension before initiation of effective antimicrobial therapy is the critical determinant of survival in human septic shock. Crit Care Med 2006;34(6):1589–96.
41. Im Y, Kang D, Ko RE, et al, Korean Sepsis Alliance KSA investigators. Time-to-antibiotics and clinical outcomes in patients with sepsis and septic shock: a prospective nationwide multicenter cohort study. Crit Care 2022;26(1):19.
42. Messacar K, Parker SK, Todd JK, et al. Implementation of rapid molecular infectious disease diagnostics: the role of diagnostic and antimicrobial stewardship. J Clin Microbiol 2017;55(3):715–23.
43. Fabre V, Davis A, Diekema DJ, et al. Principles of diagnostic stewardship: a practical guide from the society for healthcare epidemiology of America diagnostic stewardship task force. Infect Control Hosp Epidemiol 2023;44(2):178–85.
44. Lamy B, Sundqvist M, Idelevich EA, et al. Escmid study group for Bloodstream Infections E, Sepsis. Bloodstream infections - standard and progress in pathogen diagnostics. Clin Microbiol Infect 2020;26(2):142–50.
45. Miller JM, Binnicker MJ, Campbell S, et al. Guide to utilization of the microbiology laboratory for diagnosis of infectious diseases: 2024 update by the infectious diseases Society of America (IDSA) and the American Society for

microbiology (ASM). Clin Infect Dis 2024;. https://academic.oup.com/cid/advance-article/doi/10.1093/cid/ciae104/7619499.
46. Venturelli C, Righi E, Borsari L, et al. Impact of pre-analytical time on the recovery of pathogens from blood cultures: results from a large retrospective survey. PLoS One 2017;12(1):e0169466.
47. Dempsey C, Skoglund E, Muldrew KL, et al. Economic health care costs of blood culture contamination: a systematic review. Am J Infect Control 2019; 47(8):963–7.
48. Hall KK, Lyman JA. Updated review of blood culture contamination. Clin Microbiol Rev 2006;19(4):788–802.
49. Henning C, Aygul N, Dinnetz P, et al. Detailed analysis of the characteristics of sample volume in blood culture bottles. J Clin Microbiol 2019;57(8).
50. Schaumburg F, Schuler F, Fobker M, et al. Integrated decentralized blood culture incubation: a step towards a 24/7 microbiology service? J Microbiol Methods 2024;223:106973.
51. Ben-Chetrit E, Helviz Y, Levin PD. Diagnostic value of blood culture growth patterns in distinguishing contaminants from pathogens. J Clin Microbiol 2026; 64(2):e0121025.
52. Giacobbe DR, Crea F, Morici P, et al. T2Bacteria and T2Resistance assays in critically ill patients with sepsis or septic shock: a descriptive experience. Antibiotics (Basel) 2022;11(12).
53. Patel R. Matrix-assisted laser desorption ionization-time of flight mass spectrometry in clinical microbiology. Clin Infect Dis 2013;57(4):564–72.
54. Yo CH, Shen YH, Hsu WT, et al. MALDI-TOF mass spectrometry rapid pathogen identification and outcomes of patients with bloodstream infection: a systematic review and meta-analysis. Microb Biotechnol 2022;15(10):2667–82.
55. Verroken A, Defourny L, le Polain de Waroux O, et al. Clinical impact of MALDI-TOF MS identification and rapid susceptibility testing on adequate antimicrobial treatment in sepsis with positive blood cultures. PLoS One 2016;11(5):e0156299.
56. Bauer KA, Perez KK, Forrest GN, et al. Review of rapid diagnostic tests used by antimicrobial stewardship programs. Clin Infect Dis 2014;59(Suppl 3):S134–45.
57. Wang Y, Lindsley K, Bleak TC, et al. Performance of molecular tests for diagnosis of bloodstream infections in the clinical setting: a systematic literature review and meta-analysis. Clin Microbiol Infect 2025;31(3):360–72.
58. Yang M, Tao C. Diagnostic efficiency of the FilmArray blood culture identification (BCID) panel: a systematic review and meta-analysis. J Med Microbiol 2023;72(9).
59. Peri AM, Ling W, Furuya-Kanamori L, et al. Performance of BioFire blood culture identification 2 panel (BCID2) for the detection of bloodstream pathogens and their associated resistance markers: a systematic review and meta-analysis of diagnostic test accuracy studies. BMC Infect Dis 2022;22(1):794.
60. Bonnefoy C, Vannini M, Degand N, et al. Multiplex microarray PCR unyvero BCU system to accelerate relevant antimicrobial treatment in polymicrobial bloodstream infection. Eur J Clin Microbiol Infect Dis 2024;43(8):1545–57.
61. Ledeboer NA, Lopansri BK, Dhiman N, et al. Identification of gram-negative bacteria and genetic resistance determinants from positive blood culture broths by use of the verigene gram-negative blood culture Multiplex Microarray-Based molecular assay. J Clin Microbiol 2015;53(8):2460–72.
62. Wolk DM, Parrott JS, Babady NE, et al. The American Society for Microbiology's evidence-based laboratory medicine practice guidelines for the diagnosis of bloodstream infections using rapid tests: a systematic review and meta-analysis. Clin Microbiol Rev 2025;38(3):e0013724.

63. Phe K, Heil EL, Tam VH. Optimizing pharmacokinetics-pharmacodynamics of antimicrobial management in patients with sepsis: a review. J Infect Dis 2020; 222(Suppl 2):S132–41.
64. Chandrasekaran S, Abbott A, Campeau S, et al. Direct-from-Blood-Culture disk diffusion to determine antimicrobial susceptibility of gram-negative bacteria: preliminary report from the clinical and laboratory standards Institute Methods Development and Standardization Working Group. J Clin Microbiol 2018;56(3).
65. Jonasson E, Matuschek E, Kahlmeter G. The EUCAST rapid disc diffusion method for antimicrobial susceptibility testing directly from positive blood culture bottles. J Antimicrob Chemother 2020;75(4):968–78.
66. Garcia-Rivera C, Ricart-Silvestre A, Parra Grande M, et al. Evaluation of the quickmic system in the rapid diagnosis of Gram-negative bacilli bacteremia. Microbiol Spectr 2024;12(10):e0401123.
67. Kim TY, Kang M, Shim HJ, et al. Evaluation of the QMAC-dRAST System version 2.5 for rapid antimicrobial susceptibility testing of gram-negative bacteria from positive blood culture broth and subcultured colony isolates. J Clin Lab Anal 2024;38(9):e25043.
68. Ostermann G, Korber-Irrgang B, Kruger A, et al. Performance evaluation of the Specific Reveal system for rapid antibiotic susceptibility testing from positive blood cultures containing Gram-negative pathogens. J Clin Microbiol 2024;62-(12):e0069224.
69. Goransson J, Sundqvist M, Ghaderi E, et al. Performance of a System for rapid phenotypic antimicrobial susceptibility testing of gram-negative bacteria directly from positive blood culture bottles. J Clin Microbiol 2023;61(3):e0152522.
70. Pancholi P, Carroll KC, Buchan BW, et al. Multicenter evaluation of the accelerate PhenoTest BC kit for rapid identification and phenotypic antimicrobial susceptibility testing using morphokinetic cellular analysis. J Clin Microbiol 2018;56(4).
71. Cupaiolo R, Cherkaoui S, Serrano G, et al. Antimicrobial susceptibility testing determined by Alfred 60/AST (Alifax(R)) in a multi-sites lab: performance's evaluation and optimization of workflow. J Microbiol Methods 2022;194:106433.
72. Bhalodi AA, MacVane SH, Ford B, et al. Real-World impact of the accelerate PhenoTest BC kit on patients with bloodstream infections in the improving outcomes and antimicrobial stewardship Study: a quasiexperimental multicenter Study. Clin Infect Dis 2022;75(2):269–77.
73. Jacobs MR. Optimisation of antimicrobial therapy using pharmacokinetic and pharmacodynamic parameters. Clin Microbiol Infect 2001;7(11):589–96.
74. Day MR, Doumith M, Do Nascimento V, et al. Comparison of phenotypic and WGS-derived antimicrobial resistance profiles of Salmonella enterica serovars Typhi and Paratyphi. J Antimicrob Chemother 2018;73(2):365–72.
75. Harada Y, Morinaga Y, Kaku N, et al. In vitro and in vivo activities of piperacillin-tazobactam and meropenem at different inoculum sizes of ESBL-producing Klebsiella pneumoniae. Clin Microbiol Infect 2014;20(11):O831–9.
76. Weinmaier T, Conzemius R, Bergman Y, et al. Validation and application of long-read whole-genome sequencing for antimicrobial resistance gene detection and antimicrobial susceptibility testing. Antimicrob Agents Chemother 2023;67(1): e0107222.
77. Stevenson M, Pandor A, Martyn-St James M, et al. Sepsis: the LightCycler SeptiFast Test MGRADE(R), SepsiTest and IRIDICA BAC BSI assay for rapidly identifying bloodstream bacteria and fungi - a systematic review and economic evaluation. Health Technol Assess 2016;20(46):1–246.

78. Simms LA, Davies C, Jayasundara N, et al. Performance evaluation of InfectID-BSI: a rapid quantitative PCR assay for detecting sepsis-associated organisms directly from whole blood. J Microbiol Methods 2023;211:106783.
79. Chen Y, Chen C, Chen W, et al. Clinical application of metagenomic next-generation sequencing in sepsis patients with early antibiotic treatment. Infect Drug Resist 2024;17:4695–706.
80. Chien JY, Yu CJ, Hsueh PR. Utility of metagenomic next-generation sequencing for etiological diagnosis of patients with sepsis in intensive care units. Microbiol Spectr 2022;10(4):e0074622.
81. Zhang D, Li X, Wang Y, et al. The clinical importance of metagenomic next-generation sequencing in detecting disease-causing microorganisms in cases of sepsis acquired in the community or hospital setting. Front Microbiol 2024; 15:1384166.
82. Li X, Liang S, Zhang D, et al. The clinical application of metagenomic next-generation sequencing in sepsis of immunocompromised patients. Front Cell Infect Microbiol 2023;13:1170687.
83. Qin C, Zhang S, Zhao Y, et al. Diagnostic value of metagenomic next-generation sequencing in sepsis and bloodstream infection. Front Cell Infect Microbiol 2023;13:1117987.
84. Sun Q, Teng R, Shi Q, et al. Clinical implement of probe-capture metagenomics in sepsis patients: a multicentre and prospective study. Clin Transl Med 2025; 15(4):e70297.
85. Wu C, Yu X, Gai W, et al. Diagnostic value of plasma and blood cells metagenomic next-generation sequencing in patients with sepsis. Biochem Biophys Res Commun 2023;683:149079.
86. Xu F, Chen C, Lu S, et al. Impact of metagenomics next-generation sequencing on etiological diagnosis and early outcomes in sepsis. J Transl Med 2025; 23(1):394.
87. Pinzauti D, Biazzo M, Podrini C, et al. An NGS-Assisted diagnostic workflow for culture-independent detection of bloodstream pathogens and prediction of antimicrobial resistances in sepsis. Front Cell Infect Microbiol 2025;15:1656171.
88. Zhu Y, Miao H, Zhang J, et al. Role of plasma and blood-cell co-metagenomic sequencing in precise diagnosis and severity evaluation of sepsis, a prospective cohort study in sepsis patients. J Infect 2025;90(3):106434.
89. Brenner T, Decker SO, Vainshtein Y, et al, German Society of Anaesthesiology and Intensive Care GSAIC Trials Group. Improved pathogen identification in sepsis or septic shock by clinical metagenomic sequencing. J Infect 2025; 91(3):106565.
90. Brenner T, Skarabis A, Stevens P, et al, TIFOnet Critical Care Trials Group. Optimization of sepsis therapy based on patient-specific digital precision diagnostics using next generation sequencing (DigiSep-Trial)-study protocol for a randomized, controlled, interventional, open-label, multicenter trial. Trials 2021;22(1):714.
91. Dik JW, Poelman R, Friedrich AW, et al. An integrated stewardship model: antimicrobial, infection prevention and diagnostic (AID). Future Microbiol 2016; 11(1):93–102.
92. Stewardson AJ, Marimuthu K, Sengupta S, et al. Effect of carbapenem resistance on outcomes of bloodstream infection caused by enterobacteriaceae in low-income and middle-income countries (PANORAMA): a multinational prospective cohort study. Lancet Infect Dis 2019;19(6):601–10.
93. Falcone M, Tiseo G, Carbonara S, et al, Advancing knowLedge on Antimicrobial Resistant Infections Collaboration Network ALARICO Network. Mortality

attributable to bloodstream infections caused by different carbapenem-resistant gram-negative bacilli: results from a nationwide study in Italy (ALARICO network). Clin Infect Dis 2023;76(12):2059–69.

94. Reyes J, Komarow L, Chen L, et al, Antibacterial Resistance Leadership Group and Multi-Drug Resistant Organism Network Investigators. Global epidemiology and clinical outcomes of carbapenem-resistant Pseudomonas aeruginosa and associated carbapenemases (POP): a prospective cohort study. Lancet Microbe 2023;4(3):e159–70.
95. Tamma PD, Heil EL, Justo JA, et al. Infectious diseases society of America 2024 guidance on the treatment of antimicrobial-resistant gram-negative infections. Clin Infect Dis 2024;. https://academic.oup.com/cid/advance-article/doi/10.1093/cid/ciae403/7728556?login=false.
96. Paul M, Carrara E, Retamar P, et al. European Society of Clinical Microbiology and Infectious Diseases (ESCMID) guidelines for the treatment of infections caused by multidrug-resistant Gram-negative bacilli (endorsed by European society of intensive care medicine). Clin Microbiol Infect 2022;28(4):521–47.
97. Zavascki AP, Chebabo A, Cunha CA, et al. Guideline for antimicrobial treatment of multidrug-resistant Gram-negative infections: practice recommendations of the Brazilian Society of Infectious Diseases. Braz J Infect Dis 2025;29(6):104589.
98. Allel K, Peters A, Haghparast-Bidgoli H, et al. Excess burden of antibiotic-resistant bloodstream infections: evidence from a multicentre retrospective cohort study in Chile, 2018-2022. Lancet Reg Health, Am 2024;40:100943.
99. Wunderink RG, Giamarellos-Bourboulis EJ, Rahav G, et al. Effect and safety of meropenem-vaborbactam versus best-available therapy in patients with carbapenem-resistant Enterobacteriaceae infections: the TANGO II randomized clinical trial. Infect Dis Ther 2018;7(4):439–55.
100. Motsch J, Murta de Oliveira C, Stus V, et al. RESTORE-IMI 1: a Multicenter, randomized, double-blind trial comparing efficacy and safety of Imipenem/Relebactam vs Colistin plus Imipenem in patients with Imipenem-nonsusceptible bacterial infections. Clin Infect Dis 2020;70(9):1799–808.
101. Shields RK, Horcajada JP, Kamat S, et al. Ceftazidime-Avibactam in the treatment of patients with bacteremia or nosocomial pneumonia: a systematic review and meta-analysis. Infect Dis Ther 2024;13(7):1639–64.
102. Mohammad S, Al Namer Y, Rahimeh W, et al. Effectiveness and safety of meropenem-vaborbactam versus ceftazidime-avibactam in multidrug-resistant Gram-negative infections: a systematic review and meta-analysis with trial sequential analysis. Antimicrob Agents Chemother 2026;70(2):e0154625.
103. Bianco G, Boattini M, Lupo L, et al. In vitro activity and genomic characterization of KPC-producing Klebsiella pneumoniae clinical blood culture isolates resistant to ceftazidime/avibactam, meropenem/vaborbactam, imipenem/relebactam: an Italian nationwide multicentre observational study (2022-23). J Antimicrob Chemother 2025;80(2):583–92.
104. Wilhelm CM, Antochevis LC, Magagnin CM, et al. Susceptibility evaluation of novel beta-lactam/beta-lactamase inhibitor combinations against carbapenem-resistant Klebsiella pneumoniae from bloodstream infections in hospitalized patients in Brazil. J Glob Antimicrob Resist 2024;38:247–51.
105. Hsu W, Chuang MH, Tsai WW, et al. Ceftazidime-avibactam combination therapy versus monotherapy for treating carbapenem-resistant gram-negative infection: a systemic review and meta-analysis. Infection 2024;52(5):2029–42.

106. Brauncajs M, Bielec F, Malinowska M, et al. Aztreonam combinations with avibactam, relebactam, and vaborbactam as treatment for new Delhi metallo-beta-lactamase-producing Enterobacterales Infections-In vitro susceptibility testing. Pharmaceuticals (Basel) 2024;17(3).
107. Tao L, Dahlquist A, Harris H, et al. Multicenter evaluation of activity of aztreonam in combination with avibactam, relebactam, and vaborbactam against metallo-beta-lactamase-producing carbapenem-resistant gram-negative bacilli. Antimicrob Agents Chemother 2024;68(10):e0069324.
108. Carmeli Y, Cisneros JM, Paul M, et al, COMBACTE-CARE consortium REVISIT study group. Aztreonam-avibactam versus meropenem for the treatment of serious infections caused by Gram-negative bacteria (REVISIT): a descriptive, multinational, open-label, phase 3, randomised trial. Lancet Infect Dis 2025;25(2):218–30.
109. Kaye KS, Belley A, Barth P, et al. Effect of Cefepime/Enmetazobactam vs Piperacillin/Tazobactam on clinical cure and microbiological eradication in patients with complicated urinary tract infection or acute Pyelonephritis: a randomized clinical trial. JAMA 2022;328(13):1304–14.
110. Oliver A, Arca-Suarez J, Gomis-Font MA, et al. Emerging resistance mechanisms to newer beta-lactams in Pseudomonas aeruginosa. Clin Microbiol Infect 2025;31(11):1790–6.
111. Collings H, Stone M, Chrysostomou M, et al. A systematic literature review and (network) meta-analysis of the effectiveness of ceftolozane/tazobactam versus aminoglycosides/polymyxins and ceftazidime/avibactam for treating adult patients with multidrug-resistant Pseudomonas aeruginosa infections. Antimicrob Agents Chemother 2026;70(2):e0073525.
112. Pina-Sanchez M, Rua M, Lopez-Causape C, et al. Ceftazidime-avibactam plus aztreonam cocktail for the treatment of VIM-producing Pseudomonas aeruginosa infections: good enough to have another? J Antimicrob Chemother 2025;80(5):1371–6.
113. Bassetti M, Echols R, Matsunaga Y, et al. Efficacy and safety of cefiderocol or best available therapy for the treatment of serious infections caused by carbapenem-resistant Gram-negative bacteria (CREDIBLE-CR): a randomised, open-label, multicentre, pathogen-focused, descriptive, phase 3 trial. Lancet Infect Dis 2021;21(2):226–40.
114. Paterson DL, Sulaiman H, Liu PY, et al, GAME CHANGER Trial Investigators. Cefiderocol versus standard therapy for hospital-acquired and health-care-associated Gram-negative bacterial bloodstream infection (the GAME CHANGER trial): an open-label, parallel-group, randomised trial. Lancet Infect Dis 2026;26(2):148–59.
115. Risco-Risco C, Henriquez-Camacho C, Herrera-Rueda M, et al. Cefiderocol versus best available therapy in the treatment of critically ill patients with severe infections due to resistant gram-negative bacteria: a systematic review and meta-analysis. Antibiotics (Basel) 2024;13(11).
116. Onorato L, de Luca I, Monari C, et al. Cefiderocol either in monotherapy or combination versus best available therapy in the treatment of carbapenem-resistant Acinetobacter baumannii infections: a systematic review and meta-analysis. J Infect 2024;88(3):106113.
117. Harris PNA, Tambyah PA, Lye DC, et al, MERINO Trial Investigators and the Australasian Society for Infectious Disease Clinical Research Network ASID-CRN. Effect of Piperacillin-Tazobactam vs Meropenem on 30-Day mortality for patients with E coli or Klebsiella pneumoniae bloodstream infection and ceftriaxone resistance: a randomized clinical trial. JAMA 2018;320(10):984–94.

118. Lodise TP, Bhavnani SM, Ambrose PG, et al. Piperacillin/Tazobactam susceptibility Test interpretive criteria for enterobacterales: recommendations from the United States Committee on antimicrobial susceptibility testing. Clin Infect Dis 2024;79(6):1354–62.
119. Mansson TS, Askemyr A, Sunnerhagen T, et al. Piperacillin/tazobactam versus carbapenems for 30-day mortality in patients with ESBL-producing Enterobacterales bloodstream infections: a retrospective, multicenter, non-inferiority, cohort study. Infection 2025;53(5):1769–77.
120. Gatti M, Cojutti PG, Pea F. Piperacillin-tazobactam vs. carbapenems for treating hospitalized patients with ESBL-producing Enterobacterales bloodstream infections: a systematic review and meta-analysis. J Glob Antimicrob Resist 2024;39:27–36.
121. Onorato L, de Luca I, Salvati A, et al. Piperacillin/tazobactam vs. cefepime or carbapenems for the treatment of bloodstream infections due to bacteria producing chromosomal AmpC beta-lactamase: a systematic review and meta-analysis. Infection 2025;53(3):1141–53.
122. Cairns KA, Udy AA, Peel TN, et al. Therapeutics for vancomycin-resistant enterococcal bloodstream infections. Clin Microbiol Rev 2023;36(2):e0005922.
123. Tong SYC, Fowler VG Jr, Skalla L, et al. Management of Staphylococcus aureus bacteremia: a review. JAMA 2025;334(9):798–808.
124. Lakhundi S, Zhang K. Methicillin-Resistant Staphylococcus aureus: Molecular Characterization, Evolution, and Epidemiology. Clin Microbiol Rev 2018;31(4).
125. Lewis PO, Heil EL, Covert KL, et al. Treatment strategies for persistent methicillin-resistant Staphylococcus aureus bacteraemia. J Clin Pharm Ther 2018;43(5):614–25.
126. Samura M, Takada K, Hirose N, et al. Comparison of the efficacy and safety of standard- and high-dose daptomycin: a systematic review and meta-analysis. Br J Clin Pharmacol 2023;89(4):1291–303.
127. Holland TL, Cosgrove SE, Doernberg SB, et al, ERADICATE Study Group. Ceftobiprole for treatment of complicated Staphylococcus aureus bacteremia. N Engl J Med 2023;389(15):1390–401.
128. Johnson TM, Molina KC, Miller MA, et al. Combination ceftaroline and daptomycin salvage therapy for complicated methicillin-resistant Staphylococcus aureus bacteraemia compared with standard of care. Int J Antimicrob Agents 2021;57(4):106310.
129. Geriak M, Haddad F, Rizvi K, et al. Clinical data on Daptomycin plus Ceftaroline versus standard of care monotherapy in the treatment of Methicillin-Resistant Staphylococcus aureus bacteremia. Antimicrob Agents Chemother 2019;63(5).
130. Kalil AC, Holubar M, Deresinski S, et al. Is Daptomycin plus ceftaroline associated with better clinical outcomes than standard of care monotherapy for Staphylococcus aureus bacteremia? Antimicrob Agents Chemother 2019;63(11).
131. Escrihuela-Vidal F, Ong SWX, Oriol I, et al. Adjunctive fosfomycin for the treatment of Staphylococcus aureus bacteremia: a pooled post hoc analysis of individual participant data from 2 randomized trials. Clin Infect Dis 2026;82(2):238–45.
132. Pujol M, Miro JM, Shaw E, et al, MRSA Bacteremia BACSARM Trial Investigators. Daptomycin plus Fosfomycin versus Daptomycin alone for Methicillin-resistant Staphylococcus aureus bacteremia and endocarditis: a randomized clinical trial. Clin Infect Dis 2021;72(9):1517–25.

133. Raad I, Darouiche R, Vazquez J, et al. Efficacy and safety of weekly dalbavancin therapy for catheter-related bloodstream infection caused by gram-positive pathogens. Clin Infect Dis 2005;40(3):374–80.
134. Chaldoupis AE, Petrakis V, Ioannou P, et al. Dalbavancin for infective endocarditis: a systematic review of effectiveness, safety, and dosing. Eur J Clin Microbiol Infect Dis 2026;. https://link.springer.com/article/10.1007/s10096-026-05434-3.
135. Turner NA, Hamasaki T, Doernberg SB, et al, Antibacterial Resistance Leadership Group. Dalbavancin for treatment of Staphylococcus aureus bacteremia: the DOTS randomized clinical trial. JAMA 2025;334(10):866–77.
136. Texidor WM, Miller MA, Molina KC, et al. Oritavancin as sequential therapy for Gram-positive bloodstream infections. BMC Infect Dis 2024;24(1):127.
137. Jordan H, Kozierowski K, Pickles R, et al. Oritavancin for the treatment of Staphylococcus aureus Bacteremia-A retrospective single-arm cohort Study. Open Forum Infect Dis 2025;12(7):ofaf333.
138. Johnston RD, Woodall BM, Harrison J, et al. Removal of peptidoglycan and inhibition of active cellular processes leads to daptomycin tolerance in Enterococcus faecalis. PLoS One 2021;16(7):e0254796.
139. Kebriaei R, Rice SA, Singh KV, et al. Influence of inoculum effect on the efficacy of Daptomycin monotherapy and in combination with beta-Lactams against Daptomycin-Susceptible Enterococcus faecium harboring LiaSR substitutions. Antimicrob Agents Chemother 2018;62(8).
140. Chuang YC, Lin HY, Yang JL, et al. Influence of daptomycin doses on the outcomes of VRE bloodstream infection treated with high-dose daptomycin. J Antimicrob Chemother 2022;77(8):2278–87.
141. Britt NS, Potter EM, Patel N, et al. Comparative effectiveness and safety of standard-medium-and high-dose daptomycin strategies for the treatment of vancomycin-resistant enterococcal bacteremia among veterans affairs patients. Clin Infect Dis 2017;64(5):605–13.
142. Chuang YC, Lin HY, Wang JT, et al. Daptomycin area under the curve to minimum inhibitory concentration ratio by broth microdilution for predicting the outcome of vancomycin-resistant Enterococcus bloodstream infection. Biomed Pharmacother 2022;155:113710.
143. Tamma PD, Hsu AJ. Optimizing therapy for vancomycin-resistant enterococcal bacteremia in children. Curr Opin Infect Dis 2014;27(6):517–27.
144. Whang DW, Miller LG, Partain NM, et al. Systematic review and meta-analysis of linezolid and daptomycin for treatment of vancomycin-resistant enterococcal bloodstream infections. Antimicrob Agents Chemother 2013;57(10):5013–8.
145. Hayakawa K, Martin ET, Gudur UM, et al. Impact of different antimicrobial therapies on clinical and fiscal outcomes of patients with bacteremia due to vancomycin-resistant enterococci. Antimicrob Agents Chemother 2014;58(7):3968–75.
146. Hwang LE, Yang JL, Lin CY, et al. High-dose daptomycin versus linezolid for the treatment of vancomycin-resistant Enterococcus faecium bloodstream infections: role of pharmacodynamic target attainment. J Microbiol Immunol Infect 2026;59(2):237–43.
147. Serapide F, Serraino R, Spadafora L, et al. Clinical characteristics, therapy and outcome of bloodstream infections caused by vancomycin-resistant enterococci: a multicentre clinical experience. J Antimicrob Chemother 2025;80(5):1241–7.

148. Singh KV, Arias CA, Murray BE. Tedizolid as step-down therapy following Daptomycin versus continuation of Daptomycin against enterococci and Methicillin- and vancomycin-resistant Staphylococcus aureus in a rat endocarditis model. Antimicrob Agents Chemother 2020;64(5).
149. Hayden MK, Trenholme GM, Schultz JE, et al. In vivo development of teicoplanin resistance in a VanB Enterococcus faecium isolate. J Infect Dis 1993;167(5): 1224–7.
150. Zhanel GG, Calic D, Schweizer F, et al. New lipoglycopeptides: a comparative review of dalbavancin, oritavancin and telavancin. Drugs 2010;70(7):859–86.
151. Jalali S, Bhatt H, Thakkar K, et al. Management of recurrent vancomycin-resistant Enterococcus faecium bacteremia with Oritavancin: a case report. In Vivo 2024; 38(6):3106–11.
152. Di Cecco C, Monticelli J, Di Bella S, et al. Vancomycin-resistant enterococcus bloodstream infection successfully managed with oritavancin and fosfomycin as sequential treatment. J Chemother 2024;36(1):31–4.
153. 2023 Antibacterial agents in clinical and preclinical development: an overview and analysis (Internet). 2023. Available at: https://www.who.int/publications/i/item/9789240094000 (Accessed 26 April 2026).
154. Kumar A, Ellis P, Arabi Y, et al, Cooperative Antimicrobial Therapy of Septic Shock Database Research Group. Initiation of inappropriate antimicrobial therapy results in a fivefold reduction of survival in human septic shock. Chest 2009; 136(5):1237–48.
155. Kalil AC, Johnson DW, Lisco SJ, et al. Early goal-directed therapy for sepsis: a novel solution for discordant survival outcomes in clinical trials. Crit Care Med 2017;45(4):607–14.
156. Kollef MH, Sherman G, Ward S, et al. Inadequate antimicrobial treatment of infections: a risk factor for hospital mortality among critically ill patients. Chest 1999;115(2):462–74.
157. Iregui M, Ward S, Sherman G, et al. Clinical importance of delays in the initiation of appropriate antibiotic treatment for ventilator-associated pneumonia. Chest 2002;122(1):262–8.
158. Zilberberg MD, Shorr AF, Micek ST, et al. Multi-drug resistance, inappropriate initial antibiotic therapy and mortality in Gram-negative severe sepsis and septic shock: a retrospective cohort study. Crit Care 2014;18(6):596.
159. Bouza E, Sousa D, Munoz P, et al. Bloodstream infections: a trial of the impact of different methods of reporting positive blood culture results. Clin Infect Dis 2004;39(8):1161–9.
160. Timbrook TT, Morton JB, McConeghy KW, et al. The effect of molecular rapid diagnostic testing on clinical outcomes in bloodstream infections: a systematic review and meta-analysis. Clin Infect Dis 2017;64(1):15–23.
161. Lopez-Lozano JM, Lawes T, Nebot C, et al, THRESHOLDS study group. A nonlinear time-series analysis approach to identify thresholds in associations between population antibiotic use and rates of resistance. Nat Microbiol 2019; 4(7):1160–72.
162. Gupta S, Sakhuja A, Kumar G, et al. Culture-Negative severe sepsis: nationwide trends and outcomes. Chest 2016;150(6):1251–9.
163. Goncalves-Pereira J, Paiva JA. Dose modulation: a new concept of antibiotic therapy in the critically ill patient? J Crit Care 2013;28(4):341–6.
164. Goncalves-Pereira J, Martins A, Povoa P. Pharmacokinetics of gentamicin in critically ill patients: pilot study evaluating the first dose. Clin Microbiol Infect 2010; 16(8):1258–63.

165. Rybak M, Lomaestro B, Rotschafer JC, et al. Therapeutic monitoring of vancomycin in adult patients: a consensus review of the American Society of Health-System Pharmacists, the Infectious Diseases Society of America, and the Society of Infectious Diseases Pharmacists. Am J Health Syst Pharm 2009;66(1):82–98.
166. Rybak MJ, Le J, Lodise TP, et al. Therapeutic monitoring of vancomycin for serious methicillin-resistant Staphylococcus aureus infections: a revised consensus guideline and review by the American Society of Health-System Pharmacists, the Infectious Diseases Society of America, the Pediatric Infectious Diseases Society, and the Society of Infectious Diseases Pharmacists. Am J Health Syst Pharm 2020;77(11):835–64.
167. Abdul-Aziz MH, Hammond NE, Brett SJ, et al. Prolonged vs intermittent infusions of beta-Lactam antibiotics in adults with sepsis or septic shock: a systematic review and meta-analysis. JAMA 2024;332(8):638–48.
168. Dulhunty JM, Brett SJ, De Waele JJ, et al, BLING III Study Investigators. Continuous vs intermittent beta-lactam antibiotic infusions in critically ill patients with sepsis: the BLING III randomized clinical trial. JAMA 2024;332(8):629–37.
169. Roberts JA, Paul SK, Akova M, et al, DALI Study. DALI: defining antibiotic levels in intensive care unit patients: are current beta-lactam antibiotic doses sufficient for critically ill patients? Clin Infect Dis 2014;58(8):1072–83.
170. Abdul-Aziz MH, Alffenaar JC, Bassetti M, et al, Infection Section of European Society of Intensive Care Medicine ESICM, Pharmacokinetic/pharmacodynamic and Critically Ill Patient Study Groups of European Society of Clinical Microbiology and Infectious Diseases ESCMID, Infectious Diseases Group of International Association of Therapeutic Drug Monitoring and Clinical Toxicology IATDMCT, Infections in the ICU and Sepsis Working Group of International Society of Antimicrobial Chemotherapy ISAC. Antimicrobial therapeutic drug monitoring in critically ill adult patients: a Position Paper. Intensive Care Med 2020; 46(6):1127–53.
171. Ziegler I, Fagerström A, Strålin K, et al. Evaluation of a commercial multiplex PCR assay for detection of pathogen DNA in blood from patients with suspected sepsis. PLoS One 2016;11(12):e0167883.
172. Zboromyrska Y, Cillóniz C, Cobos-Trigueros N, et al. Evaluation of the magicplex™ sepsis real-time Test for the rapid diagnosis of bloodstream infections in adults. Front Cell Infect Microbiol 2019;9:56. PMID: 30931259; PMCID: PMC6423426.
173. Bloos F, Sachse S, Kortgen A, et al. Evaluation of a polymerase chain reaction assay for pathogen detection in septic patients under routine condition: an observational study. PLoS One 2012;7(9):e46003.
174. De Angelis G, Posteraro B, De Carolis E, et al. T2Bacteria magnetic resonance assay for the rapid detection of ESKAPEc pathogens directly in whole blood. J Antimicrob Chemother 2018;73(suppl_4):iv20–6. PMID: 29608753.
175. Nguyen MH, Clancy CJ, Pasculle AW, et al. Performance of the T2Bacteria Panel for diagnosing bloodstream infections: a diagnostic accuracy Study. Ann Intern Med 2019;170(12):845–52. Epub 2019 May 14. PMID: 31083728.

Sepsis and the Immunocompromised Host

Ann Zalucky, MD, MSc[a], Guillaume Dumas, MD, PhD[b],
Aleksandra Leligdowicz, MD, PhD[c], Laveena Munshi, MD, MSc[d,*]

KEYWORDS

• Sepsis • Immunocompromised • Malignancy • Transplant • Neutropenia
• Immunomodulation • ICU triage

KEY POINTS

- Immunocompromised patients are increasing, and *delayed intensive care unit admission worsens outcomes*.
- Sepsis in this group is *biologically distinct*—not just *sepsis with comorbidities*.
- *No single consensus definition/stratification* exists; immune-defect-based frameworks may be better than disease labels.
- *Diagnosis can be challenging*: fever and white blood cells (WBC) signals may be absent; midregional proadrenomedullin and computed tomography (CT)/advanced tests can help, but polymerase chain reaction positives may reflect colonization.
- Management is complex: use *early, risk-adapted antimicrobials* but also screen for *sepsis-mimicking immune syndromes*.

INTRODUCTION

Immunosuppression is a critical risk factor for infection and sepsis,[1] and as the global burden of acquired immunosuppression continues to grow,[2] optimizing care for this vulnerable population represents an urgent public health priority. The prevalence of immunosuppression within the general population is increasing, with up to one-third of all critically ill patients being immunocompromised at baseline. Three converging trends necessitate renewed focus. First, survival among patients with immunocompromising conditions has improved dramatically.[3] Contemporary data demonstrate that intensive care unit (ICU) survival in selected patients with cancer approaches that of immunocompetent patients when adjusted for organ failure severity.[4] Yet triage

[a] Department of Critical Care Medicine, University of Calgary, Calgary, Alberta, Canada; [b] Department of Critical Care Medicine, Universite Grenobles-Alpes, Grenobles, France; [c] Department of Critical Care Medicine, University of Western Ontario, London, Ontario, Canada; [d] Department of Critical Care Medicine, University of Toronto, Toronto, Ontario, Canada
* Corresponding author. Department of Medicine, Mount Sinai Hospital, 600 University Avenue, Toronto, ON, M5G1X5.
E-mail address: Laveena.munshi@sinaihealth.ca

Crit Care Clin 42 (2026) 821–837
https://doi.org/10.1016/j.ccc.2026.05.007 **criticalcare.theclinics.com**

Abbreviations	
APCs	antigen-presenting cells
CAR	chimeric antigen receptor
CRP	C-reactive protein
CRS	cytokine release syndrome
HIV	human immunodeficiency virus
HLH	hemophagocytic lymphohistiocytosis
HSCT	hematopoietic stem cell transplantation
ICANS	immune effector cell-associated neurotoxicity syndrome
ICU	intensive care unit
IL	interleukin
MR-proADM	midregional proadrenomedullin
PCR	polymerase chain reaction
PJP	pneumocystis jirovecii
SOT	solid organ transplantation

thresholds remain inconsistent, and delayed ICU transfer is associated with excess mortality.[5,6] Second, the therapeutic landscape has fundamentally altered immune function by introducing unique infectious risks and inflammatory syndromes that may mimic sepsis. Third, immunocompromised patients are underrepresented in sepsis trials. The Surviving Sepsis Campaign recommendations are derived largely from immunocompetent populations.[7] Whether fluid strategies, vasopressor thresholds, steroid responsiveness, and antimicrobial duration should differ remains uncertain. Importantly, sepsis in the immunocompromised host is not simply sepsis plus comorbidity.

Understanding the relationship between immunity and infection risk is crucial in developing personalized approaches to patient care and improving clinical outcomes. However, with prolonged survival among those with varying immunosuppressive conditions, compounded by an aging and increasingly comorbid population, this relationship is more complex than ever before. The recent seismic expansion in immunomodulating therapies, including biologics and T-cell-engaging therapies, has required physicians to recognize a new repertoire of immune toxicities, including novel infections and immune syndromes masquerading as sepsis. With clear evidence supporting an association between immune dysfunction and adverse clinical outcomes among critically ill patients, early sepsis identification, awareness of sepsis-mimickers, and tailored management strategies are of paramount importance for optimizing patient care and long-term outcomes.

This article aims to summarize the current understanding of sepsis in the immunocompromised host, highlighting diagnostic challenges and management controversies while raising awareness of important parallel immune syndromes and future research opportunities. Immunosuppression may result from primary immunodeficiencies that is, caused by genetic or congenital abnormalities, or secondary immunodeficiencies, which are acquired throughout the lifespan owing to underlying disease, comorbidities, and immunosuppressive agents. This article focuses on the latter; however, the general approaches and considerations outlined here may be applicable to the broader population. Importantly, sepsis-induced immunosuppression in critical illness is an increasingly recognized entity, underscoring the importance of viewing the immune system as a dynamic rather than static state, the kinetics of which evolve over the course of a hospital admission. Integrating temporal patterns of immune dysfunction into the care of critically ill patients represents an important area of ongoing research that, while beyond the scope of this article, has been described elsewhere.[8]

DEFINITION OF IMMUNOCOMPROMISED HOST

One of the greatest challenges facing the field is the variability in how immunocompromised patients are defined, described, and stratified. Without consistent definitions, clinical and trial populations will remain detrimentally heterogeneous, limiting the application and generalizability of findings. Unfortunately, there is no consensus definition that currently exists. Traditional disease-based categories include: hematologic malignancy, solid tumor receiving active therapy, hematopoietic stem cell transplantation (HSCT), solid organ transplantation (SOT), autoimmune or vasculitic disease, advanced human immunodeficiency virus (HIV) infection, and chronic corticosteroid exposure.

While a useful starting point, this approach is limited by a lack of granularity and obscures heterogeneity. With the rising complexity of the modern immunocompromised host, many patients carry multiple diagnoses with overlapping or competing immune defects, making it difficult to identify a single dominant immune pathology resulting in intervention uncertainty. The number of diseases and exposures that may result in an immunocompromised state are also very broad and therefore creating a comprehensive list of possible conditions may be cumbersome. For example, patients with HIV, sick cell disease or history of splenectomy, may not fit into any of the above-mentioned categories. Furthermore, these conditions are not static and may evolve and differ within the same disease state over time (eg, a patient's immunocompromised state at the time of HIV diagnosis verses at the time of follow-up after years of appropriate antiviral therapy). Importantly, immunosuppression may affect the immune system in terms of both quantity—as seen in neutropenia or lymphopenia—and quality—as seen in functional asplenia, chronic steroid use, or uremia, where cell counts may appear normal despite profound functional impairment. These important considerations remain agnostic to the disease-based classification system.

Immune Defect Classification

An alternative framework stratifies patients according to predicted baseline immune defects, categorized as[1] barrier disruption,[2] innate immune dysfunction,[3] adaptive immune suppression, and[4] immune reprogramming (**Fig. 1**, **Table 1**). This approach offers a more precise and flexible alternative to disease-based classification, compelling clinicians to consider multiple simultaneous forms of immune compromise and their associated infection risks.

Barrier disruption

The outermost layer of the host's defense system is the anatomic barrier that is, the patient's physical *envelope*, which provides both mechanical and chemical protection against pathogen entry. Barrier defense encompasses skin integrity, mucosal membrane function, mucociliary clearance, and the absence of foreign bodies breaching sterile compartments. Barrier disruption is particularly prevalent in patients with hematological malignancy or those undergoing cytotoxic chemotherapy, in whom mucositis, chemotherapy-induced colitis, and indwelling central venous catheters are common. Another important patient population that cannot be overlooked in this category are burn patients, whose mortality due to nosocomial infection are significant. These disruptions facilitate translocation of cutaneous and gastrointestinal flora into the bloodstream, where even organisms of low intrinsic virulence, such as coagulase-negative staphylococci, can cause life-threatening sepsis.

Innate immune dysfunction

The innate immune system constitutes the first cellular line of defense, providing rapid, nonspecific responses to invading pathogens. Its principal functions include

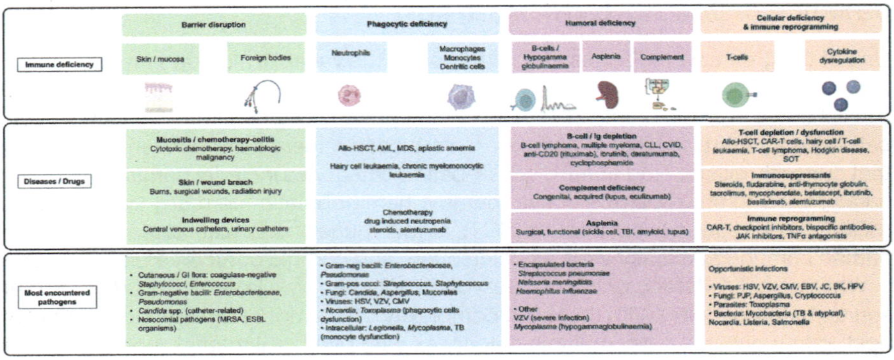

Fig. 1. Classification of immunocompromised state based upon immune deficiencies. Allo-HSCT, Allogeneic hematopoietic stem cell transplant; AML, Acute myeloid leukemia; CLL, Chronic lymphocytic leukemia; CMV, Cytomegalovirus; CVID, Common variable immune deficiency; EBV, Epstein-barr virus; ESBL, Extended spectrum beta-lactamase; HPV, Human papilloma virus; HSV, Herpes simplex virus; JAK, Janus kinase; JC, John Cunningham virus (human polyomavirus 2); MDS, Myelodysplastic syndrome; MRSA- Methicillin-resistant staphylococcus aureus; PJP, Pneumocystis jirovecii pneumonia; SOT, Solid organ transplant; TB, Tuberculosis; TNF, Tumor necrosis factor; VZV, Varicella zoster virus. (*Created in* MS Power Point and pictograms were taken from SERVIER MEDICAL ART. Servier Medical Art is licensed under CC BY 4.0.)

pathogen recognition, opsonization via complement activation, and phagocytic clearance, with neutrophils and monocytes serving as the primary effector cells. Neutrophils eliminate pathogens through phagocytosis, degranulation, and oxidative killing mechanisms. Monocytes differentiate into macrophages and dendritic cells, which not only perform phagocytosis but also serve as critical antigen-presenting cells (APCs), bridging innate and adaptive immunity by initiating downstream lymphocyte responses. Derangements may be seen in the early phase following chemotherapy, allogeneic hematopoietic stem cell transplantation, acute myeloid leukemia and aplastic anemia. Impairment of innate immune function, whether through quantitative depletion or qualitative dysfunction, increases susceptibility to both gram-positive and gram-negative bacterial infections, fungal infections including candidemia, and molds including invasive aspergillosis.

Adaptive immune suppression

Adaptive immunity comprises 2 principal arms: (1) cellular immunity, mediated by antigen-specific T lymphocytes activated through interactions with APCs; and (2) humoral immunity, mediated by B lymphocytes that differentiate into plasma cells or memory B cells and produce antigen-specific antibodies. T lymphocyte subsets, principally $CD8^+$ cytotoxic T cells and $CD4^+$ helper T cells, are activated following major histocompatibility complex-dependent antigen presentation by dendritic cells and macrophages. These subsequently proliferate to mount pathogen-specific effector responses. Cytotoxic T cells induce apoptosis of cells displaying foreign peptides on their surface, while helper T cells augment this response through macrophage activation and cytokine secretion including interferon-γ. Collectively, cellular immunity is directed primarily against intracellular pathogens-including mycobacteria, Listeria, Leishmania, and Histoplasma—and against virus-infected cells that cannot be targeted by circulating antibodies alone. The clinical consequences of cellular immune deficiency are well illustrated by HIV infection, in which progressive $CD4^+$ T cell depletion produces

Table 1
Immune defect driven risk stratification

Immune Defect	Common Causes	Infection Risk	Sepsis Phenotype	Management Implications
Barrier disruption	Chemotherapy, mucositis, lines	Gram-positive, gut translocation	Rapid bacteremia	Broad early antibiotics
Innate dysfunction	Neutropenia, steroids	Bacterial + fungal (Candida, Aspergillus)	Blunted inflammation	Consider antifungals early
Adaptive (T-cell)	HIV, calcineurin inhibitors	Viral, intracellular (TB, PJP)	Atypical presentations	Broaden to viral/opportunistic
Adaptive (B-cell)	Rituximab, myeloma	Encapsulated organisms	Recurrent infections	IVIG ± targeted antibiotics
Immune reprogramming	CAR-T, checkpoint inhibitors	Mixed (CRS vs infection)	Hyperinflammatory mimic	Immunomodulation vs antibiotics
Mixed defects	Most ICU patients	Broad spectrum	Heterogeneous	Individualized approach

Abbreviation: IVIG, intravenous immunoglobulin.

a predictable hierarchy of opportunistic infections that forms the basis of well-established prophylactic guidelines. In non-HIV immunocompromised patients however, CD4^{+} dysfunction induced by corticosteroids, calcineurin inhibitors, and purine analogs are responsible for the mechanisms of cellular immunosuppression.

Unlike T cells, B cells recognize antigens directly via surface-expressed immunoglobulins. Upon activation, B cells differentiate into plasma cells that secrete antigen-specific antibodies, which mediate pathogen elimination through complement activation, promotion of opsonization and phagocytosis, and recruitment of innate immune effectors. While a detailed review of immunoglobulin class structure and function is beyond the scope of this article, 2 clinically important causes of functional verses depletion hypogammaglobulinemia warrant specific consideration in the context of the immunocompromised host. In multiple myeloma, overproduction of a nonfunctional monoclonal paraprotein paradoxically suppresses normal antibody production, rendering patients functionally hypogammaglobulinemic despite elevated total protein levels. The use of a common biologic, Rituximab, an anti-CD20 monoclonal antibody, depletes mature B cells while sparing CD20-negative plasma cells; hypogammaglobulinemia therefore develops in a delayed fashion as the existing plasma cell pool turns over in the periphery and cannot be replenished from the depleted B cell compartment. Patients with humoral deficiency from either qualitative or quantitative mechanism are at heightened risk of infection with encapsulated bacteria, including Streptococcus pneumoniae, Haemophilus influenzae, and Neisseria meningitidis, which exploit their polysaccharide capsule to resist phagocytosis in the absence of the targeted opsonizing antibodies. Recognition of this specific vulnerability should inform prophylactic vaccination strategies and empiric antimicrobial selection in this population.

Immune reprogramming

The advent of immune effector cell therapy has created a unique category of immune dysregulation that may include cytokine excess, immune exhaustion via PD-1 axis activation and a mixed hyper and hypoinflammatory state. Of note, chimeric antigen receptor (CAR)-T cell therapy exploits the same cytotoxic mechanisms described earlier to eliminate tumor cells; however, T cell activation may simultaneously trigger pathologic cytokine release, producing sepsis-mimicking syndromes including cytokine release syndrome (CRS) and immune effector cell-associated neurotoxicity syndrome (ICANS), which add to the diagnostic complexity and ambiguity at the bedside.

Current Framework Limitations

Categorization of immunosuppression according to disease categorization versus immune dysfunction has limitations. Disease-based classification frameworks lack the mechanistic specificity required to individualize treatment decisions or inform targeted drug development. Immune defect-based frameworks aim to address this granularity, but the coexistence of multiple parallel mechanisms of immunosuppression means that the dominant immune defect precipitating infection at the time of clinical presentation currently cannot be determined. Validated biomarkers to stratify patients according to immune defect for patient enrollment in clinical trials are currently not available. Efforts to quantify immune dysfunction—monocyte human leukocyte antigen-DR isotype (HLA-DR) expression, ex vivo endotoxin challenge, cytokine profiling, programmed cell death 1/programmed cell death 1 ligand 1 (PD-1/PD-L1) expression—currently remain investigational.[9] Many immune-paralysis constructs are derived from small studies and lack longitudinal validation in immunocompromised cohorts. In addition, the fluidity of immune phenotypes with class switching observed in immunocompetent populations has not been rigorously studied in immunocompromised patients; however likely also exists.[10] An additional complexity is survivorship. When does a patient cured of lymphoma cease to be immunocompromised? These questions remain unanswered.

EPIDEMIOLOGY OF SEPSIS IN THE IMMUNOCOMPROMISED HOST

The epidemiology of sepsis is evolving in parallel with transformative advances in cancer therapeutics, transplantation, and immune-modifying agents. Current estimates indicate that 6.6% of adults in the United States were immunocompromised in 2021 based on reported health conditions, prescription medications, and medical treatments, representing a substantial increase from 2.7% in 2013.[2] Up to 15% of ICU patients in European registries carry a cancer diagnosis.[11,12] This expanding demographic is driven, in part, by the increasing use of immunosuppressive medications.

Notably, cancer-specific mortality has declined substantially, with a 33% reduction since 1991 attributable to advances in preventive strategies, alongside the development of novel therapeutics. Despite these gains, patients with cancer face a nearly ten-fold greater risk of developing sepsis compared with the general population, constituting a vulnerable and growing subpopulation with substantial health care resource needs. A large epidemiologic study by Yang and colleagues, examining emergency department utilization in the United States from 2006 to 2012, identified approximately 4 million annual adult emergency visits involving patients with active cancer diagnoses, of whom 60% were admitted primarily for severe infections and associated complications.[13]

Resource utilization and clinical outcomes are not uniform across malignancy types however, with considerable heterogeneity even within the hematological malignancy population. Among patients with solid organ tumors, sepsis-related mortality accounts for approximately 9% of all deaths, with the highest mortality rates (5%–13%) observed in the context of severe infections complicating postchemotherapy neutropenia. In contrast, 12% to 27% of patients with hematological malignancies develop sepsis within the first year of diagnosis, with an associated in-hospital mortality rate of 14%.[14,15] The incidence of severe sepsis is approximately 5 times higher among recipients of hematopoietic stem cell transplantation compared with hospitalized patients without a history of hematopoietic stem cell or solid organ transplantation.[16] Collectively, these data underscore the growing public health significance of immunosuppression.

UNDERSTANDING THE PATHOPHYSIOLOGY OF SEPSIS IN IMMUNOCOMPROMISED PATIENTS

The pathophysiology of sepsis is characterized by a dysregulated immune response to infection, involving the synchronized activation and cross-talk between the innate and adaptive immune systems. The rapid, nonspecific effector functions of innate immunity followed by the sophisticated and targeting adaptive immune response, are both amplified by proinflammatory cascades mediated by cytokines, coagulation factors, and markers of endothelial and epithelial injury. This inflammatory cascade underlies the immune dysregulation hypothesis central to sepsis pathobiology and has been implicated in driving deleterious vasodilation, microvascular leak, microthrombotic formation, and acute organ injury. A concurrent anti-inflammatory response also exists, which may, when persistently dysregulated, contribute to subacute adaptive immune exhaustion and heightened susceptibility to secondary infections.

The determinants of the host immune response to infection are numerous and likely encompass a broad range of endogenous and exogenous factors, including genetic composition, age, biological sex, comorbidities, metabolic state, prior microbial exposure, and concurrent medications. The interplay of these variables gives rise to profound interindividual heterogeneity in immune response. Over the past decade, significant progress has been made in characterizing this heterogeneity through the discovery of molecular phenotypes of sepsis. Approaches leveraging plasma protein biomarkers, transcriptomics, and metabolomics combined with unsupervised clustering techniques have identified biologically distinct patient subgroups with differential risks of adverse outcomes and heterogeneity in treatment effects with supportive and targeted therapies. Collaborative efforts, such as the Subtyping in Sepsis and Critical Illness Consortium, aim to harmonize findings across independent research groups to define generalizable patient cohorts characterized by distinct molecular pathways and immune cell-specific dysregulation.[17] These initiatives hold promise for a biology-driven classification framework that may inform future prospective targeted trials to test novel and supportive interventions. However, phenotypic frameworks have been derived in immunocompetent patient cohorts shaped by carefully curated inclusion criteria and therefore may not be generalizable immunocompromised patients.

Efforts to address this gap are nonetheless emerging. Notably, studies by Ronner and colleagues and Weingart and colleagues have investigated how baseline perturbations in host immune function may influence molecular phenotype assignment and its generalizability.[18,19] Both studies examined the performance of the inflammatory subphenotypes of sepsis, developed by Calfee and colleagues. Weingart and colleagues examined the relationship between immunocompromised status and subphenotype assignment, demonstrating that patients with hematological malignancies were disproportionately classified as hyperinflammatory and that this phenotype was significantly associated with impaired survival. Interestingly, elevated cytokine levels of interleukin (IL)-8, a powerful neutrophil chemoattractant, emerged as a key determinant of phenotype assignment in this population, highlighting retained mechanistic relevance even in patients who are often plagued by neutropenia. Ronner and colleagues found that unlike in immunocompetent cohorts, parsimonious models incorporating IL-6 and IL-8 inconsistently predicted hospital mortality and discordantly classified patients by inflammatory phenotype, particularly among those with leukemia. Collectively, these studies suggest that immunocompromised patients may not easily mirror existing sepsis phenotypes. Simply put, the assumption that immunocompromised patients are uniformly hypoinflammatory is overly simplistic. In reality, what may exist is a phenotypic spectrum that spans various categories including hyperinflammatory, hypoinflammatory, mixed hyper–hypo and immunoparalysis. Temporal evolution likely occurs, but longitudinal data in immunocompromised cohorts are sparse.

DIAGNOSTICS AND CHALLENGES

Early recognition of sepsis in immunocompromised patients is fraught with challenges. Clinical presentations may differ substantially from that of immunocompetent patients leading to delays in diagnosis and initiation of time-sensitive interventions. Immune-modulating medications can further distort or mask the cardinal features of infection. Classic findings such as fever and leukocytosis become unreliable diagnostic markers in this context: corticosteroids may suppress fever, while lymphoproliferative disorders can produce noninfectious pyrexia. Similarly, the hallmark local inflammatory signs of erythema, pain, warmth, and swelling may be attenuated due to an impaired inflammatory response. Neutropenia may both minimize the clinical manifestations of infection and paradoxically worsen during the recovery phase—a phenomenon most prominently described in patients with hematological malignancy with acute respiratory failure.[20]

Conventional biomarkers, including C-reactive protein (CRP), procalcitonin, and leukocyte count, although lacking robust evidence even in the immune competent patient, may be even less sensitive and specific for signaling infection in immunocompromised patients. Alternative biomarkers, such as midregional proadrenomedullin (MR-proADM) however may represent a potentially valuable emerging biomarker in this population. Adrenomedullin is a potent vasodilator and endothelial barrier stabilizer that regulates vascular tone, reduces vascular permeability, and modulates inflammation. During sepsis, circulating levels rise dramatically within hours, reflecting a compensatory response to endothelial dysfunction, vascular leak, and vasodilation. MR-proADM has demonstrated superior performance compared with CRP for the prediction of bloodstream infection and sepsis in immunocompromised patients with cancer,[21] and has also shown prognostic utility in predicting clinical outcomes and treatment response.[22]

Pulmonary infections are the most common source of sepsis in immunocompromised patients and carry significant implications for morbidity and mortality. Accordingly, diagnostic strategies aimed at early identification of pulmonary infection and causative pathogen should be prioritized in this population. Radiographical assessment using chest X-ray imaging has limited sensitivity and specificity for detecting pulmonary infiltrates and may be difficult to distinguish from competing diagnosis that is, drug-related toxicity or radiation injury; therefore, low-dose computed tomography has demonstrated superior diagnostic performance.[23] Evidence behind the utility of lung ultrasound in this population is currently lack. The diagnostic yield of noninvasive testing has improved substantially with the introduction of more sensitive molecular diagnostics, including polymerase chain reaction (PCR)-based assays. However, these tests are characterized by high sensitivity at the expense of specificity, and the clinical significance of a positive result is thus not always certain. This is well illustrated by PCR detection of pneumocystis jirovecii (PJP) and Aspergillus species, both of which may yield positive results even when the burden of these organisms are very low. Asymptomatic colonization with both PJP and Aspergillus is well documented in immunocompromised patients, particularly in the presence of structural lung disease or recent corticosteroid exposure, rendering the distinction between colonization and active infection clinically challenging. Identifying the underlying etiology of acute respiratory failure remains undetermined in 10% to 15% of cases and is of paramount importance as it is independently associated with increased mortality.[24] While fiberoptic bronchoscopy is one invasive diagnostic strategy often employed when noninvasive tests fail to identify a diagnosis, it may be limited by low yield to assist in narrowing down antimicrobials if broad spectrum antimicrobials have already commenced or be associated with clinical deterioration in the setting of high oxygen requirements.[25] Its utility is maintained if ruling out noninfectious causes (such as diffuse alveolar hemorrhage) or identifying organisms that may not be covered by traditional broad spectrum antimicrobials (ie, Stenotrophomonas, PJP, fungal infections, Cytomegalovirus). The pursuit of tissue pathology to make a diagnosis using lung biopsy has been explored in a limited number of studies. Although some studies report achieving a diagnostic yield exceeding 60%, this is balanced with a complication rate of approximately 10% even with careful patient selection (and as high as 25% in ventilated patients).[26–28] This diagnostic yield is further reduced in patients receiving invasive ventilation. Given this unfavorable risk-benefit profile, lung biopsy is generally not recommended in critically ill patients who are ventilated.

Finally, several noninfectious conditions may closely mimic sepsis, presenting with fever, multi-organ dysfunction, and elevated inflammatory biomarkers. These include CRS following CAR-T cell or bispecific antibody therapy, tumor lysis syndrome, hemophagocytic lymphohistiocytosis, and engraftment syndrome. Careful clinical and laboratory evaluation is essential to differentiate these entities from true infectious sepsis, as their management differs substantially (**Fig. 2**).

EARLY IDENTIFICATION OF SEPSIS

Early identification of sepsis in immunocompromised patients is particularly challenging, yet critically important, because delayed recognition may rapidly translate into irreversible organ dysfunction and excess mortality. Compared with immunocompetent patients, immunocompromised hosts often have reduced physiologic reserve and atypical clinical manifestations, narrowing the window in which timely intervention can alter outcomes.

Timing of ICU referral is a major determinant of prognosis. Patients initially considered "too well" for ICU admission but subsequently transferred after deterioration have significantly worse outcomes, with mortality rates reported as high as 62% in delayed admissions compared with substantially lower rates among those admitted earlier in the disease course.[4,5] Each additional day spent on the ward before ICU transfer is associated with incremental increases in mortality, underscoring the importance of early recognition and proactive triage.[5]

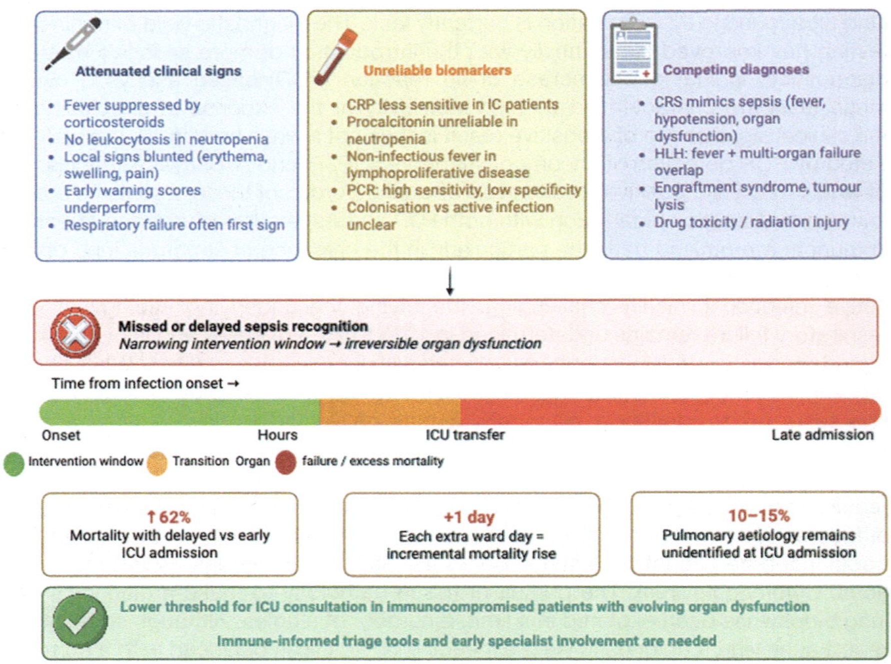

Fig. 2. Challenges and considerations in the identification of sepsis in immunocompromised patients. CRP, C reactive protein; CRS, cytokine release syndrome; ICU, intensive care unit; PCR, polymerase chain reaction. (*Created in* MS Power Point and pictograms were taken from SERVIER MEDICAL ART. Servier Medical Art is licensed under CC BY 4.0.)

Conventional early warning tools may underperform in immunocompromised populations. In patients with hematologic malignancies, deterioration is often driven by early respiratory failure rather than circulatory collapse, and traditional triggers such as fever or leukocytosis may be absent. Modified scoring systems incorporating oxygenation parameters, such as the peripheral oxygen saturation (SpO_2)/fraction of inspired oxygen (FiO_2) ratio, have demonstrated improved discrimination in this population.[29]

Taken together, these data support a lower threshold for ICU consultation and admission in immunocompromised patients with evolving organ dysfunction. Future work should focus on developing and validating triage tools tailored specifically to this population.

SEPSIS MANAGEMENT-UNIQUE CONSIDERATIONS

The fundamental principles of sepsis management remain applicable in immunocompromised patients; however, each domain is complicated by altered pathogen range, competing diagnoses, and uncertainty regarding optimal immunosuppression management.

Empiric antimicrobial therapy: Empiric therapy is typically broader, reflecting increased risk of resistant bacterial pathogens, invasive fungal infections, and viral reactivation. Given this, it remains imperative to obtain microbiologic samples to identify the culprit pathogen before or soon after the initiation of antimicrobial therapy to tailor treatment and minimize excess duration of broad therapy. Risk-adapted strategies for invasive fungal infection diagnosis and prevention in immunocompromised hosts have been advocated in this population,[30] while epidemiologic data highlight the substantial burden of opportunistic infections in transplant and oncology populations.[31,32] Broader therapy; however, must be balanced against risks of microbiome disruption, resistance, drug–drug interactions and organ toxicities. This is particularly relevant for azole antifungals, which interact with calcineurin inhibitors and other immunosuppressants. Evidence supporting biomarker-guided de-escalation (eg, procalcitonin) remains limited in neutropenic populations, and extrapolation from immunocompetent cohorts should be approached cautiously.[7]

Hemodynamic and organ support: Optimal fluid and vasopressor strategies in immunocompromised patients are not well defined. Current practice is extrapolated from general sepsis guidelines (Surviving Sepsis Campaign).[7] Mortality increases significantly once organ failure develops—particularly among patients with cancer—highlighting the importance of early recognition, timely hemodynamic support, adequate resuscitation, and supporting consideration of early ICU admission.

Immunosuppression management: Balancing continuation versus interruption of immunosuppressive therapy is complex and highly context-dependent. Data from rheumatologic populations suggest that continuation of certain immunomodulators during infection may be safe in selected patients[33] although extrapolation to transplant and malignancy populations remains uncertain. Abrupt withdrawal may precipitate graft rejection, or autoimmune flare whereas continuation may impair pathogen clearance. In the setting of cancer, if subsequent rounds of chemotherapy were scheduled—these may be delayed until infection clearance. Engaging the specialist in the immunocompromised subspecialty is necessary to guide decision making regarding immunosuppression management.

Corticosteroids: Major trials of corticosteroids in septic shock included few profoundly immunocompromised patients, and subgroup data are lacking.[7] Whether steroid responsiveness differs by immune phenotype or baseline immunosuppression remains unknown.

Growth-colony stimulating factor (G-CSF): Meta-analyses have not demonstrated consistent mortality benefit in sepsis with the use of G-CSF, although faster neutrophil recovery is observed.[34] Current oncology guidelines recommend selective use in high-risk febrile neutropenia,[35] rather than routine use in all septic patients.

Granulocyte transfusions: While evidence remains limited, preliminary studies demonstrate the possible role of granulocyte transfusions in select patients with severe neutropenia with refractory infection and anticipated marrow recovery.[36] Their role in critically ill patients is uncertain.

Immune modulation: Emerging strategies—including interferon-γ, checkpoint modulation, and immune adjuvant therapies—aim to restore immune competence. However, without validated tools to define immune state, the risk of misaligned therapy (eg, augmenting inflammation in hyperinflammatory states) remains possible.[37] Current phenotyping strategies remain incompletely validated and as a result, not yet ready for routine bedside use.

Future trials should prioritize biomarker-guided and phenotype-driven designs rather than syndromic enrollment.

SEPSIS MIMICKERS

A major diagnostic challenge is distinguishing infection from noninfectious inflammatory syndromes. Conditions such as CRS, hemophagocytic lymphohistiocytosis (HLH), engraftment syndrome, and tumor lysis syndrome may closely mimic sepsis, presenting with fever, shock, and multiorgan dysfunction. These syndromes are particularly relevant in patients receiving modern immunotherapies, including CAR-T cell therapy.[38] Failure to distinguish these entities may result in inappropriate therapy. For example, CRS requires immunomodulatory treatment (eg, tocilizumab), whereas delayed antimicrobial therapy in true sepsis is associated with worse outcomes.

Given the overlap, diagnosis requires integration of clinical trajectory, treatment exposure, microbiologic data, and disease-specific biomarkers. In many cases, early management may require simultaneous empiric antimicrobial therapy and investigation for immune-mediated syndromes (**Table 2**).

OUTCOMES

Outcomes following sepsis in immunocompromised patients have improved but remain heterogeneous. ICU mortality in patients with malignancy ranges from approximately 40% to 60% depending on disease type and severity of organ failure.[6,39] One-year mortality remains high, particularly among patients with hematologic malignancies. Importantly, contemporary data challenge the perception that critical illness in these patients is uniformly futile. Selected patients may achieve outcomes comparable to immunocompetent populations when adjusted for illness severity.[39] Survival alone, however, is insufficient as an endpoint. Functional recovery, quality of life, and ability to resume disease-directed therapy are increasingly recognized as critical outcomes.[40] These considerations are particularly relevant in oncology populations, where ICU survival may serve as a bridge to further treatment. Prognostication should therefore incorporate not only acute illness severity but also reversibility of the underlying condition and patient-centered goals. Delayed ICU admission and therapeutic nihilism may adversely influence outcomes, reinforcing the importance of timely and individualized care. Future research priorities can assist in improving ICU outcomes of this population (**Table 3**).

Table 2
Sepsis mimickers in the immunocompromised host

Syndrome	Clinical Context	Key Clinical Features	Distinguishing Clues	Diagnostic Tests	Initial Management
CRS	CAR-T, bispecific antibodies	Fever, hypotension, hypoxia	Temporal relationship to immunotherapy; very high ferritin/CRP	IL-6 (if available), ferritin	Tocilizumab ± steroids
HLH	Heme malignancy, infection, autoimmune disease	Fever, cytopenias, organ failure	Ferritin often >10,000; hepatosplenomegaly; hypertriglyceridemia	Ferritin, triglycerides, sCD25	Steroids ± etoposide
Engraftment Syndrome	Post-HSCT (neutrophil recovery phase)	Fever, rash, pulmonary edema	Occurs at neutrophil recovery; noninfectious	Clinical diagnosis	Steroids
Tumor Lysis Syndrome	Hem malignancy, high tumor burden	AKI, arrhythmia, metabolic abnormality	Hyperuricemia, hyperkalemia, hyperphosphatemia	Electrolytes, uric acid	Fluids, rasburicase
Drug Reaction (DRESS, SJS/TEN)	New medication	Fever, rash, organ dysfunction	Eosinophilia, skin findings	Clinical ± biopsy	Stop drug ± steroids
Vasculitis Flare	Autoimmune disease	Fever, organ dysfunction	Known disease; ANCA or complement abnormalities	Autoimmune panel	Immunosuppression
Leukemic progression	Hem malignancy	Cytopenias, fever	Blasts on smear, marrow progression	Peripheral smear, bone marrow	Disease-directed therapy
Immune checkpoint toxicity	ICI therapy	Pneumonitis, colitis, hepatitis	Subacute course, exposure to ICI	Imaging, labs	Steroids

Abbreviations: AKI, acute kidney injury; ANCA, anti-neutrophil cytoplasmic antibody; CART, Chimeric antigen receptor T cell therapy; DRESS, Drug reaction with eosinophilia and systemic symptoms; ICI, immune checkpoint inhibitor; SJS/TEN, Stevens-Johnson syndrome/Toxic epidermal necrolysis.

Table 3
Research gaps

Domain	Key Gap	Why It Matters	Proposed Direction
Definitions of immunocompromise	No consensus classification	Heterogeneous cohorts limit trials	Standardized, immune-based taxonomy (beyond disease labels)
Immune phenotyping	Static, single time-point measures	Immune state is dynamic	Longitudinal profiling (transcriptomics, biomarkers)
Trial inclusion	Underrepresentation in randomized controlled trial (RCTs)	Poor generalizability of guidelines	Dedicated trials or enriched subgroups
Precision antimicrobials	Overuse vs under-treatment	Resistance, toxicity, microbiome disruption	Biomarker-guided duration and de-escalation
Infection vs inflammation	Poor discrimination (eg, CRS vs sepsis)	Delayed or inappropriate therapy	Integrated diagnostic frameworks
Steroid strategies	One-size-fits-all approach	Variable immune phenotypes	Immune-aligned steroid use (phenotype-guided)
Microbiome preservation	Antibiotic-driven dysbiosis	Secondary infection risk	Microbiome-sparing strategies
ICU triage tools	Existing tools underperform	Delayed ICU admission worsens outcomes	Tailored prediction models (eg, oxygenation-based)
ICU admission thresholds	Variable across centers	Impacts mortality	Early escalation strategies
Prognostication	Survival-focused metrics	Ignores functional recovery	Long-term, patient-centered outcomes

SUMMARY

In summary, sepsis in immunocompromised patients represents a fundamentally distinct clinical entity, shaped by altered host defenses, unique pathogen profiles, and competing risks related to the underlying disease and its treatment. These differences challenge conventional sepsis paradigms and underscore the need for tailored diagnostic, prognostic, and therapeutic approaches. Advancing care in this population will require integration of clinical insight with biologic understanding to move toward more precise and individualized management strategies.

CLINICS CARE POINTS

- Pearl: Early ICU referral is often more important than the underlying immunocompromising diagnosis in determining outcome.

- Pitfall: Excluding sepsis because fever, leukocytosis, or elevated inflammatory biomarkers are absent.
- Pearl: Frame the patient according to their dominant immune defect (barrier disruption, innate dysfunction, adaptive dysfunction, or immune reprogramming) to guide diagnostic testing and empiric therapy.
- Pitfall: Attributing all fever and shock to infection without considering immune-mediated syndromes such as CRS or HLH.
- Pearl: In acute respiratory failure, prioritize early high-yield diagnostics and pursue a microbiologic diagnosis whenever possible before prolonged exposure to broad-spectrum antimicrobials.

DISCLOSURE

No conflicts to declare.

REFERENCES

1. Deinhardt-Emmer S, Chousterman BG, Schefold JC, et al. Sepsis in patients who are immunocompromised: diagnostic challenges and future therapies. Lancet Respir Med 2025;13(7):623–37.
2. Martinson ML, Lapham J. Prevalence of immunosuppression among US adults. JAMA 2024;331(10):880–2.
3. Boomer JS, To K, Chang KC, et al. Immunosuppression in patients who die of sepsis and multiple organ failure. JAMA 2011;306(23):2594–605.
4. Thiéry G, Azoulay E, Darmon M, et al. Outcome of cancer patients considered too well for intensive care unit admission. J Clin Oncol 2005;23(19):4404–9.
5. Metaxa V, Anandanadesan R, Hussain A, et al. Outcome of critically ill patients with haematological malignancies referred to critical care: impact of timing of admission. J Intensive Care Soc 2015;16(3):195–202.
6. Dumas G, Darmon M, Kouatchet A, et al. Intensive care unit outcomes in patients with malignancies. Crit Care Med 2014;42(7):1586–95.
7. Prescott HC, Antonelli M, Alhazzani W, et al. Surviving sepsis campaign: international guidelines for management of sepsis and septic shock 2026. Crit Care Med 2026;54(4):725–812.
8. Torres LK, Pickkers P, van der Poll T. Sepsis-induced immunosuppression. Annu Rev Physiol 2022;84:157–81.
9. van der Poll T, Shankar-Hari M, Wiersinga WJ. The immunology of sepsis. Immunity 2021;54(11):2450–64.
10. Shankar-Hari M, Bos L, Derde L, et al. Defining and categorizing immunocompromised patients in critical care. Lancet Respir Med 2025;13(7):e45–58.
11. Taccone FS, Artigas AA, Sprung CL, et al, SOAP Study Investigators. Characteristics and outcomes of cancer patients in European ICUs. Crit Care 2009; 13(1):R15.
12. Puxty K, McLoone P, Quasim T, et al. Survival in solid cancer patients following intensive care unit admission. Intensive Care Med 2014;40(10):1409–28.
13. Rivera DR, Gallicchio L, Brown J, et al. Emergency department visits among cancer patients in the United States, 2006–2012. PLoS One 2018;13(8):e0201465.
14. Williams MD, Azoulay E, Dabbagh O, et al. Cancer patients in the intensive care unit: outcomes and predictors of mortality. Crit Care Clin 2010;26(1):1–20.

15. Kuderer NM, Dale DC, Crawford J, et al. Clinical impact of febrile neutropenia in patients with cancer. Cancer 2006;106(10):2258–66.
16. Kumar G, Ahmad S, Taneja A, et al. Severe sepsis in hematopoietic stem cell transplant recipients. Crit Care Med 2015;43(2):411–21.
17. Moore AR, Zheng H, Ganesan A, et al. A consensus immune dysregulation framework for sepsis and critical illnesses. Nat Med 2025;31(12):4084–96.
18. Ronner L, Giannini HM, Miano TA, et al. Inflammatory phenotypes in immunocompromised patients with sepsis. Crit Care Med 2024;52(5):e321–32.
19. Weingart MF, Willmore A, Zhuo H, et al. Hyperinflammatory and hypoinflammatory subphenotypes in immunocompromised sepsis. Crit Care Med 2024;52(8): e457–68.
20. Gudiol C, Royo-Cebrecos C, Laporte-Amargós J, et al. Clinical features, etiology and outcomes of infections in neutropenic cancer patients. Front Med 2021;8: 660088.
21. Debiane L, Hachem RY, Al Wohoush I, et al. Prognostic value of proadrenomedullin in critically ill patients with cancer and sepsis. Crit Care Med 2014;42(12): 2503–11.
22. Christ-Crain M, Morgenthaler NG, Stolz D, et al. Pro-adrenomedullin to predict severity and outcome in community-acquired pneumonia. Crit Care 2005;9(6): R816–24.
23. Self WH, Courtney DM, McNaughton CD, et al. High discordance of chest x-ray and computed tomography for detection of pulmonary opacities in ED patients: implications for diagnosing pneumonia. AJEM (Am J Emerg Med) 2013;31(2): 401–5.
24. Azoulay E, Russell L, Van de Louw A, et al. Diagnosis of severe respiratory infections in immunocompromised patients. Intensive Care Med 2020;46(2):298–314.
25. Bauer PR, Chevret S, Yadav H, et al. Diagnostic yield and safety of bronchoscopy in immunocompromised patients with acute respiratory failure: a secondary analysis of the EFRAIM study. Intensive Care Med 2019;45(5):638–49.
26. Azoulay E, Mokart D, Lambert J, et al. Diagnostic strategy for hematology and oncology patients with acute respiratory failure: randomized clinical trial (EPIC). JAMA 2015;314(16):1711–9.
27. Papazian L, Doddoli C, Chetaille B. Diagnostic yield and safety of open lung biopsy in ICU patients with acute respiratory failure. Crit Care Med 2007;35(1): 103–7.
28. Wong AK, Walkey AJ. Open lung biopsy in critically ill patients with diffuse lung disease: a systematic review. Ann Thorac Surg 2015;100(6):1976–82.
29. Lee JR, Jung YK, Kim HJ, et al. Modified early warning score with SpO_2/FiO_2 ratio predicts ICU admission in hematologic malignancy patients. Korean J Intern Med 2020;35(6):1424–33.
30. Wahab A. Diagnosis and prevention of invasive fungal infections in the immunocompromised host. Chest 2022;162(6):1416–30.
31. Neofytos D, Fishman JA, Horn D, et al. Epidemiology and outcome of invasive fungal infections in transplant recipients. Transpl Infect Dis 2019;21(5):e13214.
32. Pagano L, Busca A, Candoni A, et al. Risk stratification for invasive fungal infections in patients with hematological malignancies: SEIFEM recommendations. Blood Rev 2017;31(2):17–29.
33. Clinical Infectious Diseases Study Group. Continuation versus temporary interruption of immunomodulatory therapy during infection in rheumatoid arthritis. Clin Infect Dis 2025;80(3):e210–8.

34. Clark OA, Lyman GH, Castro AA, et al. Colony-stimulating factors for chemotherapy-induced febrile neutropenia: a meta-analysis. J Clin Oncol 2005; 23(18):4198–214.
35. Lehrnbecher T, Robinson P, Fisher B, et al. Guideline for the management of fever and neutropenia in children with cancer and hematopoietic stem-cell transplantation recipients. J Clin Oncol 2017;35(18):2082–94.
36. Price TH, Boeckh M, Harrison RW, et al. Efficacy of transfusion with granulocytes from G-CSF/dexamethasone–treated donors in neutropenic patients with infection (RING study). Blood 2015;126(18):2153–61.
37. Cafferkey J, Shankar-Hari M. Informative subtyping of patients with sepsis. Semin Respir Crit Care Med 2024;45(4):516–22.
38. Chemaly RF. Viral infections in immunocompromised hosts. Hematology Am Soc Hematol Educ Program 2021;2021(1):173–80.
39. Azoulay E, Soares M, Darmon M, et al. Intensive care of the cancer patient: recent achievements and remaining challenges. Ann Intensive Care 2011;1(1):5.
40. Benguerfi S, Messéant O, Painvin B, et al. Factors associated with cancer treatment resumption after ICU stay in patients with solid tumors. Ann Intensive Care 2024;14(1):135.

Real-time Subgrouping of Sepsis and Systemic Inflammatory Syndromes

Ross McMullan, MB BCh, BAO[a,*],
Sivasubramanium V. Bhavani, MD[b],
Pratik Sinha, MB ChB, PhD, FFICM, FRCEM[c]

KEYWORDS

• Sepsis • Phenotype • Precision medicine • Biomarkers • Decision support systems • Clinical • Machine learning

KEY POINTS

- Syndromic definitions aggregate biologically distinct patients which dilute treatment effects and undermines bedside actionability.
- Reproducible sepsis subgroups exist across clinical, protein biomarker-based, omics, and microbiology-informed dimensions.
- Trajectory-based subtyping may provide additional dynamic insights beyond static subgroups.
- A 2-stage pipeline can combine real-time assessment of sepsis subgroup eligibility with continually updated subgroup classification.
- Prospective validation of real-time subtyping pipelines is required to enable robust precision medicine.

INTRODUCTION

Despite decades of investment in therapeutics, guidelines and management pathways,[1] sepsis remains a leading cause of death worldwide.[2] A central barrier to progress is the marked biological and clinical heterogeneity encompassed by the syndromic label of sepsis,[3] such that patients meeting the same clinical definition can differ substantially in upstream drivers such as infection site and pathogen burden. Patients also exhibit distinct downstream pathophysiological processes

[a] School of Medicine, Dentistry and Biomedical Sciences, Wellcome-Wolfson Institute for Experimental Medicine, Queen's University of Belfast, Belfast, UK; [b] Department of Medicine, Emory University, Atlanta, GA, USA; [c] Department of Anesthesia, Washington University in St. Louis, St Louis, MO, USA
* Corresponding author.
E-mail address: rmcmullan07@qub.ac.uk

Crit Care Clin 42 (2026) 839–855
https://doi.org/10.1016/j.ccc.2026.05.008 **criticalcare.theclinics.com**

Abbreviations	
AKI	acute kidney injury
ARDS	acute respiratory distress syndrome
EHR	electronic health record
PCM	parsimonious classifier model
SRS	sepsis response signature

including dysregulated inflammation, endothelial injury and dysregulated coagulation, with different clinical trajectories and outcomes.[4–6] This profound heterogeneity attenuates treatment effects in trials and has contributed to repeated failures of broadly applied interventions.[7] Consequently, the label of sepsis has limited bedside utility for mechanistic stratification.

A precision medicine approach to sepsis requires moving beyond broad syndromic labels toward clinically actionable subgroups. The aim of subgroup discovery is to identify reproducible patient cohorts that are associated with differences in outcomes and treatment response, and ideally, have distinct biology that would permit targeted intervention. Over the past decade, data-driven analyses have consistently identified such subgroups using disparate datatypes.[8,9] Importantly, analytical frameworks have employed multivariate modeling to identify these subgroups, which logically, given that sepsis is a systems biology problem, is advantageous compared to the use of a single variable, which had been the historical approach to stratifying sepsis. Most of the described subtyping approaches have leveraged data from a single cross-sectional timepoint, yet sepsis is highly dynamic and phasic.[10,11] A growing body of work is using longitudinal data to identify subgroups, seeking to leverage the phasic changes seen in sepsis to identify trajectory-based subgroups. However, most work in this space has been retrospective, relied on research-grade assays, and/or required high-fidelity data at multiple timepoints. Therefore, a central challenge in realizing the clinical potential of sepsis subgrouping is deploying these complex multivariable models to assign patients to subgroups early, reliably and at scale.

This article summarizes evidence for sepsis subgroups, examines longitudinal subtyping methods, and describes the practical requirements for real-time subtyping implementation. Terminology in this field is inconsistently applied, and nascent. For clarity and simplicity, throughout this article, subgroup is used as an umbrella term for reproducible patient subtypes. When discussing individual studies, the terminology used by the original authors is retained. Key terms used throughout this article are summarized in **Table 1**.

OVERVIEW OF SEPSIS SUBGROUPS

Reproducible sepsis subgroups have been described using clinical data, protein biomarker-based approaches, transcriptomics, and microbiology-informed dimensions (**Fig. 1**). This section summarizes key evidence and feasibility for real-time assignment.

Clinical-Data Derived Subgroups

Clinical phenotyping assigns subgroups using routinely available bedside and electronic health record (EHR) variables including demographic data, comorbidities, vital signs, and standard laboratory tests. Seymour and colleagues derived 4 clinical sepsis phenotypes using early physiologic, laboratory, and organ dysfunction features.[8] In a

Table 1
Standardized terminology

Term	Definition
Subgroup	Umbrella term for a reproducible patient cluster identified within a defined population
Phenotype	A group of patients with a shared set of observable or measurable characteristics[12]
Subphenotype	A subgroup that shares features distinguishing it from other patients within a phenotype[12]
Endotype	Subgroup defined by a distinct underlying biological mechanism or pathway that helps explain the observed clinical pattern[12]
Cross-sectional subtyping	Single-time-point subgroup assignment using a prespecified early time window, without subsequent updating[13]
Trajectory-based subtyping	Trajectory-based subgroup assignment using longitudinal data, where membership can change as physiology and biomarkers evolve[14]

septic shock trial cohort, Aldewereld and colleagues identified 5 baseline clinical phenotypes using vital signs, routine laboratory tests, and organ dysfunction measures with 14-day all-cause mortality ranging from 7.9% to 36.3% across phenotypes and reported differences in clinical course.[15]

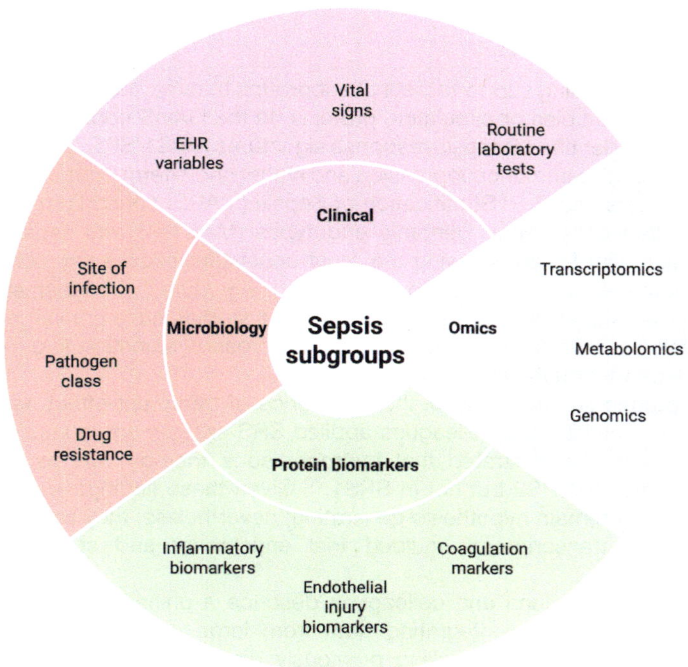

Fig. 1. Sepsis subgroups by framework and inputs. Clinical, protein biomarker-based, omics data and microbiology-informed approaches derive reproducible sepsis subgroups. Frameworks differ in input availability and mechanistic resolution supporting integrated real-time assignment. (*Created in* BioRender. O'Kane, C. (2026) https://BioRender.com/s77esnc.)

Clinical phenotypes offer the theoretic advantage of a simpler pathway to clinical implementation, albeit their lack of tethering to underlying biology may make identifying targeted therapy more challenging. Prospective implementation of clinical subgroups has nevertheless been limited.

Protein-Derived Subgroups

Biomarker-based subtyping has been used to define sepsis subgroups using early circulating markers of the host response that capture variation in systemic inflammation, endothelial injury and coagulopathy. In a representative analysis spanning 2 prospective cohorts, Sinha and colleagues identified a 2-class structure comprising Hyperinflammatory and Hypoinflammatory molecular phenotypes.[16] The Hyperinflammatory phenotype was characterized by higher cytokine concentrations associated with inflammation, coagulopathy, and endothelial dysfunction, greater shock severity, and worse outcomes.[16] Phenotypes were then assigned in PROWESS-SHOCK and VASST using validated classifier models applied to available biomarkers and clinical variables. Notably, treatment effect differed by phenotype for activated protein C in PROWESS-SHOCK, where treatment appeared to harm patients in the Hypoinflammatory phenotype and benefit patients in the Hyperinflammatory phenotype.[16] In a subsequent study of approximately 8000 mechanically ventilated patients with sepsis, the same investigators observed that gram-negative bacteraemia was one of the biggest predictors of the Hyperinflammatory signature, which in turn was contingent on the pathogen's burden, site of infection, and virulence.[17] In the secondary analysis of a prior trial, they observed differential treatment response in the phenotypes with polymyxin B hemoperfusion.[17]

Transcriptomic Subgroups

Transcriptomic profiling supports distinct subgroups that may not be fully captured by routine clinical variables or circulating proteins. In the GAinS consortium, Davenport and colleagues identified 2 sepsis response signatures (SRS1/SRS2), with SRS1 characterised by relative immunosuppression and higher short-term mortality.[18] In the Molecular Diagnosis and Risk Stratification of Sepsis (MARS) consortium, Scicluna and colleagues derived 4 sepsis genomic endotypes (Mars1–4) with separation in 28-day mortality, with Mars1 showing the most consistent excess risk across cohorts and characterized by an immune-suppressed signature.[9] Complementing these cohort-derived signatures, cross-cohort classifier studies have converged on broad immunobiological subgroups with separation in organ dysfunction and mortality risk across independent datasets.[19]

Transcriptomic subgroups also show evidence of treatment-effect heterogeneity. For example, Antcliffe and colleagues applied SRS assignment in septic shock trial participants and demonstrated that hydrocortisone therapy was associated with worse outcomes in SRS2 but not in SRS1.[20] Given these findings were in a subset of patients, they remain hypothesis-generating; nevertheless, they provide a foundation for future transcriptomic guided trial enrichment and stratified treatment evaluation.

More recently, Scicluna and colleagues describe a unified blood transcriptomic framework for sepsis by integrating data from large, well-characterized cohorts (MARS and GAinS) and reconciling previously disparate classification systems.[21] Through cross-cohort harmonization and network-based clustering, the authors identified 3 reproducible consensus transcriptomic subgroups (CTS1–3), each defined by distinct biological programs, including inflammatory/neutrophilic activation, heme and coagulopathic pathways, and interferon-driven adaptive immune responses. Notably, exploratory analyses suggested treatment heterogeneity in one subgroup (CTS2) with corticosteroids, once again in the VANISH trial.

Microbiology-Informed Subgroups

Microbiology-informed subtyping recognizes that sepsis heterogeneity is partly determined by upstream factors related to the infection. Zhao and colleagues compared a host-only model with a host–pathogen model that added 3 microbiology variables: site of infection, pathogen class and drug resistance. Inclusion of microbiology variables altered phenotype assignment and was associated with differences in outcomes and treatment-response signals.[22]

Candidate microbiology inputs for host–pathogen subtyping include infection site, organism class and measures of burden where available; however, culture-derived features are often delayed and show context-dependent associations with outcome, supporting their use as incremental evidence rather than stand-alone real-time stratifiers.[23,24]

SUBGROUPS ACROSS SYSTEMIC INFLAMMATORY SYNDROMES

Many actionable biological processes, such as inflammation, endotheliopathy, coagulopathy and immune dysfunction transcend syndromic labels,[25] and are also observed in acute respiratory distress syndrome (ARDS),[26] and acute kidney injury (AKI).[27] This cross-syndrome overlap raises the spectre of a unified prediction and subtyping approach across systemic inflammatory syndromes.

Acute Respiratory Distress Syndrome

ARDS subgroups are well described, with consistent identification of Hyperinflammatory and Hypoinflammatory subphenotypes in multiple studies with biological differences similar to those described above in sepsis.[26,28] These biological differences translate into clinically meaningful outcomes. Hyperinflammatory ARDS is associated with fewer ventilator-free days, fewer organ-failure–free days and higher mortality compared with the Hypoinflammatory subphenotype.[26] ARDS subtyping has also been used to explore heterogeneity of treatment effect. In secondary analyses of randomized trials, simvastatin therapy is associated with improved survival in the Hyperinflammatory subphenotype but not in the Hypoinflammatory subphenotype.[28] Differential treatment responses were also observed in these molecular phenotypes with positive end-expiratory pressure (PEEP) strategy in secondary analysis of a randomized trial[26] and an observational study.[29] While such analyses should be interpreted cautiously and require prospective confirmation, they have motivated phenotype-informed trial designs.

To make this phenotyping schema clinically actionable, parsimonious classifiers have been developed that combine small biomarker sets with routine physiology to approximate latent class membership.[30] Machine learning–based variable selection identified 6 key classifier variables (IL-8, IL-6, protein C, soluble TNF receptor-1, bicarbonate and vasopressor use) from which 3-variable and 4-variable logistic models were derived. The best-performing models reproduced latent class assignment with high accuracy in an independent validation cohort and preserved separation in clinical outcomes and treatment-response signals.

Acute Kidney Injury

AKI provides further proof-of-concept for biologically informed subtyping. In critically ill adults with AKI, latent class analysis identified two reproducible molecular subphenotypes distinguished primarily by endothelial dysfunction and inflammation, with the higher-risk subphenotype showing a greater risk of 7-day renal nonrecovery, defined as death, incident dialysis, or lack of resolution of AKI by day 7.[27] Parsimonious classifiers enabled practical assignment of subphenotype membership. In VASST, these subphenotypes showed differential response to vasopressin, with lower 90-day mortality in the lower-risk subphenotype.

In pediatric septic shock, the PERSEVERE biomarker panel has been used to identify patients at risk of severe sepsis-associated AKI and to distinguish those more likely to recover renal function.[31] Although this approach is better viewed as prognostic enrichment than subgroup discovery, it further supports the principle that early host-response profiling can refine renal risk stratification beyond conventional clinical variables alone.

Extending a parsimonious biomarker model derived from prior AKI subphenotyping work, Kiernan and colleagues applied it in a secondary analysis of CLOVERS and identified a sepsis subphenotype with greater endotheliopathy and inflammation that had higher 28-day mortality and fewer organ-support–free days with a liberal versus restrictive fluid strategy.[32]

CLINICAL IMPLEMENTATION OF CROSS-SECTIONAL SUBTYPING SCHEMES

Clinical Implementation of Molecular Phenotypes

Arguably, among the multivariate subtyping schemes described above, the Hyperinflammatory and Hypoinflammatory molecular phenotypes are closest to being operationalized in the clinical space. There are 2 specific challenges that needed overcoming for the clinical implementation of these phenotypes. First, the phenotypes were originally identified using latent class analysis models that comprised 20 to 35 variables that were standardized to the population mean.[16,26] Second, these models also comprise 6 to 8 protein biomarkers with almost all lacking clinical-grade assays.

To address this problem, investigators used unbiased variable selection approaches to identify several 3- to 4-variable parsimonious classifier models (PCMs) to help identify the phenotypes at the bedside.[30] The PCMs showed high performance metrics in validation sets comprising adult and pediatric ARDS[33–35] and in adult critically ill patients with sepsis.[16]

The reproducibility of these PCMs across multiple cohorts has motivated prospective evaluation of near-real-time implementation of molecular phenotypes. In the PHenotypes IN the Acute Respiratory Distress Syndrome trial (PHIND), plasma interleukin-6 (IL-6) and soluble tumor necrosis factor receptor-1 (sTNFR-1) were measured at enrollment using the Evidence MultiSTAT (Randox) near-patient immunoassay and combined with arterial bicarbonate in a validated parsimonious model to assign Hyperinflammatory and Hypoinflammatory ARDS subphenotypes in real-time.[36] Prospectively assigned Hyperinflammatory patients had substantially higher 60-day mortality than Hypoinflammatory patients, supporting the clinical relevance of bedside classification. Similar feasibility work is underway in the Sub-Phenotypes of ARDS using Rapid Prospective Classification study, embedded within the United States-based I-SPY network, which is evaluating real-time prospective biologic subphenotype assignment in severe acute respiratory failure using rapid biomarker testing on the Evidence MultiSTAT (Randox) and Ella (Bio-Techne) platforms (NCT04488081).[37] Building on this feasibility work, PANTHER is a Bayesian adaptive platform trial in acute hypoxaemic respiratory failure that incorporates real-time biologic classification at enrollment to enable phenotype-stratified evaluation of candidate therapies (ISRCTN81435672).[38]

While these innovations have enabled advancing molecular phenotype-informed trials, the tests are relatively expensive and may not be ubiquitously available. Novel approaches to molecular diagnostics and protein quantification, such as plasmonic fluor lateral flow assays,[39] electrochemical biosensors,[40] and microfluidics[41] are promising bioengineering innovations that may provide rapid and relatively inexpensive protein quantification (**Table 2**).

A second challenge to the translation of these models is inconsistent availability of technology that quantifies protein biomarkers at the bedside. To circumvent the need for rapid quantification of research protein biomarkers, Sinha and colleagues used only readily available clinical data to classify molecular phenotypes using a machine learning algorithm called XGBoost.[42] This model was trained to predict the Hyperinflammatory phenotype and showed good performance metrics in validation cohorts, including differential treatment responses in the 2 phenotypes for multiple therapies that included PEEP,[29] fluid management,[42] activated protein C,[16] and polymyxin B.[17]

Clinical Implementation of Transcript-Derived Subgroups

As with molecular phenotypes, transcriptomic subtyping studies have sought to compress high-dimensional clustering solutions into parsimonious gene sets that enable more rapid clinical classification.

Hector Wong arguably pioneered this field through a series of studies in pediatric sepsis that delineated a translational pathway from transcriptomic endotyping discovery to clinical applicability. Initial work identified 2 reproducible pediatric septic shock endotypes (A and B) based on coordinated gene-expression programs, with endotype A characterized by repression of adaptive immunity and glucocorticoid signaling and associated with higher mortality.[43] Subsequent studies demonstrated that these

Table 2
Emerging approaches for rapid protein quantification relevant to near-patient biomarker testing

Method	Principle of Protein Quantification	Relevance to Near-Patient Use
Plasmonically enhanced fluorescent lateral-flow assay	Antibody-based capture on a lateral-flow strip with plasmonically amplified fluorescent detection; signal intensity is related to protein concentration by calibration.	Rapid and potentially suitable for near-patient deployment
Electrochemical biosensor	Protein binding generates an electrical signal, such as amperometric, voltammetric, or impedimetric change, that is converted to concentration by calibration.	Offers high analytical sensitivity and strong potential for compact, miniaturized point-of-care formats, although clinical standardization and validation remain ongoing.
Automated microfluidic cartridge-based immunoassay	Automated cartridge-based sandwich immunoassay in microfluidic channels with fluorescent readout and assay-specific calibration.	Supports relatively rapid and standardized protein measurement with minimal hands-on processing, although platform-specific cartridges and instrumentation may limit flexibility and increase cost.

endotypes are biologically conserved and clinically relevant, extending across age groups and aligning with independently derived adult transcriptomic signatures such as the sepsis response signature (SRS).[44,45]

Sweeney and colleagues used large-scale transcriptomic integration to develop parsimonious classifiers of sepsis heterogeneity. In a multicohort meta-analysis across infectious and sterile inflammatory states, an 11-gene host-response signature was derived that distinguished infection from noninfectious inflammation across platforms and populations.[10] They subsequently used unsupervised transcriptomic analysis to identify 3 reproducible sepsis subgroups (Inflammopathic, Adaptive, and Coagulopathic) that were conserved across independent cohorts and associated with distinct immune and coagulation pathways, clinical severity and outcomes.[46] Together, these studies establish a coherent strategy in which cross-cohort harmonization can be used to identify sepsis signatures that are in turn identifiable via parsimonious gene-sets, bridging high-dimensional discovery with scalable clinical translation.

Likewise, the above-mentioned SRS, MARS, and CTS signatures of sepsis have all described parsimonious gene-sets that would theoretically allow rapid classification of the subgroups in critically ill patients. The residual challenge for the field for translating transcriptomics signatures to the bedside in sepsis involves using high-throughput molecular analysis that is rapid, reproducible, and relatively inexpensive that would allow prospective evaluation of therapies in transcriptomic subgroups in clinical trials. Antcliffe and colleagues have shown feasibility of prospective deployment of a parsimonious gene-set derived classifier across 17 intensive care units (ICUs) in Europe in 357 patients using an 11-gene panel measured on the FilmArray system at multiple timepoints after ICU admission, which they used to stratify patients into *high-risk* and *low-risk* groups.[47]

Notably, there are several commercial point-of-care platforms that appear to have the technical capabilities using reverse transcription with either loop-mediated isothermal amplification or polymerase chain reaction to quantify gene-expression rapidly at the bedside for the purpose of sepsis recognition and management, but not real-time phenotyping. Specifically, the Inflammatix TriVerity system, an FDA-cleared platform uses a 29-gene mRNA panel and machine learning algorithm to distinguish bacterial from viral infections. Similarly, the SeptiCyte RAPID utilizes a focused 4-gene signature to provide a *SeptiScore*, helping clinicians differentiate sepsis from noninfectious systemic inflammation. Other emerging technologies, such as the Sepset *lab-on-a-chip* microfluidic device, aim to automate the process further, offering a potentially scalable way to identify high-risk endotypes directly in the emergency department or ICU. Together, these tools demonstrate the potential of moving sepsis management toward a model of real-time precision medicine. All these tools, however, require prospective evaluation of validity and clinical utility.

TRAJECTORY-BASED SUBTYPING

In sepsis, host-response and organ dysfunction are dynamic and likely evolve over minutes to hours to days, influenced by source control, supportive care, and disease progression. Trajectory-based subtyping, therefore, aims to identify within-patient trajectories, which could support time-updated subgroup assignment.

Subgroups determined at single cross-sectional timepoints can be useful at presentation but cannot disambiguate whether the patient is improving or deteriorating, as similar signatures may be experienced despite different underlying risk. Trajectory-based approaches address this limitation by explicitly modeling direction and rate of change to identify underlying subgroups.

Vital Signs Trajectory Subgroups

Routinely captured vital signs can support dynamic subtyping in early sepsis.[14] Bhavani and colleagues derived 4 reproducible subphenotypes using vital signs recorded over the first 8 hours of hospital presentation and demonstrated meaningful separation in vasopressor use and 30-day mortality.[14] In secondary analyses using SMART trial data, subphenotype membership modified the association between balanced crystalloids and saline with Group D patients (hypotensive without accompanying elevations in heart rate, temperature, and respiratory rate) demonstrating lower 30-day mortality with balanced crystalloids than saline.[14] Based on these findings, there is now a prospective trial underway that is evaluating the efficacy of crystalloids versus saline among Group D patients in a randomized controlled trial.[48]

Temperature Trajectory Subgroups

Temperature is a high-frequency, near-universal signal that can inform dynamic subtyping in sepsis. Four externally validated 72-hour temperature trajectory subphenotypes (hyperthermic fast resolvers, hyperthermic slow resolvers, normothermic, hypothermic) have been shown to differ in comorbidity burden and mortality.[49] Subsequent work has linked these temperature trajectories to distinct cytokine profiles, with hyperthermic fast resolvers showing more rapid decline of several inflammatory mediators than hyperthermic slow resolvers.[49] These studies suggest temperature may be a pragmatic input for dynamic subtyping, although a subgrouping window shorter than 72 hours may be required to enhance clinical relevance.

Time-Updated Membership

A key distinction in dynamic subtyping is between assigning patients to trajectory-defined groups after observing a fixed window and continuously updating subgroup probabilities as information accrues. Early data can support an initial assignment that is refined as additional physiology and organ dysfunction are captured. Transcriptomic studies demonstrate temporal variation in gene expression,[50] supporting models that update subgroup membership over time rather than assuming stability. A similar principle appears to apply to molecular phenotypes. In multicohort analyses of critically ill patients, the Hyperinflammatory and Hypoinflammatory phenotypes were not temporally fixed: the proportion classified as Hyperinflammatory declined over the first several days of illness and transition from Hyperinflammatory to Hypoinflammatory was associated with lower mortality than persistent Hyperinflammatory classification.[11] An enticing prospect for temporally dynamic subgrouping is the use of a valid measurement system that dynamically captures disease resolution as a potential endpoint for treatment efficacy in randomised trials and obviates the use of mortality and organ-support days which are frequently unrelated to the disease in critically ill patients.[51,52]

INPUTS AND PIPELINES FOR ELECTRONIC HEALTH RECORD–EMBEDDED REAL-TIME SUBGROUP ASSIGNMENT

For real-time subphenotype assignment, the initial priority is not establishing the syndromic label of sepsis per se but identifying when a patient has entered the clinical state in which subphenotypic classification becomes meaningful. In bedside use, this upstream task comprises 3 dynamic considerations: (1) identifying patients currently within the target population for subgrouping; (2) estimating the likelihood that they will enter that population within a defined window; and (3) detecting deterioration that should trigger reassessment and updating of subgroup probabilities.

Most real-time models require a label for training and evaluation. In EHR studies, *sepsis* is inferred from proxies determined by local clinical workflow and documentation practices, such as culture ordering and antibiotic administration. This has 2 important implications. First, even when Sepsis-3 is the conceptual target, heterogeneity persists because studies differ in how infection is defined and timed. Second, information leakage occurs when predictors capture signals that arise primarily because clinicians have already recognized possible sepsis and initiated investigations or therapies. For instance, a model may use lactate as a predictor, and of course, a clinician ordering lactate may already suspect sepsis. Together, these factors can inflate retrospective performance while shrinking prospective utility, which may explain the consistent failure in translating strong retrospective results outside the development setting.[53] A practical safeguard is to restrict predictors to data only available at the intended decision time and to data that would not *leak* clinical suspicion.[54]

A Practical 2-Stage Detection and Subtyping Pipeline for Deployment

EHR embedded classifier models commonly use physiology, updated routine laboratories, time-stamped microbiology results and clinical text as inputs.[55–57] A deployable architecture that keeps the clinical logic clear is a 2-stage pipeline (**Fig. 2**). Stage 1 ascertains eligibility, estimating whether a patient has entered the clinical state in which subgroup assignment becomes clinically meaningful, only using inputs available at the decision time. For example, stage 1 asks whether a patient meets criteria for sepsis. Stage 2 estimates the probability of subgroup membership in patients who have crossed the stage 1 threshold. When used for clinical decision making, probabilities could be updated as new model input data arrive. This design supports clinicians by first addressing whether subgroup assignment is appropriate, and only then, refining subgroup probabilities over time.

Evaluation and Monitoring Standards

Subtyping systems should be evaluated in ways that reflect intended use, including prospective validation across multiple sites (**Fig. 3**).

Reporting of model development and evaluation should follow established guidance for prediction models, with transparent specification of intended use, timing and evaluation design.[58] Performance can vary as practice, measurement and populations change so monitoring for dataset shift and calibration drift is an essential maintenance requirement.[59,60]

IMPLEMENTATION

Using Subgroups in Trial Design

Enrichment of clinical trials through subgroup assignment theoretically improves alignment between the enrolled population and the tested intervention.[13] Subgroup information could either support prognostic enrichment, where patients with higher baseline risk of the study are preferentially enrolled,[13,61] or predictive enrichment, where selected patients are more likely to benefit from the intervention, based on subgroup characteristics,[13] or both.

Real-time phenotyping promises to enable a fundamental redesign of clinical trials in critical care by allowing patients to be stratified according to biological state at the point of enrollment. In umbrella designs, multiple therapies would be tested in the same subgroup.[25] Conversely, in basket designs, the same therapies could be tested across multiple subgroups.[25] When integrated into adaptive platform trials, these approaches allow dynamic allocation, early stopping for futility or efficacy, and iterative

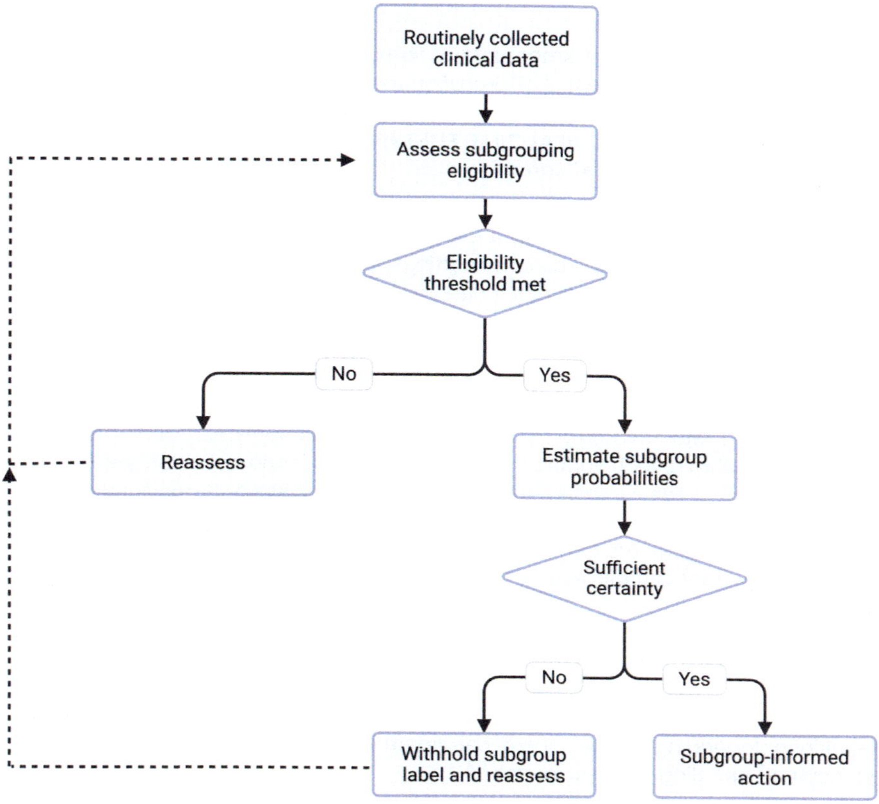

Fig. 2. A proposed 2-stage pipeline for real-time detection and subtyping. At a defined decision time, routinely collected clinical data are used to assess subtyping eligibility. If the eligibility threshold is met, the system estimates subgroup probabilities and supports subgroup-informed actions only when certainty is sufficient. If the eligibility threshold is not met, or if certainty is insufficient, the system prompts reassessment as new data arrive and withholds a subgroup label until confidence is adequate. (*Created in* BioRender. O'Kane, C. (2026) https://BioRender.com/3lyrq97.)

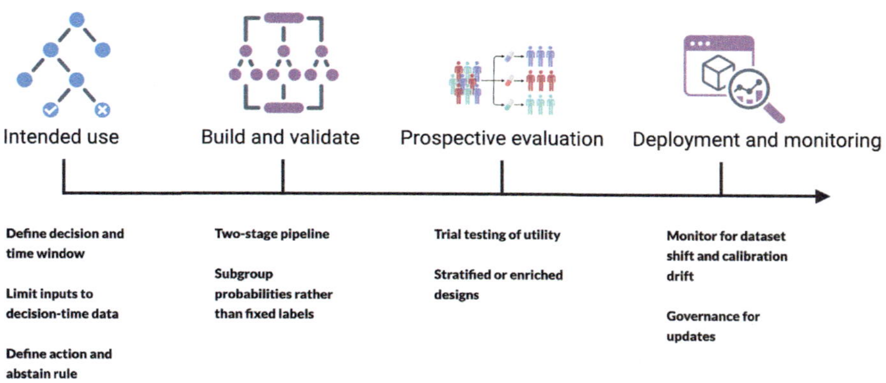

Fig. 3. Lifecycle for development, evaluation, and maintenance of real-time subtyping systems. A staged framework spanning intended use definition, model building and validation, prospective evaluation, and deployment. (*Created in* BioRender. O'Kane, C. (2026) https://BioRender.com/cafhuk6.)

refinement of phenotype–treatment interactions. Therefore, real-time phenotyping is integral to realizing the potential of precision therapeutics in critical illness.

BARRIERS AND PITFALLS TO REAL-TIME SUBTYPING

Practical and Methodological Constraints

Biomarker-informed subtyping faces biases due to measurement platform heterogeneity, including assay-specific calibration differences and batch effects. These biases will likely be amplified in low-resource settings, where near-patient platforms may be unavailable, unaffordable, and with limited troubleshooting capacity.

For EHR-embedded or trajectory-based clinical subtyping, reliable capture and temporal alignment of model inputs, stable pipelines and integration across bedside monitoring systems, laboratory information systems and EHR systems are essential. Delayed charting, inconsistent reporting units, and nonstandardized nomenclature can introduce systematic error. Missingness threatens subtyping generalizability, as missing data often reflect workflow pressures, local ordering behavior, and/or transfer between clinical areas. Crucially, differences in missingness patterns across hospitals can drive calibration drift when models are deployed across sites. By contrast, biologically measured classifiers may depend less on dense time-stamped clinical data, but are constrained by sample timing, assay turnaround time, and inconsistent platform standardisation.

Overfitting and weak external validation remain pervasive risks in subgroups derived in one dataset. Guidance for latent class analysis highlights common pitfalls, including sensitivity to modeling choices and the need to report uncertainty rather than forcing deterministic labels.[62] Trajectory methods introduce parallel issues with subgroup definitions depending on the chosen candidate variables, time window, sampling frequency and handling of missingness.[63]

Funding and Incentives

A major barrier to routine deployment is limited funding for prospective subtyping trials and implementation beyond discovery. The costs of real-time subtyping extend beyond model development to include EHR integration, interface design, training, governance and model maintenance.[59,60]

Ethics and Equity

Equity is central to safe implementation because subtyping systems can perform differently across demographic and clinical subgroups, and these differences can translate into unequal access to trials or targeted therapies.[64] Algorithms trained in narrow populations can amplify inequalities when deployed in settings with different demographic or comorbidity profiles and proxy targets can embed structural bias.

FUTURE WORK

A major impediment to progress is that *subgroup* labels are not yet sufficiently standardized for direct comparison across cohort and modeling frameworks. Priority work should therefore focus on harmonizing subgroup definitions, minimum candidate variable sets and reporting standards so that models are comparable across studies. It is probably beyond question that technology for implementing biological or clinical classifiers currently exists; however, engagement with industry, through prospective demonstration of feasibility and utility are critical to accelerating the bedside implementation of these technologies, which are likely only feasible with academic-industry partnership.

SUMMARY

Reproducible subgroups exist across sepsis, ARDS, AKI, and other inflammatory critical illnesses, with meaningful separation in biology and outcomes. Subgroup implementation depends on early and reliable subgroup assignment with time-updated probabilities and demonstrable validity across sites, platforms, and time. A probabilistic 2-stage pipeline can combine identification of patients eligible for subtyping with subgroup probability estimation, enabling uncertainty management by allowing the system to abstain when subgroup probabilities are imprecise. Priorities include harmonized definitions and reporting standards, hybrid pipelines combining pragmatic EHR signals with decision-critical biomarker panels and prospective multicenter evaluation of whether acting on subgroup probabilities improves outcomes and trial efficiency.

CLINICS CARE POINTS

- Subgroups recur in sepsis across clinical, protein biomarker-based, omics and microbiology-informed dimensions.
- Subtyping has the potential to reduce heterogeneity in conventional trials through enrichment and stratified randomization.
- Trajectory-based subtyping has the benefit of updating subgroup probabilities over time rather than relying on a single snapshot.
- Subtyping methods require prospective multicenter validation before routine clinical deployment.

DISCLOSURE

Dr R. McMullan has nothing to disclose. Dr S.V. Bhavani was funded by grants from the National Institutes of Health, United States (K23GM144867 and R01HL175626). Dr P. Sinha was funded by grants from the National Institutes of Health (R35GM142992, R01HL173531) and the Department of Defense, United States (PR241420). He receives consulting fees from AstraZeneca and has equity ownership in Prenosis Inc for consultancy, that are unrelated to the current work. The other author discloses no conflicts.

REFERENCES

1. Prescott HC, Antonelli M, Alhazzani W, et al. Surviving Sepsis campaign: international guidelines for management of sepsis and septic shock 2026. Crit Care Med 2026;54:725–812.
2. Rudd KE, Johnson SC, Agesa KM, et al. Global, regional, and national sepsis incidence and mortality, 1990–2017: analysis for the global burden of disease study. Lancet 2020;395:200–11.
3. Singer M, Deutschman CS, Seymour C, et al. The third international consensus definitions for sepsis and septic shock (Sepsis-3). JAMA 2016;315:801–10.
4. van der Poll T, van de Veerdonk FL, Scicluna BP, et al. The immunopathology of sepsis and potential therapeutic targets. Nat Rev Immunol 2017;17:407–20.
5. McMullan RR, McAuley DF, O'Kane CM, et al. Vascular leak in sepsis: physiological basis and potential therapeutic advances. Crit Care 2024;28:97.
6. Levi M, van der Poll T. Coagulation and sepsis. Thromb Res 2017;149:38–44.

7. Marshall JC. Why have clinical trials in sepsis failed? Trends Mol Med 2014;20: 195–203.
8. Seymour CW, Kennedy JN, Wang S, et al. Derivation, validation, and potential treatment implications of novel clinical phenotypes for sepsis. JAMA 2019;321: 2003–17.
9. Scicluna BP, van Vught LA, Zwinderman AH, et al. Classification of patients with sepsis according to blood genomic endotype: a prospective cohort study. Lancet Respir Med 2017;5:816–26.
10. Sweeney TE, Shidham A, Wong HR, et al. A comprehensive time-course-based multicohort analysis of sepsis and sterile inflammation reveals a robust diagnostic gene set. Sci Transl Med 2015;7:287ra71.
11. van Amstel RBE, Bartek B, Vlaar APJ, et al. Temporal transitions of the hyperinflammatory and hypoinflammatory phenotypes in critical illness. Am J Respir Crit Care Med 2025;211:347–56.
12. Reddy K, Sinha P, O'Kane CM, et al. Subphenotypes in critical care: translation into clinical practice. Lancet Respir Med 2020;8:631–43.
13. Prescott HC, Calfee CS, Taylor Thompson B, et al. Toward smarter lumping and smarter splitting: rethinking strategies for sepsis and acute respiratory distress syndrome clinical trial design. Am J Respir Crit Care Med 2016;194:147–55.
14. Bhavani SV, Semler M, Qian ET, et al. Development and validation of novel sepsis subphenotypes using trajectories of vital signs. Intensive Care Med 2022;48: 1582–92.
15. Aldewereld ZT, Zhang LA, Urbano A, et al. Identification of clinical phenotypes in septic patients presenting with hypotension or elevated lactate. Front Med 2022; 9:794423.
16. Sinha P, Kerchberger VE, Willmore A, et al. Identifying molecular phenotypes in sepsis: an analysis of two prospective observational cohorts and secondary analysis of two randomised controlled trials. Lancet Respir Med 2023;11:965–74.
17. Chanderraj R, Bartek B, Stringer KA, et al. Pathogen characteristics are key determinants of distinct host response phenotypes of sepsis. J Clin Invest 2026;136: e197346.
18. Davenport EE, Burnham KL, Radhakrishnan J, et al. Genomic landscape of the individual host response and outcomes in sepsis: a prospective cohort study. Lancet Respir Med 2016;4:259–71.
19. Sweeney TE, Liesenfeld O, Wacker J, et al. Validation of inflammopathic, adaptive, and coagulopathic sepsis endotypes in coronavirus disease 2019. Crit Care Med 2021;49:E170–8.
20. Antcliffe DB, Burnham KL, Al-Beidh F, et al. Transcriptomic signatures in sepsis and a differential response to steroids. From the VANISH randomized trial. Am J Respir Crit Care Med 2019;199:980–6.
21. Scicluna BP, Cano-Gamez K, Burnham KL, et al. A consensus blood transcriptomic framework for sepsis. Nat Med 2025;31:4119–30.
22. Zhao H, Kennedy JN, Wang S, et al. Revising host phenotypes of sepsis using microbiology. Front Med 2021;8:775511.
23. Hsieh YC, Chen HL, Lin SY, et al. Short time to positivity of blood culture predicts mortality and septic shock in bacteremic patients: a systematic review and meta-analysis. BMC Infect Dis 2022;22:142.
24. Paquette K, Sweet D, Stenstrom R, et al. Neither blood culture positivity nor time to positivity is associated with mortality among patients presenting with severe manifestations of sepsis: the FABLED cohort study. Open Forum Infect Dis 2021;8:ofab321.

25. Gordon AC, Alipanah-Lechner N, Bos LD, et al. From ICU syndromes to ICU subphenotypes: consensus report and recommendations for developing precision medicine in the ICU. Am J Respir Crit Care Med 2024;210:155–66.
26. Calfee CS, Delucchi K, Parsons PE, et al. Subphenotypes in acute respiratory distress syndrome: latent class analysis of data from two randomised controlled trials. Lancet Respir Med 2014;2:611–20.
27. Bhatraju PK, Zelnick LR, Herting J, et al. Identification of acute kidney injury subphenotypes with differing molecular signatures and responses to vasopressin therapy. Am J Respir Crit Care Med 2019;199:863–72.
28. Calfee CS, Delucchi KL, Sinha P, et al. Acute respiratory distress syndrome subphenotypes and differential response to simvastatin: secondary analysis of a randomised controlled trial. Lancet Respir Med 2018;6:691–8.
29. Maddali MV, Churpek M, Pham T, et al. Validation and utility of ARDS subphenotypes identified by machine-learning models using clinical data: an observational, multicohort, retrospective analysis. Lancet Respir Med 2022;10:367–77.
30. Sinha P, Delucchi KL, McAuley DF, et al. Development and validation of parsimonious algorithms to classify ARDS phenotypes: secondary analyses of randomised controlled trials. Lancet Respir Med 2020;8:247–57.
31. Stanski NL, Stenson EK, Cvijanovich NZ, et al. PERSEVERE biomarkers predict severe acute kidney injury and renal recovery in pediatric septic shock. Am J Respir Crit Care Med 2020;201:848–55.
32. Kiernan E, Zelnick LR, Khader A, et al. Molecular phenotyping of sepsis and differential response to fluid resuscitation. Am J Respir Crit Care Med 2025;211: 1681–8.
33. Dahmer MK, Yang G, Zhang M, et al. Identification of phenotypes in paediatric patients with acute respiratory distress syndrome: a latent class analysis. Lancet Respir Med 2022;10:289–97.
34. Flori HR, Zhang M, Xie J, et al. Subphenotypes assigned to pediatric acute respiratory failure patients show differing outcomes. Am J Respir Crit Care Med 2023;208:331–3.
35. Sinha P, Neyton L, Sarma A, et al. Molecular phenotypes of acute respiratory distress syndrome in the ROSE trial have differential outcomes and gene expression patterns that differ at baseline and longitudinally over time. Am J Respir Crit Care Med 2024;209:816–28.
36. Reddy K, Sinha P, Antcliffe DB, et al. Bedside identification of subphenotypes in acute respiratory failure (PHIND): a multicentre, observational cohort study. Lancet Respir Med 2026. https://doi.org/10.1016/S2213-2600(26)00040-8.
37. Files DC, Gibbs K, Matthay MA, et al. Real-time prospective classification of biologic sub-phenotypes in severe acute respiratory failure: an interim report on the SPARC study. Am J Respir Crit Care Med 2024;209:A5512.
38. Reddy K, Aggarwal N, Alipanah-Lechner N, et al. Building an international precision medicine platform trial for the acute respiratory distress syndrome (ARDS): an expert consensus project report. Efficacy Mech Eval 2025. https://doi.org/10.3310/TTND8896.
39. Gupta R, Gupta P, Wang S, et al. Ultrasensitive lateral-flow assays via plasmonically active antibody-conjugated fluorescent nanoparticles. Nat Biomed Eng 2023;7:1556–70.
40. Guo L, Zhao Y, Huang Q, et al. Electrochemical protein biosensors for disease marker detection: progress and opportunities. Microsyst Nanoeng 2024;10:65.

41. Dysinger M, Marusov G, Fraser S. Quantitative analysis of four protein biomarkers: an automated microfluidic cartridge-based method and its comparison to colorimetric ELISA. J Immunol Methods 2017;451:1–10.
42. Sinha P, Churpek MM, Calfee CS. Machine learning classifier models can identify acute respiratory distress syndrome phenotypes using readily available clinical data. Am J Respir Crit Care Med 2020;202:996–1004.
43. Wong HR, Cvijanovich NZ, Anas N, et al. Developing a clinically feasible personalized medicine approach to pediatric septic shock. Am J Respir Crit Care Med 2015;191:309–15.
44. Wong HR, Sweeney TE, Hart KW, et al. Pediatric sepsis endotypes among adults with sepsis. Crit Care Med 2017;45:e1289–91.
45. Wong HR, Hart KW, Lindsell CJ, et al. External corroboration that corticosteroids may be harmful to septic shock endotype A patients. Crit Care Med 2021;49: E98–101.
46. Sweeney TE, Azad TD, Donato M, et al. Unsupervised analysis of transcriptomics in bacterial sepsis across multiple datasets reveals three robust clusters. Crit Care Med 2018;46:915–25.
47. Antcliffe DB, Peronnet E, Pène F, et al. An international observational study validating gene-expression sepsis immune subgroups. Crit Care 2025;29:98.
48. Bhavani SV, Holder A, Miltz D, et al. The precision resuscitation with crystalloids in sepsis (PRECISE) trial: a trial protocol. JAMA Netw Open 2024;7:e2434197.
49. Bhavani SV, Wolfe KS, Hrusch CL, et al. Temperature trajectory subphenotypes correlate with immune responses in patients with sepsis. Crit Care Med 2020; 48:1645–53.
50. Burnham KL, Davenport EE, Radhakrishnan J, et al. Shared and distinct aspects of the sepsis transcriptomic response to fecal peritonitis and pneumonia. Am J Respir Crit Care Med 2017;196:328–39.
51. Mayr VD, Dünser MW, Greil V, et al. Causes of death and determinants of outcome in critically ill patients. Crit Care 2006;10:R154.
52. Torres LK, Hoffman KL, Oromendia C, et al. Attributable mortality of acute respiratory distress syndrome: a systematic review, meta-analysis, and survival analysis using targeted minimum loss-based estimation. Thorax 2021;76:1176–85.
53. Wong A, Otles E, Donnelly JP, et al. External validation of a widely implemented proprietary sepsis prediction model in hospitalized patients. JAMA Intern Med 2021;181:1065–70.
54. Matheny ME, Davis SE. Avoiding label leakage in AI risk models—a shared responsibility for a pervasive problem. JAMA Netw Open 2025;8:e2550464.
55. Shashikumar SP, Wardi G, Malhotra A, et al. Artificial intelligence sepsis prediction algorithm learns to say "I don't know.". npj Digit Med 2021;4:134.
56. Boussina A, Shashikumar SP, Malhotra A, et al. Impact of a deep learning sepsis prediction model on quality of care and survival. npj Digit Med 2024;7:14.
57. Goh KH, Wang L, Yeow AYK, et al. Artificial intelligence in sepsis early prediction and diagnosis using unstructured data in healthcare. Nat Commun 2021;12:711.
58. Collins GS, Moons KGM, Dhiman P, et al. TRIPOD+AI statement: updated guidance for reporting clinical prediction models that use regression or machine learning methods. BMJ 2024;385:e078378.
59. Finlayson SG, Subbaswamy A, Singh K, et al. The clinician and dataset shift in artificial intelligence. N Engl J Med 2021;385:283–6.
60. Davis SE, Greevy RA, Lasko TA, et al. Detection of calibration drift in clinical prediction models to inform model updating. J Biomed Inf 2020;112:103611.

61. Saha R, Pham T, Sinha P, et al. Estimating the attributable fraction of mortality from acute respiratory distress syndrome to inform enrichment in future randomised clinical trials. Thorax 2023;78:990–1003.
62. Sinha P, Calfee CS, Delucchi KL. Practitioner's guide to latent class analysis: methodological considerations and common pitfalls. Crit Care Med 2021;49: e63–79.
63. Nagin DS. Group-based trajectory modeling: an overview. Ann Nutr Metab 2014; 65:205–10.
64. Obermeyer Z, Powers B, Vogeli C, et al. Dissecting racial bias in an algorithm used to manage the health of populations. Science 2019;366:447–53.

The Immunometabolic Architecture of Sepsis

Bridging Cellular Bioenergetics and Systemic Immune Dysregulation

Valentim Rodrigues, MBBS[a], Duarte Abecasis, MBBS[a],
Luis F. Moita, MD, PhD[b,*]

KEYWORDS

• Sepsis-3 • MODS • PICS • Immunometabolism • Mitochondrial dysfunction

KEY POINTS

- Definitions: Sepsis (Sepsis-3) is life-threatening organ dysfunction from a dysregulated host response to infection; septic shock requires vasopressors (mean arterial pressure ≥ 65 mm Hg) and lactate greater than 2 mmol/L despite fluids.
- Coexisting immune states: Modern models reject a simple *hyperinflammation then immunosuppression* sequence—both proinflammatory and immunosuppressive processes can occur simultaneously, driving multiple organ dysfunction syndrome.
- Immunometabolism as a core driver: Metabolic reprogramming is central to sepsis biology; metabolites regulate immune signaling and inter-organ communication, and survival depends on balance between resistance and disease tolerance.
- Endothelial dysfunction: Endothelial barrier breakdown, vasoplegia, microthrombosis, and mitochondrial/oxygen utilization failure (cytopathic dysoxia) together impair tissue perfusion contributing to organ failure.
- Diagnosis and future therapy direction: Diagnosis is probabilistic; emerging approaches emphasize biomarker-driven immunometabolic phenotyping and metabolic resuscitation rather than one-size-fits-all treatment.

INTRODUCTION

Critical illness represents one of the major challenges of contemporary medicine, with sepsis standing out as one of its most complex and prevalent manifestations, responsible for countless deaths worldwide. Defined by the Sepsis-3 consensus as a life-threatening organ dysfunction caused by a dysregulated host response to infection,[1]

[a] Faculdade de Medicina da Universidade de Lisboa, Lisboa, Portugal; [b] Center for Disease Mechanisms Research, Medicine ULisboa for Health Clinical Research and Innovation (MUH-CRI), Faculdade de Medicina da Universidade de Lisboa, Lisboa, Portugal
* Corresponding author.
E-mail address: lmoita@medicina.ulisboa.pt

Crit Care Clin 42 (2026) 857–874
https://doi.org/10.1016/j.ccc.2026.05.009 **criticalcare.theclinics.com**

Abbreviations	
2-DG	2-deoxy-D-glucose
CARS	compensatory anti-inflammatory response syndrome
DAMP	damage-associated molecular pattern
HAMP	homeostasis-altering molecular process
IL-6	interleukin-6
IL-10	interleukin-10
IL-1β	interleukin-1β
MAP	mean arterial pressure
MODS	multiple organ dysfunction syndrome
NET	neutrophil extracellular trap
NEWS2	National Early Warning Score
NF-κB	nuclear factor-κB
PAMP	pathogen-associated molecular pattern
PCT	procalcitonin
PICS	persistent inflammation, immunosuppression, and catabolism syndrome
POCUS	point-of-care ultrasound
PRR	pattern recognition receptor
qSOFA	quick Sequential Organ Failure Assessment
ROS	reactive oxygen species
SIRS	systemic inflammatory response syndrome
SOFA	Sequential Organ Failure Assessment
TNF-α	tumor necrosis factor-α

it is estimated to account for approximately 20% of global deaths,[2] maintaining a guarded prognosis despite advances in therapy. Its most severe form, septic shock, is defined by the need for vasopressors to maintain a mean arterial pressure (MAP) $\geq$ 65 mm Hg and a serum lactate level greater than 2 mmol/L despite adequate fluid resuscitation and is associated with significantly higher mortality.[1]

The pathophysiology of sepsis has historically been conceptualized as a sequence of phases: a proinflammatory peak followed by compensatory immunosuppression. However, current models propose that hyperinflammation and immunosuppression coexist simultaneously across different biological compartments and even within the same tissue.[3] This overlap promotes multiple organ dysfunction syndrome (MODS), and in survivors of the acute phase, may evolve into persistent inflammation, immunosuppression, and catabolism syndrome (PICS), a state of chronic vulnerability associated with high subacute/chronic mortality.[4,5] Metabolic reprogramming has emerged as a central axis for the pathophysiology of sepsis: beyond serving as energy sources, metabolites act as regulators of interorgan communication. Host survival depends on the balance between mechanisms of resistance and disease tolerance, which is often impaired and leads to high morbidity and mortality.[6]

Given the clinical heterogeneity and the immunometabolic complexity of this syndrome (which serves as an umbrella term for a vast array of pathology), here we analyze the pathophysiological mechanisms of sepsis, integrating the coexistence of opposing immune states, the signaling role of metabolism, and emerging clinical diagnostic metrics and therapeutic targets.

Historically, the pathophysiology of sepsis has been focused almost exclusively on *resistance*.[7] This is the host's ability to detect, engage, and eliminate pathogens through the activation of classic immune effector responses. This defense strategy is energetically very demanding and often leads to collateral tissue damage and the development of MODS. A critical, emerging paradigm is *disease tolerance*: the host's ability to maintain physiologic function and survive an infectious burden without necessarily reducing the pathogen load.[7] The metabolic reprogramming observed in sepsis might not merely be a failure of bioenergetics, but a potential adaptive mechanism to preserve cell viability under extreme stress. Survival to sepsis may rely on a dynamic and delicate balance between resistance (driven by rapid metabolic shifts that support high-energy effector functions to clear the pathogen) and disease tolerance (characterized by a *quiescent* metabolic state that minimizes oxidative damage and prevents the transition from reversible organ dysfunction to permanent failure). Reframing sepsis through the lens of disease tolerance allows us to better understand the *immunometabolic double-edged sword*. Therapeutic success may depend not just on how well we assist the host in fighting the pathogen, but on how effectively we support the metabolic pathways that protect the host from its own dysregulated immune response.

FUNDAMENTAL CONCEPTS

The key definitions in this essay reflect the evolution from earlier consensus frameworks—Sepsis-1 and Sepsis-2, which centered on the systemic inflammatory response syndrome (SIRS)—toward the current Sepsis-3 paradigm, which repositions organ dysfunction as the defining feature of the syndrome and leaves the concept of SIRS behind.[1] Throughout this article, sepsis and septic shock are defined and described according to the Sepsis-3 criteria, with organ dysfunction quantified by the Sequential Organ Failure Assessment (SOFA) score incorporating the 2025 update, and the Phoenix Sepsis Score applied where the pediatric population is specifically considered. MODS and the immunosuppressive component of the host response—historically termed compensatory anti-inflammatory response syndrome (CARS), though increasingly framed within the broader concept of sepsis-induced immune dysregulation—are introduced in the following subsections as the principal syndromic expressions of the pathophysiological processes this article examines.

MODS: It is the clinical expression of a sustained and dysregulated response of the host to a stressor, leading to the progressive failure of 2 or more organ systems. It develops when the body can no longer properly control its response to a major insult, involving complex interactions between the immune system, the endothelium, metabolism, and coagulation, leading to a loss of response regulation and ultimately gravely affecting the host's tissues.[8] While it is most commonly associated with sepsis, MODS can also occur in noninfectious conditions such as noninfectious shock, severe trauma, acute pancreatitis, or extensive burns, among many other scenarios. Its pathophysiology is complex and not yet fully understood.[8] Rather than being simply a state of excessive inflammation, MODS reflects a dynamic imbalance between proinflammatory and anti-inflammatory processes, which often occur simultaneously.[8] Key mechanisms include endothelial dysfunction, microcirculatory impairment, immune dysregulation, mitochondrial dysfunction, and disturbances in coagulation.[8] In addition, factors such as pathogen-derived endotoxins and the translocation of gut bacteria and toxins into the bloodstream can further drive disease progression.[8] Together, these processes impair tissue perfusion and cellular function, ultimately leading to organ failure—mechanisms that will be explored in more detail in the following sections.[8]

CARS and PICS: CARS is an immunosuppressive state that occurs in sepsis, characterized by profound immune dysfunction.[9] Although classically described as following SIRS (in the biphasic model of immune activity in sepsis), current consensus is that it occurs alongside hyperinflammatory states in the host. Over time, this condition has been characterized by features such as cutaneous energy, lymphocyte depletion through apoptosis, reduced cytokine production by monocytes in response to stimulation, decreased expression of human leukocyte antigen (HLA) antigen–presenting molecules on monocytes, and increased production of anti-inflammatory cytokines such as interleukin-10 (IL-10).[9] At this point, the individual enters a stage of relative immunosuppression, becoming susceptible to secondary or nosocomial infections, thus perpetuating the sepsis cascade and possibly leading to his death.

PICS: It refers to a prolonged clinical phenotype in which patients present low-grade chronic inflammation, persistent immunosuppression (with associated recurrent infections and prolonged hospital stays) and a catabolic metabolism resulting in, among other phenomena, severe sarcopenia.[5] It is thought of as a long-term consequence of an ill-resolved septic episode and can cause severe morbidity and mortality, and its self-perpetuating nature poses severe challenges to its treatment.

PATHOPHYSIOLOGICAL MECHANISMS

Immune Responses Initiation: The recognition of the infectious agent constitutes the initial and determining event in the pathophysiology of sepsis, establishing the transition from a localized infection to a dysregulated systemic inflammatory response, which is what usually poses a fatal threat to the host. Although classically centered on the detection of microbial components, the current paradigm acknowledges that this process involves a complex integration of signals derived from the pathogen, the host, and disturbances in cellular homeostasis, followed by profound metabolic and functional reprogramming.[3] The simple recognition of a pathogen by immune cells as the starting point is not only too simplistic as it is often simply not the case.

The Signal Triad: *Pathogen-associated molecular patterns (PAMPs), damage-associated molecular patterns (DAMPs), and homeostasis-altering molecular processes (HAMPs):* The primary initial stimuli are PAMPs, conserved microbial structures—such as bacterial lipopolysaccharide, viral RNA, or fungal β-glucans. These are recognized by pattern recognition receptors (PRRs), notably toll-like receptors, nucleotide-binding oligomerization domain (NOD)-like receptors, and retinoic acid-inducible gene - I (RIG-I)-like receptors (**Fig. 1**).[10] Activation of these receptors triggers intracellular signaling cascades, centered on pathways such as nuclear factor-κB (NF-κB) and MAP kinases, culminating in the nuclear genetic transcription of pro-inflammatory cytokines and mediators of the innate immune response.[11]

However, the inflammatory response is not strictly exogenous. Infection-induced tissue injury releases damage-associated molecular patterns (DAMPs), such as mitochondrial DNA, histones, and heat shock proteins.[10] These endogenous agonists amplify immune activation through the same PRRs, establishing a self-propagating inflammatory feedback loop.[10] This way, our *threat sensors* not only react to external pathogens that may pose a threat to the individual but also to actual signs of cellular damage. A critical event at this stage is the activation of the NLRP3 inflammasome, which processes pro-interleukin-1β (IL-1β) and pro-interleukin-18 into their active forms and may induce pyroptosis, a highly inflammatory form of programmed cell death that exacerbates the progression of organ dysfunction.[12]

More recently, the concept of HAMPs has redefined surveillance immunity.[13] HAMPs are not discrete molecules but rather states of functional deviation—such as mitochondrial dysfunction, endoplasmic reticulum stress, and inhibition of protein synthesis.[14] The detection of these alterations, frequently involving cellular stress-response pathways such as the integrated stress response,[15] allows the immune system to monitor and fine-tune the magnitude of its response by integrating signals of perceived damage with the presence of a pathogen, thereby perfecting the response,

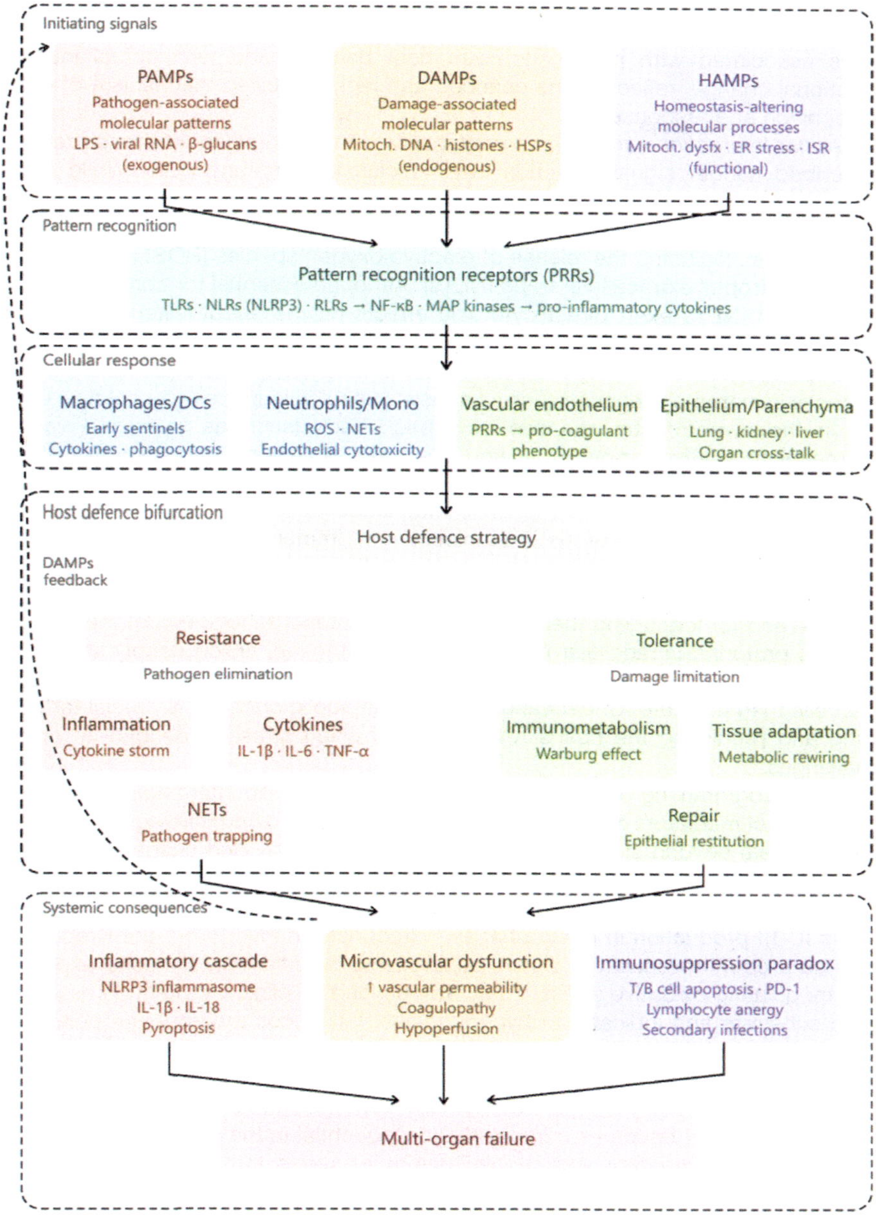

Fig. 1. Pathogen recognition and early immune signaling in sepsis. PRRs on innate immune cells, including toll-like receptors and NOD-like receptors sense PAMPs on invading microorganisms. This recognition triggers intracellular signaling cascades that activate transcription factors such as NF-κB and interferon regulatory factors (IRFs), and lead to the production of proinflammatory cytokines, chemokines, and interferons. The resulting response promotes pathogen clearance but may contribute to systemic inflammation and organ dysfunction characteristic of sepsis. Created using Inkscape.

although sepsis is one of many examples of this system leading to deleterious consequences on the host. This way, the current signaling model includes molecular patterns associated with pathogens, with host damage and with actual states of functional change, reflecting the nuanced and highly detailed mechanism of danger recognition and response.[13]

Cellular Interactions and Immunometabolism: The recognition of these previously described *danger* signals extends beyond classical immune cells. While macrophages and dendritic cells act as early sentinels (given their initial role as antigen-presenting cells), the recruitment of neutrophils introduces potent amplification mechanisms, including the release of reactive oxygen species (ROS) and the formation of neutrophil extracellular traps (NETs). Although essential for controlling microbial burden, NETs exert direct cytotoxic effects on the endothelium and promote immunothrombosis, representing a critical interface between innate immunity and vascular injury, exemplifying the somewhat maladaptive nature of many of these responses in extreme scenarios such as sepsis; vascular injury being absolutely essential in the symptomatic changes of septic shock (such as increased vascular permeability, relative hypovolemia, and effective hypotension), this response is highly mechanistically important.[16]

The calibration of immune response magnitude described above is inseparable from the metabolic state of the cells executing it. Immunometabolism—the study of how metabolic programs shape and are shaped by immune function—has emerged as a central organizing framework in sepsis research, both for understanding host damage and for identifying therapeutic targets. Instead, recognition of these signals induces profound intracellular metabolic reprogramming, which deeply shapes and determines the nature, magnitude, and duration of the inflammatory response that the cells then promote. Understanding these metabolic changes is crucial for evaluating and predicting the host's response to a given stressor, despite its obvious challenges.

This reprogramming operates through specific metabolic intermediates that function as direct mediators of intercellular communication and immune regulation.[6] Metabolism exists beyond simple processes for energy supply and usage and is critical for appropriate cell-to-cell communication and coordinating responses. Succinate, released from mitochondria under inflammatory conditions, stabilizes HIF-1α and amplifies IL-1β production in macrophages.[17] Itaconate, derived from the Krebs cycle, acts as a counter-regulatory signal, suppressing proinflammatory gene expression and modulating oxidative stress.[18] Lactate, beyond its clinically vital role as a metabolic substrate and indicator of hypoperfusion, influences macrophage polarization and T-cell function, connecting the bioenergetic state of the cell to its immunologic output.[3] These relationships establish an indissociable link between the metabolic state of immune cells, the nature of the host response, and the clinical phenotype of sepsis—a link that becomes particularly consequential in the context of the simultaneous hyperinflammatory and hypoinflammatory states that characterize the syndrome, and which will be explored in detail in subsequent sections.

Endothelial dysfunction and microcirculation: Endothelial dysfunction represents a central component in the pathophysiology of sepsis, constituting a critical junction between systemic inflammatory activation and progression to multiorgan failure.[19] Far from being a passive mechanical barrier, the endothelium functions as a dynamic organ with immunologic, metabolic, and hemostatic properties.[20] During systemic infection, profound endothelial reprogramming plays a decisive role in the loss of vascular homeostasis, with very consequential effects on the whole immune response.

Endothelial activation is triggered early by exposure to PAMPs and DAMPs, which are recognized by PRRs expressed on endothelial cells.[10] This response is further amplified by proinflammatory cytokines such as tumor necrosis factor-α (TNF-α) and IL-1β, driving a phenotypic transition. Activated endothelial cells upregulate adhesion molecules, produce inflammatory mediators, and actively modulate vascular tone and coagulation pathways.[8] While this activated state contributes to pathogen containment, it simultaneously initiates maladaptive alterations in systemic vascular regulation. In a way, this is the *natural story* of the immune response in sepsis: although adaptive at first, its dysregulation and consequences result in life-threatening danger to the host.

One of the earliest consequences of this phenotypic endothelial reprogramming is the disruption of endothelial barrier integrity.[8] This process frequently begins with shedding of the endothelial glycocalyx, a proteoglycan-rich luminal layer that plays a key role in mechano-transduction and permeability regulation.[8] Glycocalyx degradation, alongside the disorganization of cell-to-cell junctions, results in a marked increase in vascular permeability.[8] The ensuing extravasation of fluid into the interstitial space leads to diffuse tissue edema, a reduction in effective intravascular volume, and impaired oxygen diffusion to tissues, with the characteristic hypotension leading to severe tissue hypoxia and eventually shock.[8]

Concurrently, a profound dysregulation of the vascular tone develops, characterized by excessive production of nitric oxide and other vasodilatory mediators.[8] The result is systemic vasodilation with reduced peripheral vascular resistance resulting in hypotension.[8] This state is compounded by vascular hyporesponsiveness to catecholamines, reflecting a failure of both endogenous and exogenous vasoconstrictive mechanisms and interconnecting vascular collapse with endocrine changes.[21] This phenomenon represents a key pathophysiological hallmark of septic shock (hence its alternative name *vasoplegic shock*) and critically limits hemodynamic compensation. Many of the problems in the medical management of septic shock are caused not only by the affected vascular tone but fundamentally from the vascular tissues hyporesponsiveness.

In parallel, the endothelium acquires a procoagulant phenotype, characterized by increased expression of tissue factor and inhibition of physiologic anticoagulant and fibrinolytic pathways.[8] These changes promote the formation of microthrombi within the capillary network, leading to obstruction of the microcirculation.[8] Consequently, a dissociation between macrocirculatory parameters and effective tissue perfusion emerges, whereby systemic hemodynamic variables may appear stabilized despite persistent and heterogeneous microvascular dysfunction.[8] This is the way DIC is so common in septic shock.

The combined effects of increased permeability, vasoplegia, and microvascular thrombosis culminate in impaired oxygen delivery and utilization at the cellular level.[8] This condition, often referred to as cytopathic hypoxia, is frequently associated with mitochondrial dysfunction, in which cells are unable to effectively utilize available oxygen for energy production. In addition, the injured endothelium acts as an amplifier of the inflammatory response by facilitating leukocyte recruitment and promoting further release of DAMPs, thereby contributing to a self-sustaining cycle of inflammation. This persistent inflammatory state may subsequently transition into prolonged immunosuppression, contributing to increased susceptibility to secondary infections and adverse clinical outcomes.

From an integrative perspective, endothelial dysfunction represents a pivotal transition from adaptive host defense mechanisms toward a maladaptive systemic response. When endothelial activation becomes excessive or sustained, the failure to restore vascular homeostasis drives the progression to multiorgan dysfunction.

Thus, the endothelium is not merely a passive bystander in sepsis but an active mediator linking the initial infectious insult to the circulatory and metabolic failure that defines its most severe forms and eventually leads to catastrophic consequences on the host.

MITOCHONDRIAL DYSFUNCTION AND METABOLISM

Mitochondrial dysfunction represents a critical node in the pathophysiology of sepsis, linking microcirculatory disturbances to cellular bioenergetic failure and exemplifying how sepsis, rather than simply a systemic disturbance, causes and is caused by severe cellular dysfunction. Rather than a passive consequence of critical illness, it is increasingly recognized as a central component of immunometabolic reprogramming that influences both immune responses and organ function—and contributes to the multi-organ dysfunction and excess mortality that characterize the most severe presentations of the syndrome.

During early sepsis, inflammatory signaling induces a shift toward aerobic glycolysis in immune cells, supporting rapid effector functions.[22] This occurs alongside a reprogramming of mitochondrial metabolism, with reduced pyruvate oxidation and impaired oxidative phosphorylation.[22] The resulting state—often termed cytopathic dysoxia—reflects a condition in which oxygen utilization for adenosine triphosphate (ATP) generation is compromised despite apparently adequate systemic delivery.[22] This distinction is important: microcirculatory heterogeneity in sepsis means that regional oxygen availability is frequently impaired even when global delivery parameters appear preserved, and the two phenomena likely coexist and reinforce one another. Therefore, normal oxygenation patterns do not mean that there is no cellular damage. Mitochondrial dysfunction itself manifests through alterations in respiratory chain activity, loss of mitochondrial membrane potential, and reduced coupling efficiency—that is, increased proton leak relative to ATP production—ultimately leading to bioenergetic insufficiency. While challenging, this creates chances for drugs targeting mitochondria to be repurposed for sepsis if their effect helps fight back against this organelle's dysfunction.[22]

Sepsis also disrupts mitochondrial quality control. Excessive production of ROS, combined with impaired antioxidant defenses, promotes oxidative damage to mitochondrial components.[22] Concurrently, mitochondrial dynamics shift toward fragmentation, while mitophagy—initially protective—becomes insufficient and impaired under sustained stress.[22] Reduced mitochondrial biogenesis, partly linked to decreased expression of regulators such as PGC-1α, further contributes to the accumulation of dysfunctional organelles.[23] Importantly, mitochondrial DNA released into the cytosol can act as a damage-associated molecular pattern, activating the cGAS–STING pathway and amplifying intracellular inflammatory signaling.[24] When released into the extracellular space, it may engage TLR9 on immune cells, extending this proinflammatory signal to the systemic level.[24] These mechanisms are complementary but distinct, and both appear operative in sepsis and working toward prolonging the response.

Importantly, mitochondrial dysfunction may not solely represent irreversible injury. In certain contexts, reduced mitochondrial activity appears to reflect an adaptive metabolic downregulation aimed at preserving cellular viability under stress.[22] In organs such as the kidney, heart, and brain, this has been conceptualized as a reversible *cellular shutdown*, which may limit activation of apoptotic and potentially ferroptotic cell death pathways, allowing functional recovery following resolution of the septic insult. However, when prolonged or dysregulated, this adaptive response may itself become pathologic—contributing to persistent organ dysfunction, failure to recover renal tubular function, and the broader syndrome of chronic critical illness seen in patients who survive the acute phase but do not return to baseline organ function. The limit between the adaptive mitochondrial downregulation and the overly extensive harmful prolongation, although very nuanced and challenging, is nevertheless a potential target for study and therapeutics.

The transition from cellular biology to therapeutic implications is, in this domain, particularly consequential. Due to their bacterial ancestry, mitochondrial ribosomes are susceptible to inhibition by antibiotics targeting bacterial protein synthesis.[25] Of the agents used to treat infection, oxazolidinones—linezolid in particular—carry the most well-established clinical signal of mitochondrial toxicity, primarily through inhibition of mitochondrial translation with prolonged use.[26] Tetracyclines and macrolides share this theoretic susceptibility, but clinically relevant mitochondrial toxicity at standard exposures appears limited, and the risk should not be overstated for these classes before further studies. In all cases, the potential for mitochondrial effects is most relevant in the setting of prolonged exposure. Conversely, preclinical studies suggest that partial inhibition of mitochondrial function may induce adaptive stress responses, including mitohormesis, promoting cellular resilience.[25,27] While such effects remain experimental and have not been translated into clinical practice, they hold substantial potential.

Accordingly, antimicrobial therapy in sepsis should remain guided by established principles—early administration, appropriate coverage, and source control—rather than attempts to modulate mitochondrial function. Nevertheless, awareness of potential mitochondrial effects is clinically relevant in selected scenarios, most notably in patients with prolonged illness in whom persistent lactic acidosis despite adequate resuscitation and source control prompts consideration of a metabolic rather than purely circulatory etiology. Given the metabolic importance of mitochondria, it is critical to understand how these drugs affect this organelle.

Despite growing insights, key uncertainties persist. Mitochondrial dysfunction is consistently associated with disease severity, but its precise role—whether causal, contributory, or adaptive—remains context-dependent.[22] Moreover, interventions targeting mitochondrial metabolism have shown biochemical improvements without consistent benefit in clinical outcomes. These findings highlight the heterogeneity of sepsis and underscore the need for biomarker-driven approaches to better define metabolic phenotypes and guide targeted therapies. Among the candidates under investigation, the lactate-to-pyruvate ratio, circulating mitochondrial DNA levels, NAD^+/NADH redox state, and plasma succinate have each demonstrated mechanistic relevance, though none has yet achieved validated clinical utility.

Immune reprogramming and immunosuppression—Host defense against infection involves a complex interplay between innate and adaptive immune responses, supported by the profound metabolic reprogramming as discussed above. Building on the established framework of PAMPs, DAMPs, and HAMPs recognition, what follows describes how the downstream immune response unfolds at the cellular level—and how the metabolic state of immune cells shapes its trajectory, magnitude, and ultimate consequences for the host.

In sepsis, immune cells—particularly leukocytes—mount an intense response aimed at rapid pathogen clearance.[28] Activation of major inflammatory pathways, including NF-κB and the inflammasome, drives rapid cellular activation, proliferation, and the production of early proinflammatory cytokines including TNF-α, IL-1β, and interleukin-6 (IL-6). These processes impose substantial metabolic demands, driving increased glucose utilization and extensive remodeling of amino acid metabolism to sustain effector functions.

At the cellular level, this early response is characterized by a shift toward aerobic glycolysis and enhanced nutrient uptake—a state that prioritizes speed of activation over energetic efficiency.[3] When sustained, this metabolic configuration contributes to mitochondrial dysfunction, impaired oxidative phosphorylation, and reduced fatty acid oxidation. The resulting decline in ATP availability, together with persistent inflammatory signaling, progressively impairs immune cell function and creates the conditions for the immunosuppressive transition described below.

Concurrently, regulatory mechanisms are activated to limit excessive inflammation. These include the upregulation of anti-inflammatory mediators such as IL-10 and transforming growth factor-β, immune cell reprogramming, lymphocyte apoptosis, dendritic cell dysfunction, and increased expression of immune checkpoint molecules—notably PD-1 and PD-L1—which attenuate T-cell activation and have emerged as relevant therapeutic targets in the context of sepsis-induced immunosuppression. Collectively, these processes contribute to a state of impaired pathogen clearance and increased susceptibility to secondary and nosocomial infections. Both sides of this immune double edge sword pose a significant threat to the host but nevertheless offer therapeutic options.

Importantly, contemporary models reject the notion of a strictly sequential transition from hyperinflammation to immunosuppression.[3] Instead, these processes occur simultaneously across different biological compartments, reflecting a dynamic and dysregulated host response in which inflammatory and anti-inflammatory pathways coexist and interact throughout the course of the illness, in different organs and tissues at the same time.[3]

Neuroendocrine Axis: Sepsis both affects and is influenced by the neuroendocrine system, reflecting a tightly integrated and bidirectional interplay between inflammation and hormonal regulation. This interaction is inseparable from the immunometabolic reprogramming described above: inflammatory mediators disrupt hormonal signaling pathways, while neuroendocrine alterations reciprocally modulate immune cell function and systemic metabolic homeostasis. Microbial products and cytokine signaling profoundly reshape the host endocrine profile, contributing to global physiologic dysregulation and organ dysfunction.[21] Accordingly, the identification of biomarkers that capture this axis—such as copeptin, a surrogate marker of vasopressin secretion—represents a promising approach for improved risk stratification in severe illness.[29]

At a mechanistic level, sepsis disrupts neuroendocrine function through both intracellular signaling alterations and intercellular dysregulation across endocrine axes. Proinflammatory cytokines, including interleukin-1, TNF-α, and IL-6, impair hypothalamic–pituitary signaling, reduce peripheral hormone receptor sensitivity, and alter hormone metabolism at the tissue level. These effects are compounded by direct adrenal cytotoxicity, microcirculatory dysfunction affecting endocrine organs, and cytokine-mediated downregulation of receptor expression. In parallel, mitochondrial dysfunction and metabolic reprogramming further compromise the energetically demanding processes of hormone synthesis and intracellular signal transduction, reinforcing endocrine failure.[21]

Clinically, sepsis is associated with a characteristic pattern of endocrine derangements. Relative vasopressin deficiency contributes to vasodilatory shock and underpins the use of vasopressin in norepinephrine-refractory states.[21] The early stage of sepsis includes the mass-release of hypophyseal reserves of vasopressin, leading to this deficiency. The nonthyroidal illness syndrome—also referred to as sick euthyroid syndrome—reflects impaired peripheral thyroid hormone metabolism and is consistently associated with worse outcomes, although its adaptive versus maladaptive nature remains unresolved.[21] Impaired adrenal responsiveness despite elevated adrenocorticotropic hormone levels defines critical illness-related corticosteroid insufficiency, providing the rationale for adjunctive corticosteroid therapy in refractory shock, although the use of corticosteroids in sepsis is still a controversy in critical care medicine.[30] Insulin resistance and stress-induced hyperglycemia, beyond their metabolic consequences, directly impair innate immune function—including neutrophil activity and complement efficiency—thereby linking neuroendocrine dysfunction to the immunosuppressive phenotype observed in sepsis.[21]

Collectively, these alterations represent a maladaptive neuroendocrine response that amplifies hemodynamic instability, perpetuates metabolic dysfunction, and impairs recovery, directly and indirectly affecting the immune system. Importantly, several components of this axis are therapeutically actionable, positioning the neuroendocrine system as both a mediator of disease severity and a potential target for precision-based interventions.

DIAGNOSIS AND CLINICAL APPROACH TO SEPSIS

Clinical recognition: Sepsis is a clinically heterogeneous syndrome that frequently presents with non-specific manifestations, contributing to delayed recognition. Rather than a single defining phenotype, patients exhibit a constellation of abnormalities reflecting systemic dysregulation. Early features may be subtle and difficult to assimilate clinically, including mild tachycardia, diaphoresis, or nonspecific clinical decline, whereas advanced disease is characterized by tachypnea, altered mental status, and hypotension. Classical signs such as fever may be absent or attenuated in vulnerable populations, including older adults and immunocompromised patients. Importantly, hypothermia may represent an equally significant, often overlooked, manifestation in these groups. These features necessitate a high index of suspicion and continuous reassessment, particularly in emergency and intensive care settings, in which sepsis must always be in the differential diagnosis.

Diagnostic criteria: Sepsis is a time-sensitive condition in which diagnosis remains inherently probabilistic. The current framework, as described previously, is defined by Sepsis-3, which characterizes sepsis as life-threatening organ dysfunction resulting from a dysregulated host response to infection. Organ dysfunction is operationalized using the SOFA score, with an acute increase of two or more points defining sepsis.[1] This approach shifts emphasis from the inflammatory response itself to its physiologic consequences, providing a more mechanistically coherent conceptual model, guiding treatment and clinical approaches.

Septic shock represents a distinct and more severe subset, defined by the requirement for vasopressor therapy to maintain a MAP $\geq$ 65 mm Hg and a serum lactate greater than 2 mmol/L despite adequate fluid resuscitation, a combination associated with substantially increased mortality. It is the most common type of distributive shock, a category that also includes anaphylactic and neurogenic shock.

Diagnostic strategies integrate clinical evaluation, organ dysfunction assessment, and laboratory data. Bedside tools such as the National Early Warning Score (NEWS2) and the quick SOFA (qSOFA) are widely used. However, their roles have evolved: NEWS2 is favored for early screening owing to its higher sensitivity, particularly outside the intensive care unit, whereas qSOFA is better interpreted as a marker of disease severity and adverse prognosis rather than an early diagnostic tool.[31]

Point-of-care ultrasound (POCUS) has emerged as an important extension of the bedside examination, enabling real-time assessment of hemodynamic status and early identification of potential infectious sources.[1] By integrating physiologic assessment with focused imaging, POCUS reduces diagnostic uncertainty and informs early resuscitation and management decisions and is quickly becoming one of the cornerstones of intensive care medicine.

Biomarkers: Biomarkers such as C-reactive protein, procalcitonin (PCT), and lactate remain central to the evaluation and monitoring of sepsis.[32] However, these markers largely reflect downstream consequences of the host response—namely inflammation and global metabolic stress, alongside cardiovasculatory collapse—rather than the underlying pathophysiological processes.

Lactate, known to all health care professionals as the laboratory hallmark of shock, warrants consideration. Traditionally interpreted as a marker of anaerobic metabolism secondary to tissue hypoxia, it is now understood as a multifactorial metabolic intermediate. Hyperlactatemia in sepsis (besides merely a result of tissue hypoperfusion) arises from increased aerobic glycolysis driven by catecholaminergic and inflammatory signaling, impaired hepatic clearance, and mitochondrial dysfunction, rather than solely reflecting oxygen debt.[33] This distinction is clinically relevant: persistent lactate elevation following adequate resuscitation may indicate ongoing immunometabolic dysregulation rather than unresolved circulatory failure. Beyond its role as a biomarker, lactate exerts immunomodulatory effects, influencing macrophage polarization and T-cell function[34]; its role is not merely as a byproduct of metabolism; it exerts effects as a cell modulator.

In addition to these classical markers, the diagnostic landscape is expanding to include indicators of specific host-response patterns. Emerging tools such as heparin-binding protein, monocyte distribution width, and presepsin have shown promise for early risk stratification and diagnosis.[32] Furthermore, discriminating between bacterial and viral etiologies—particularly in conditions such as severe COVID-19 or acute respiratory distress syndrome (ARDS), where lactate levels may remain within normal ranges despite severe disease—increasingly relies on interferon-related proteins and myxovirus resistance protein A.

Emerging diagnostic approaches are increasingly focused on immunometabolic profiling, reflecting a shift from isolated inflammatory markers toward integrated characterization of host response dynamics and the underlying physiologic changes. Molecules involved in substrate transport and cellular metabolism—including glucose transporter GLUT1, amino acid transporters such as SLC7A5, and lipid transporters such as CD36 or the SLC27 family of fatty acid transport proteins—are under investigation as indicators of metabolic state and may well be in their way to becoming part of the sepsis standard lab work. These candidates provide a mechanistic link between immunometabolic dysfunction and the development of organ failure. At present, these markers remain within preclinical and early translational domains and should be regarded as components of an evolving research framework rather than tools for routine clinical use.[6]

Identification of the Infectious Source

Identification of the infectious source is a cornerstone of sepsis management, guiding both antimicrobial therapy and the need for procedural intervention.[35] Common sources include the respiratory tract, intra-abdominal cavity, urinary tract, and intravascular devices. A systematic approach is required to exclude less apparent foci such as endocarditis, epidural abscess, or deep-seated soft tissue infection, which may well be at the root cause of sepsis.

Equally critical is timely source control, which should be pursued in parallel with initial resuscitation rather than sequentially.[36] Interventions such as abscess drainage, debridement of necrotic tissue, removal of infected devices, and surgical management of visceral perforation are essential, as antimicrobial therapy alone is often insufficient to prevent the worsening of symptoms. Observational data support achieving source control within 6 to 12 hours for most infections, with more urgent intervention required in rapidly progressive conditions such as necrotizing soft tissue infections, in which timely intervention is key.[37]

Failure to improve despite appropriate antimicrobial therapy and resuscitation should prompt reassessment of source control adequacy. In this context, biomarker trajectories—particularly serial lactate and PCT—may provide indirect evidence of ongoing infection or inadequate control, reinforcing the integration between diagnostic assessment and therapeutic response.

Initial Treatment and Individual Specific Approach

The management of sepsis is centered on early antimicrobial therapy, hemodynamic resuscitation, source control, and organ support. Prompt administration of appropriate antibiotics remains one of the most impactful interventions, with delays consistently associated with increased mortality, particularly in septic shock. Although the *1-hour bundle* remains debated—particularly in the context of diagnostic uncertainty—the principle of avoiding treatment delay in patients with suspected sepsis and hemodynamic compromise is well established. Empirical therapy should provide broad-spectrum coverage tailored to the suspected source and local resistance patterns, with subsequent de-escalation guided by microbiological data. This way, it is usually advised that the patient is started on broad-spectrum antibiotics, adjusted to the suspected infection source, before cultures guide treatment more specifically.

The primary goal of antimicrobial therapy in sepsis is rapid pathogen clearance. However, many effective antibiotics can inadvertently inhibit mitochondrial function due to the *bacterial ancestry* of mitochondria. Clinicians should maintain a high index of suspicion when a patient exhibits persistent hyperlactatemia despite adequate hemodynamic resuscitation and source control. In such cases, the etiology may be metabolic (drug-induced mitochondrial interference) rather than circulatory. Attention is warranted especially to oxazolidinones (Linezolid), tetracyclines and macrolides. Oxazolidinones pose the most significant clinical risk because they can inhibit mitochondrial protein synthesis and potentially lead to lactic acidosis that mimics worsening shock in patients receiving prolonged therapy. Also, tetracyclines and macrolides may cause mitochondrial dysfunction at standard doses, even if this remains a subject of ongoing study. Interestingly and counterintuitively, they have demonstrated *mitohormetic* (adaptive stress) protective effects in preclinical models and deserve to be tested in randomized clinical trial (RCT) for their potential to improve sepsis outcomes.[25,38]

Fluid resuscitation strategies have evolved substantially. Protocolized early goal-directed therapy has been supplanted by a more individualized approach, informed by trials such as PROCESS, ARISE, and ProMISe, and more recently the CLASSIC trial, which demonstrated that a restrictive fluid strategy is not inferior to standard care and may reduce fluid overload.[39] Current practice favors balanced crystalloids, early initiation of vasopressors when indicated, and dynamic assessment of fluid responsiveness.

Norepinephrine remains the first-line vasopressor in septic shock, with vasopressin commonly used as an adjunct in refractory cases.[36] In patients with persistent shock despite adequate resuscitation, low-dose corticosteroids represent an established adjunctive therapy, supported by randomized trials including ADRENAL and APROCCHSS, although optimal patient selection continues to be refined and the clinical practice remains skeptic toward corticosteroid use in sepsis.[40]

Beyond these established interventions, the paradigm of uniform treatment is increasingly challenged by the recognition of biological heterogeneity in sepsis. Data-driven analyses have identified reproducible clinical subphenotypes characterized by distinct patterns of organ dysfunction, inflammatory profiles, and differential responses to therapy. Although these subphenotypes have not yet been prospectively validated for clinical decision-making, they provide a conceptual framework for precision medicine approaches. Future advances will depend on the integration of biomarker-based stratification with adaptive trial designs, enabling therapies to be aligned with the dominant pathophysiological mechanisms in individual patients, although techniques to divide patients in these categories are still very much being worked on.[41]

Multiorgan Failure

Sepsis-induced acute failure of multiple organ systems markedly increases mortality risk. The degree of organ dysfunction can range from mild and reversible injury to complete failure, particularly when necrosis or gangrene develops. Because of the close physiologic interconnection between organs, isolated dysfunction is rare. Impairment in one system typically triggers widespread failure, as seen in MODS.

Clinically, patients with sepsis present multiorgan disturbances—including circulatory, respiratory, and neurologic abnormalities such as ischemia, dyspnea, altered mental status and hypotension.

These manifestations result from an uncontrolled immune response to infection. Excessive cytokine release (IL-6, IL-1β, TNF-α) creates a self-sustaining inflammatory loop, promoting widespread immune activation and tissue injury. The overproduction of ROS and reactive nitrogen species damages mitochondria, leading to cytopathic hypoxia, energy failure, and apoptosis. Mitochondrial dysfunction—including structural damage, redox imbalance, and extracellular mitochondrial DNA release—has been observed in the liver, skeletal and cardiac muscle, and immune cells. Restoring mitochondrial respiration may improve recovery in sepsis.

In parallel, endothelial dysfunction critically contributes to sepsis-induced organ failure. Loss of vascular integrity leads to hypoperfusion, vasodilation, microthrombosis, and dysregulated blood flow, culminating in tissue hypoxia. These changes manifest clinically as skin mottling, delayed capillary refill, peripheral ischemia, and oliguria.

Together, mitochondrial and endothelial impairments form the pathologic core of sepsis-induced multiple organ failure by jointly disrupting cellular metabolism, oxygen delivery, and systemic homeostasis, affecting the system besides impairing cell functioning at the individual level.

IMMUNOMETABOLIC REPROGRAMMING AND TARGETING AS A THERAPEUTIC TOOL

The accumulation of evidence that sepsis is guided and perpetuated by intense and dysfunctional changes in immune cell metabolism creates a window of opportunity to develop tools to improve outcome in patient survival and morbidity.[41] This strategy has the advantage of approaching the core of sepsis and its self-perpetuating nature instead of merely targeting its effects on the host.

The opportunities, as described by Velho and collaborators,[42] are twofold: firstly, it could help better understand the complexity of the syndrome and develop actual individual-based approaches, perhaps by developing specific host-response classifications to divide patients and to then approach them with more knowledge of how they would actually benefit from medical treatment. As described in their perspective, this approach has already been used for prognosis, as impairment in several metabolic pathways has been linked to higher sepsis mortality.[42]

Furthermore, key metabolic regulatory nodes are great targets for approaches aimed at reprogramming metabolic reactions. Targeting metabolism in sepsis can involve broad pharmacologic approaches that shift key metabolic pathways. For example, 2-deoxy-D-glucose (2-DG), a glycolysis inhibitor, has improved survival in preclinical models of sepsis, although clinical translation is still missing. Long-term metabolic therapies such as statins and metformin may also enhance outcomes by chronically reprogramming cellular metabolism. However, effectively managing opposing metabolic states across different tissues is, quite evidently, challenging, given it will require reliable, noninvasive biomarkers to monitor local metabolic and inflammatory conditions in real time. Additionally, after monitoring ability is achieved, given the heterogeneous metabolic profile of sepsis, varying wildly between tissues (often in antagonistic manners) advanced therapies are needed—such as pH-sensitive prodrugs that activate specifically in acidic environments associated with high glycolytic activity.[42]

Recent research into immunometabolic targeting has focused on inhibiting *overactive* pathways, including using 22-DG decrease excessive glycolysis. However, metabolic reprogramming offers extensive transformative opportunities to improve sepsis outcomes. The concept of metabolic resuscitation[43] proposes that instead of just suppressing inflammation, clinicians need to *fuel* specific immune phenotypes to promote the resolution of inflammation and the restoration of organ function. There are several strategies under investigation, including substrate supplementation, mitochondrial protection, and precision phenotyping. Substrate supplementation aims to drive macrophage polarization from a proinflammatory M1-like state toward a proresolving M2-like phenotype using specific nutrients like glutamine or omega-3 fatty acids, not merely as caloric support but as signaling molecules. To move beyond circulatory resuscitation to focus on *bioenergetic resuscitation* and achieve mitochondrial protection requires the use of agents that stabilize the mitochondrial membrane or reduce oxidative damage to the respiratory chain. Going forward, it is critical to move away from a *one-size-fits-all* approach. Precision phenotyping using real-time biomarkers, including the lactate-to-pyruvate ratio or plasma succinate levels, may allow to transition toward a model where metabolic therapies are tailored to the host's specific temporal and functional phenotype. This transition from reactive support to active metabolic guidance represents the next frontier in sepsis therapy, aiming to bridge the gap between systemic hemodynamic stability and cellular functional recovery. Although still quite far from the short-term clinical future, it is nevertheless vital that basic and clinical research is focused on the development of appropriate monitoring and interventive techniques aimed at the core of immunometabolic septic changes.

SUMMARY AND FUTURE PROSPECTS

Overall, critical inflammation and critical illness, and their expression in SIRS, CARS, sepsis, and MODS remain great unresolved challenges. Current treatment lacks solid large-scale evidence to show that it is in fact the best approach. Best prospects include individual-based therapy, especially those in the field of the modulation of immunometabolism. One highly promising way forward may be to invest in developing pharmacologic tools to modulate the host's immune and metabolic response. With this strategy, instead of using a merely supportive and reactive response to sepsis, these unresolved conditions can be targeted at its pathophysiological core.

As the basic and clinical research on the topics of sepsis, particularly the molecular alterations of homeostasis in the host, continue to add more knowledge into the scientific world, it becomes critical to review this knowledge and organize it in a way that is focused on clinical application. Even if the new literature does not yet have clinical implications, it is crucial for physicians to be aware of the new possibilities, so that when clinical approaches start being implemented and become available to physicians, they can be swiftly implemented and are met with excitement.

Due to the high significance and impact of sepsis on mortality, the need of additional mechanistic research of human sepsis is critical. For decades the continuous stride for improvement in this area has been driven mainly by clinicians and their efforts to mitigate the death toll that comes from sepsis. Despite the efforts and improving results, the management of sepsis continues to fall short of the need to save lives and limit sepsis-associated morbidity. The way forward must be inspired by human basic research, with much attention being paid to translation science, that can help add better therapeutic weapons to the ever-lasting war against sepsis.

CLINICS CARE POINTS

- Distinguish Circulatory vs. Metabolic Etiologies in Persistent Hyperlactatemia.
- Monitor Antibiotic-Induced Mitochondrial Toxicity During Prolonged Therapy.
- Implement Early and Simultaneous Source Control.
- Utilize Biomarkers and Screening Tools Contextually.
- Incorporate Individualized Resuscitation Strategies.

ACKNOWLEDGMENTS

The work in the Ferreira Moita laboratory is supported by the “la Caixa” Foundation (LCF/PR/HR23/52430007).

DISCLOSURE

The authors have no financial disclosures or conflicts of interest to disclose.

REFERENCES

1. Singer M, Deutschman CS, Seymour CW, et al. The third international consensus definitions for sepsis and septic shock (Sepsis-3). JAMA 2016;315:801–10.
2. Rudd KE, Johnson SC, Agesa KM, et al. Global, regional, and national sepsis incidence and mortality, 1990–2017: analysis for the global burden of disease study. Lancet 2020;395:200–11.
3. Willmann K, Moita LF. Physiologic disruption and metabolic reprogramming in infection and sepsis. Cell Metab 2024;36:927–46.
4. Efron PA, Brakenridge SC, Mohr AM, et al. The persistent inflammation, immunosuppression, and catabolism syndrome 10 years later. J Trauma Acute Care Surg 2023;95:790–9.
5. Mira JC, Brakenridge SC, Moldawer LL, et al. Persistent inflammation, immunosuppression and catabolism syndrome. Crit Care Clin 2017;33:245–58.
6. Paul SN, Nessel I, Puthucheary Z, et al. Sepsis and the immunometabolic inflammatory response. NPJ Metabolic Health Dis 2026;4:4.

7. Soares MP, Teixeira L, Moita LF. Disease tolerance and immunity in host protection against infection. Nat Rev Immunol 2017;17.
8. Hotchkiss RS, Moldawer LL, Opal SM, et al. Sepsis and septic shock. Nat Rev Dis Primers 2016;2:16045.
9. Ward NS, Casserly B, Ayala A. The compensatory anti-inflammatory response syndrome (CARS) in critically ill patients. Clin Chest Med 2008;29:617–25, viii.
10. Kumar V, Stewart Iv JH. Pattern-recognition receptors and immunometabolic reprogramming: what we know and what to explore. J Innate Immun 2024;16:295–323.
11. Cicchinelli S, Pignataro G, Gemma S, et al. PAMPs and DAMPs in sepsis: a review of their molecular features and potential clinical implications. Int J Mol Sci 2024;25.
12. Vigneron C, Py BF, Monneret G, et al. The double sides of NLRP3 inflammasome activation in sepsis. Clin Sci (Lond) 2023;137:333–51.
13. Willmann K, Moita LF. Biological and clinical implications of a model of surveillance immunity. J Clin Investig 2025;135.
14. Liston A, Masters SL. Homeostasis-altering molecular processes as mechanisms of inflammasome activation. Nat Rev Immunol 2017;17:208–14.
15. Kubelkova K, Bostik V, Joshi L, et al. Innate immune recognition, integrated stress response, infection, and tumorigenesis. Biology 2023;12.
16. Zhu S, Yu Y, Qu M, et al. Neutrophil extracellular traps contribute to immunothrombosis formation via the STING pathway in sepsis-associated lung injury. Cell Death Discov 2023;9:315.
17. Tannahill GM, Curtis AM, Adamik J, et al. Succinate is an inflammatory signal that induces IL-1β through HIF-1α. Nature 2013;496:238–42.
18. Pålsson-McDermott EM, O'Neill LAJ. Gang of 3: how the Krebs cycle-linked metabolites itaconate, succinate, and fumarate regulate macrophages and inflammation. Cell Metab 2025;37:1049–59.
19. Tang F, Zhao X-L, Xu L-Y, et al. Endothelial dysfunction: pathophysiology and therapeutic targets for sepsis-induced multiple organ dysfunction syndrome. Biomed Pharmacother 2024;178:117180.
20. Amersfoort J, Eelen G, Carmeliet P. Immunomodulation by endothelial cells - partnering up with the immune system? Nat Rev Immunol 2022;22:576–88.
21. Wahab F, Atika B, Oliveira-Pelegrin GR, et al. Recent advances in the understanding of sepsis-induced alterations in the neuroendocrine system. Endocr Metab Immune Disord Drug Targets 2013;13:335–47.
22. Singer M. The role of mitochondrial dysfunction in sepsis-induced multi-organ failure. Virulence 2014;5:66–72.
23. Lira Chavez FM, Gartzke LP, van Beuningen FE, et al. Restoring the infected powerhouse: mitochondrial quality control in sepsis. Redox Biol 2023;68:102968.
24. Harrington JS, Choi AMK, Nakahira K. Mitochondrial DNA in sepsis. Curr Opin Crit Care 2017;23:284–90.
25. Colaço HG, Barros A, Neves-Costa A, et al. Tetracycline antibiotics induce host-dependent disease tolerance to infection. Immunity 2021;54:53–67.e7.
26. De Vriese AS, Van Coster R, Smet J, et al. Linezolid-induced inhibition of mitochondrial protein synthesis. Clin Infect Dis 2006;42:1111–7.
27. Cheng Y-W, Liu J, Finkel T. Mitohormesis. Cell Metab 2023;35:1872–86.
28. Li Y, Chen M, Li J, et al. The role of pattern recognition receptors in epigenetic and metabolic reprogramming: insights into trained immunity. J Inflamm Res 2025;18:7795–811.

29. Huang J, Niu T, Shi H. Efficacy of blood copeptin level for the prediction of mortality of adult patients with sepsis: a meta-analysis. Front Med 2025;12:1686137.
30. Rochwerg B, Oczkowski S, Siemieniuk RA, et al. Corticosteroids in sepsis: an updated systematic review and meta-analysis (protocol). BMJ Open 2017;7:e016847.
31. Proctor LJ, Aarons GA, Dubowitz H, et al. Trajectories of maltreatment re-reports from ages 4 to 12:: evidence for persistent risk after early exposure. Child Maltreat 2012;17:207–17.
32. Bourika V, Rekoumi E-A, Giamarellos-Bourboulis EJ. Biomarkers to guide sepsis management. Ann Intensive Care 2025;15:103.
33. Garcia-Alvarez M, Marik P, Bellomo R. Sepsis-associated hyperlactatemia. Crit Care 2014;18:503.
34. Choi EJ, Jang YY, Choi EJ, et al. The role of lactate in immune regulation: a metabolic rheostat via transporters, receptors, and epigenetic modifiers. Cells 2025;14.
35. Guo X, Li C, Wu J, et al. The association of TNF-α -308G/A and -238G/A polymorphisms with type 2 diabetes mellitus: a meta-analysis. Biosci Rep 2019;39.
36. Cecconi M, Evans L, Levy M, et al. Sepsis and septic shock. Lancet 2018;392:75–87.
37. Guliyeva G, Huayllani MT, Sharma NT, et al. Practical review of necrotizing fasciitis: principles and evidence-based management. Plast Reconstr Surg Glob Open 2024;12:e5533.
38. Velho TR, Raquel H, Figueiredo N, et al. Immunomodulatory effects and protection in sepsis by the antibiotic moxifloxacin. Antibiotics (Basel) 2024;13.
39. Early, goal-directed therapy for septic shock — a patient-level meta-analysis. N Engl J Med 2017;376:2223–34.
40. Postow MA, Sidlow R, Hellmann MD. Immune-related adverse events associated with immune checkpoint blockade. N Engl J Med 2018;378:158–68.
41. Cao M, Wang G, Xie J. Immune dysregulation in sepsis: experiences, lessons and perspectives. Cell Death Discov 2023;9:465.
42. Payen D, Velho TR, Moita LF. Beyond inflammation: the role of metabolic dysregulation in sepsis diagnosis and treatment. Intensive Care Med 2025;51:1359–62.
43. Leite HP, de Lima LFP. Metabolic resuscitation in sepsis: a necessary step beyond the hemodynamic? J Thorac Dis 2016;8:E552–7.

Immunosuppression in the Pathophysiology of Sepsis

Tristan Couwenbergh, MD[a,*],
Wouter A. van der Heijden, MD, PhD[b,c], Mihai G. Netea, MD, PhD[a,c]

KEYWORDS

- Sepsis immunosuppression • Sepsis-induced immunoparalysis
- Immune dysregulation • Immunotherapy

KEY POINTS

- Mechanisms of immunosuppression in sepsis include dysregulated programmed cell death, epigenetic and transcriptional reprogramming, metabolic defects, and neuroimmune interactions.
- Immunosuppression in sepsis leads to both short-term and long-term clinical consequences, including heightened susceptibility to secondary infections, which can affect survivors for years after recovery.
- Therapeutic approaches are under investigation to restore immune function, although their clinical efficacy remains uncertain.

INTRODUCTION

Sepsis occurs when infection leads to life-threatening organ dysfunction due to a dysregulated host response.[1] This definition highlights 3 key pillars in the pathophysiology and management of sepsis. First, infection is the primary driver of sepsis, and early appropriate antimicrobial treatment and source control are crucial. Second, life-threatening organ dysfunction is the main cause of morbidity and mortality, and this is mitigated by intensive supportive care of failing organs. Finally, the dysregulated host response links the infection to organ function, and its rebalancing may benefit the host. However, standardized and effective immunomodulatory treatments are still lacking. This reflects both the incomplete understanding of the complex pathophysiology of sepsis, and the profound heterogeneity of the disease.

---

[a] Department of Internal Medicine, Radboud Center for Infectious Diseases, Radboud University Medical Center, Nijmegen, the Netherlands; [b] Department of Intensive Care, Radboud Center for Infectious Diseases, Radboud University Medical Center, Nijmegen, the Netherlands; [c] Department of Immunology and Metabolism, Life and Medical Sciences Institute (LIMES), University of Bonn, Germany
* Corresponding author. Department of Internal Medicine, Radboud University Medical Center, Geert Grooteplein 10, Postbus 9101, Huispostnummer 669, 6500 HB Nijmegen, Nijmegen, The Netherlands.
E-mail address: tristan.couwenbergh@radboudumc.nl

Crit Care Clin 42 (2026) 875–889
https://doi.org/10.1016/j.ccc.2026.05.010 **criticalcare.theclinics.com**

Abbreviations	
BCG	Bacille Calmette-Guérin
CMV	cytomegalovirus
GM-CSF	granulocyte–macrophage colony-stimulating factor
HLA-DR	human leukocyte antigen–DR
IVIg	intravenous immunoglobulin
LPS	lipopolysaccharide
MALS	macrophage activation–like syndrome
MDSCs	*myeloid-derived suppressor cells*
mHLA-DR	monocytic HLA-DR
MSCs	mesenchymal stem cells
PD-1	programmed cell death-1
RCTs	randomized clinical trials
sPD-L1	soluble programmed death ligand 1
TLR4	toll-like receptor 4
Tregs	regulatory T-cells
Tα1	thymosin α1

Immune dysregulation in sepsis is complex. While local production of proinflammatory cytokines is essential for pathogen clearance, excessive cytokine release causes systemic inflammation, leading to endothelial dysfunction, coagulopathy, tissue damage and multi-organ failure.[2] However, immune dysregulation in sepsis is highly heterogeneous. It may result in exaggerated inflammation and systemic organ failure, or in immunosuppression, reducing control of the primary infection and increasing vulnerability to secondary infections.[3] These immune endotypes vary between patients, depending on pathogen type, infection site, disease stage, and patient characteristics. In some patients hyperinflammation and immunosuppression occur simultaneously, whereas in others they change over time.[2]

Over the past century, advances like antibiotics and intensive care units have substantially reduced sepsis-related mortality. More recently, specific improvements in supportive care, as bundled in the Surviving Sepsis Campaign,[4] have increased sepsis survival. Despite these gains, overall sepsis mortality remains unacceptably high at 30% to 40%.[5] This underscores the need for therapies that rebalance immune responses and improve outcomes. While both hyperinflammation and immunosuppression can occur in sepsis, this article focuses on immunosuppression, its underlying mechanisms, and potential therapeutic approaches.

THE INNATE AND ADAPTIVE IMMUNE SYSTEMS IN SEPSIS

Sepsis often involves immune suppression that is associated with early mortality and increased vulnerability to secondary infections, including opportunistic pathogens and viral reactivation.[3,6] As shown in **Fig. 1**, this suppression affects both the innate and adaptive immune system.

Defects in the Innate Immune Cells

In sepsis, suppression of innate immunity is marked by the functional reprogramming of myeloid cells. Monocytes from sepsis patients produce fewer proinflammatory cytokines (tumor necrosis factor [TNF]α, interleukin [IL]-1α, IL-1β, IL-6, IL-12) after lipopolysaccharide (LPS) stimulation, while anti-inflammatory cytokines like IL-1RA and IL-10 are preserved or increased.[7] This suggests altered intracellular signaling that limits proinflammatory cytokines while promoting anti-inflammatory responses.[7] This anti-inflammatory reprogramming extends beyond circulating monocytes to

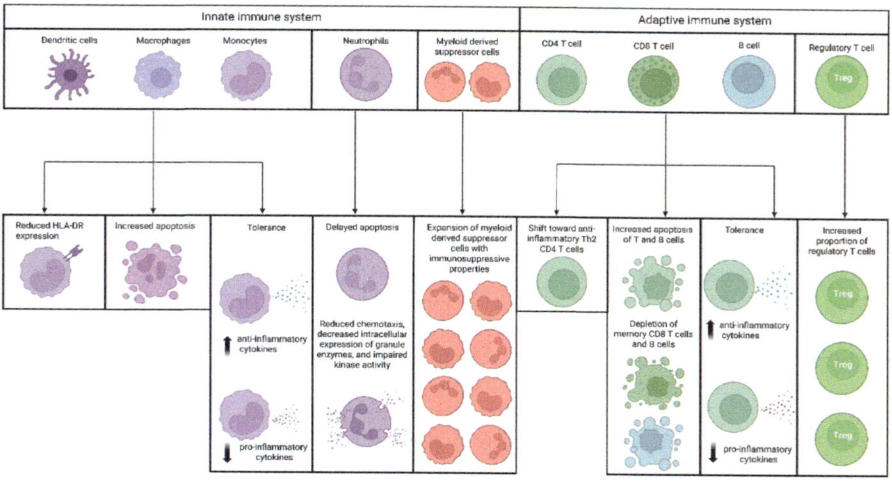

Fig. 1. Defects in innate and adaptive immune cells in sepsis. (*Created in* BioRender. Research, I. (2026) https://BioRender.com/k818b60.)

dendritic cells and tissue macrophages with reduced proinflammatory cytokine production and enhanced IL-10 production.[3,8] Macrophages are pushed into a tolerant phenotype, secreting IL-10 and TGF-β.[9] Altogether, this altered state of myeloid cells in sepsis patients is also referred to as tolerance. Although tolerance may reduce antimicrobial activity in sepsis, it is also part of a physiologic response to severe stress. Balancing antimicrobial activity with tolerance to limit tissue damage is crucial for favorable outcomes.[7]

In addition to tolerance, myeloid cells in sepsis exhibit reduced antigen-presenting capacity, reflected by decreased surface expression of human leukocyte antigen–DR (HLA-DR), which is essential for antigen presentation to T cells. This reduction is observed in monocytes as well as in peripheral blood dendritic cells from sepsis patients.[10,11] Decreased monocytic HLA-DR (mHLA-DR), assessed by flow cytometry, has become the most important biomarker of sepsis-induced immunosuppression and has been successfully used in randomized clinical trials (RCTs).[12] Reduced mHLA-DR expression reflects monocyte dysfunction and is associated with impaired cytokine production in response to LPS.[11] Persistently low mHLA-DR expression in sepsis patients correlates with an increased risk of secondary infections and higher mortality.[13,14]

Beyond inhibition and reprogramming of the myeloid cell populations in blood and organs, increasing evidence supports the presence of immunosuppressive cells termed *myeloid-derived suppressor cells* (MDSCs) in sepsis. MDSCs are a heterogeneous group of immature myeloid cells including progenitors of monocytes, neutrophils and dendritic cells, that expand during inflammation or infection.[15] During chronic inflammation, dysregulated myelopoiesis drives the accumulation of MDSCs.[16] MDSCs suppress both innate and adaptive immune cells, particularly by inhibiting T-cell responses through L-arginine consumption and IL-10 production.[15] MDSCs also promote the expansion of regulatory T-cells (Tregs).[15] Studies have shown that MDSC numbers remain elevated for up to 28 days post sepsis and are associated with increased secondary infections, prolonged ICU stays, and poor outcomes.[17,18] In surgical sepsis survivors, MDSCs remained elevated for 6 weeks post sepsis. Furthermore, their suppressive activity developed around 14 days post sepsis, suggesting that MDSCs may acquire immune-suppressive functions over time.[19] It is important to note however that MDSCs may also play a beneficial role by limiting hyperinflammation during early sepsis and protecting against organ dysfunction.[15]

Defects in Adaptive Immune Cells

Sepsis-induced immunosuppression also affects adaptive immune cells, particularly T lymphocytes, which undergo anti-inflammatory reprogramming similar to innate immune cells. T cells from peripheral blood, as well as spleen and lung tissue from postmortem sepsis patients, show altered cytokine production. Reduced production of cytokines includes IFN-γ, TNF, and IL-2, while IL-4 and IL-10 remain largely unchanged.[3,20] B cells show decreased HLA-DR expression and increased IL-10 production.[2] Antigen presentation defects further impair T cell activation, with reduced expression of costimulatory and signaling molecules, like CD28[21] and CD3.[22]

Sepsis causes lymphopenia, increasing susceptibility to secondary infections and late mortality.[23] This depletion results from widespread apoptosis in B cells, natural killer (NK) cells, and CD4/CD8 T cells in clinical and postmortem studies.[24,25] CD4 T cell numbers decrease but typically recover in survivors, while failure to restore CD4 counts correlates with poor prognosis.[26] Sepsis also disrupts immunologic memory by depleting memory CD8 T cells, altering their composition and reducing their diversity,[27] while memory B cells are also disproportionately affected by apoptosis.[28]

Sepsis alters CD4 T cell subsets, shifting the balance from proinflammatory Th1 cells to anti-inflammatory Th2 cells.[29] This shift, marked by increased Th2-associated cytokines IL-4 and IL-10 and reduced Th1 cytokines TNF-α, IFN-γ, and IL-2, is driven in part by impaired IL-12 production and associated with diminished antimicrobial defense.[30,31] Persistently elevated Th2/Th1 ratios correlate with higher ICU-acquired infections and 28-day mortality.[32] Additionally, Th17 cells, important for defense against fungal pathogens, are increased in sepsis patients but decline after day 7 in nonsurvivors, while survivors maintain higher levels.[33] This may, in part, explain the increased susceptibility to secondary fungal infections in sepsis.[34]

During sepsis, Tregs increase relative to effector T cells, especially in nonsurvivors.[35] This phenomenon is best interpreted not as an absolute expansion of Tregs, but rather as a relative increase resulting from the loss of other T cell populations.[36] One possible explanation is that Tregs have increased resistance to apoptosis, potentially due to elevated BCL-2 expression.[37] Tregs promote monocyte apoptosis in septic shock,[38] and exert broad immunosuppressive effects, including production of inhibitory cytokines.[39] Increases in Treg proportions may also be beneficial, as they help limit excessive inflammation and promote tissue repair, particularly in conditions such as acute lung injury.[39]

MECHANISMS OF IMMUNOSUPPRESSION

As shown in **Fig. 2**, immunosuppression in sepsis is influenced by several mechanisms.

Induction of Immunosuppression by Initial Hyperinflammation

Sepsis-induced hyperinflammation paradoxically drives immunosuppression, promoting tolerance of innate and adaptive immune cells. Supporting this concept, patients who developed secondary infections exhibited a more dysregulated host response during the first days after ICU admission, characterized by heightened inflammation, coagulation, endothelial activation, and vascular disruption.[40] These changes are partly driven by epigenetic and metabolic reprogramming. In parallel,

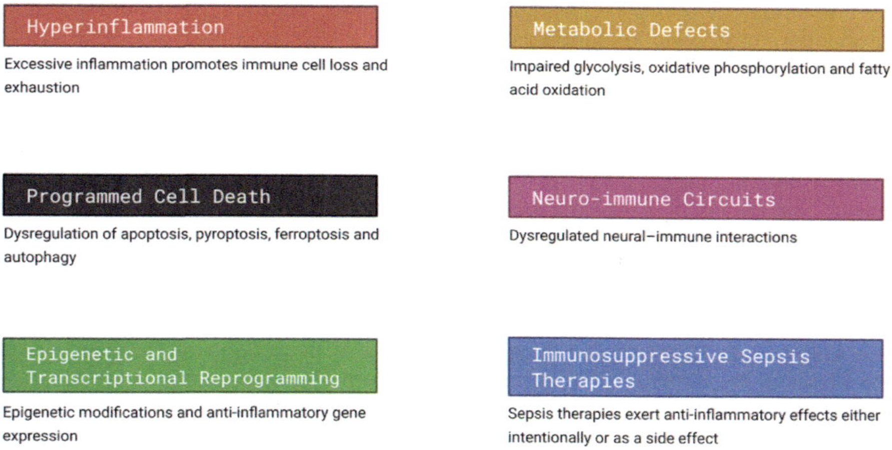

Fig. 2. Mechanisms of immunosuppression in sepsis. (*Created in* BioRender. Research, I. (2026) https://BioRender.com/sl8twii.)

overwhelming inflammation induces immune cell loss through dysregulated activation of programmed cell death.

Dysregulation of Programmed Cell Death Mechanisms

Sepsis-induced apoptosis involves both death-receptor and mitochondrial pathways, initiated by inflammatory and cellular stress signals.[2,24] There is evidence that checkpoint regulators, such as programmed cell death-1 (PD-1), contribute to apoptosis of T cells. The interaction of PD-1 and its ligands PD-L1 and PD-L2 on antigen-presenting cells results in T cell suppression and increases susceptibility to apoptosis.[3,34] The expression of PD-1 on T cells and PD-L1 on antigen presenting cells is associated with lymphopenia, T cell anergy, and T cell apoptosis.[3,41] Increased expression was also associated with occurrence of secondary infections and mortality.[42] Ex vivo PD-1 blockade in $CD8^+$ T cells from sepsis patients reduces apoptosis and enhances IFN-γ production.[41] Other checkpoint regulators like cytotoxic T-lymphocyte–associated protein 4 (CTLA-4) may contribute to immunosuppression. CTLA-4 is a negative checkpoint regulator that suppresses T cell activity, promotes apoptosis, and its expression on T cells increases during sepsis.

Sepsis induces dendritic cell apoptosis, linked to secondary infections and higher mortality.[43,44] Apoptosis of circulating monocytes also increases.[45] Macrophages remove apoptotic cells from inflamed tissues, promoting IL-10 and TGF-β release, suppressing HLA-DR expression, and inducing endotoxin tolerance.[46] In contrast to other innate immune cells, apoptosis of neutrophils is delayed in sepsis.[47] Neutrophils during sepsis also undergo functional changes, including reduced chemotaxis, decreased intracellular expression of myeloperoxidase and lactoferrin, and impaired kinase activity, which may contribute to immunosuppression.[2] Furthermore, IFN-γ–stimulated neutrophils in experimental endotoxemia suppress T cells proliferation through expression of PD-L1.[48]

Alternative forms of programmed cell death, including pyroptosis and ferroptosis, also contribute to immune dysregulation in sepsis, with pyroptosis causing macrophage loss.[9] Similarly, ferroptosis drives macrophage death and skews the immune response toward a more tolerant phenotype.[9] Autophagy, a key process for maintaining homeostasis and supporting antigen presentation, is impaired in sepsis. In a murine model, defective T-cell autophagy accelerates apoptosis and increases IL-10 production, promoting immunosuppression.[49]

Epigenetic and Transcriptional Reprogramming in Sepsis

Epigenetic modifications are another mechanism affecting immunosuppression by influencing gene expression. In experimental models of endotoxin tolerance, sepsis-induced immunosuppression has been characterized by loss of activating histone marks, accumulation of repressive marks, and increased histone deacetylation at promoters of proinflammatory genes, leading to sustained transcriptional repression.[34]

Epigenetic changes also affect adaptive immune cells, promoting repressive histone modifications at key cytokine and transcription factor genes in T cells and favoring regulatory T-cell differentiation.[34] Evidence from murine models suggests that these epigenetic changes can originate in bone marrow progenitor cells, resulting in long-lasting impairment of macrophage inflammatory responses after sepsis.[34] Although less studied than chromatin modifications, posttranscriptional regulation by microRNAs also contributes to immune regulation in sepsis, although their role in immunosuppression remains unclear.[50]

Epigenetic reprogramming in sepsis leads to profound changes in blood leukocyte transcriptomes, affecting 70% to 80% of RNA transcripts compared to healthy controls.[34,51] These changes, likely also influences by shifts in leukocyte composition, encompass proinflammatory and anti-inflammatory programs, reflecting the heterogeneity of immune dysregulation in sepsis. Most of these transcriptional alterations appear independent of the source of infection or pathogen, supporting sepsis as a host-driven syndrome.[52] Hypoxia-inducible factor-1α (HIF-1α) is a key regulator of this host response. HIF-1α is upregulated and transcriptionally active in sepsis monocytes driving reprogramming toward an endotoxin-tolerant, immunosuppressive phenotype.[53] In addition, early repression of the antiapoptotic gene BCL2 in circulating mononuclear cells is linked to increased lymphocyte apoptosis, $CD4^+$ and $CD8^+$ T-cell lymphopenia, and poor outcomes in sepsis.[54] The sepsis transcriptomic response also overlaps with severe blunt trauma or noninfectious respiratory failure, indicating an intrinsic response to inflammatory stimuli.[51]

Metabolic Defects of Immune Cells During Sepsis

Alterations in the metabolism of immune cells play a key role in immunosuppression. Usually during inflammation, immune cells shift from oxidative phosphorylation to aerobic glycolysis despite sufficient oxygen (Warburg effect) to meet energy demands. However, this metabolic program is not universal: pathogen- and context-specific stimulation can induce more complex metabolic rewiring in myeloid cells, characterized by increased glycolysis with variable, and in some cases enhanced, oxidative phosphorylation.[34] Warburg-like metabolic reprogramming promotes HIF-1α–dependent transcription of proinflammatory genes, whereas this pathway is dysregulated during LPS-induced tolerance.[34] Tolerant monocytes produce less lactate than nontolerant cells, reflecting an impaired ability to induce Warburg-like glycolysis.[55] Beyond defective glycolysis, these cells also display reduced oxidative phosphorylation and impaired fatty acid oxidation, consistent with a state of immunometabolic paralysis.[55] These metabolic defects were associated with impaired mTOR signaling.[34,55]

Neuroimmune Circuits

Dysregulation of central nervous system–immune interactions might contribute to immunosuppression. Sepsis-associated encephalopathy, driven by neuroinflammation and cerebral ischemia, suppresses peripheral immune responses, including impaired function of monocytes, dendritic cells, neutrophils, and T cells, although most evidence derives from animal models.[34] The vagus nerve's cholinergic anti-inflammatory reflex can suppress innate immune responses in animal sepsis.[34] Similarly, the sympathetic nervous system may promote immunosuppression through stimulation of β-adrenergic receptors on immune cells.[34] However, the exact role of these neuroimmune mechanisms in human sepsis remains unclear.[34]

Therapies Used in Sepsis with Immunosuppressive Effects

The β-adrenergic receptor also plays a role in therapies used in sepsis, such as norepinephrine, which, in addition to its vasopressor function, can exert anti-inflammatory effects by suppressing proinflammatory cytokine production and increasing IL-10 in experimental sepsis models and in humans, mediated largely through β-adrenergic signaling.[34] Glucocorticoids, like hydrocortisone, are used in sepsis after improving outcomes in an RCT.[56] While beneficial during the hyperinflammatory phase, their anti-inflammatory effects can worsen immunosuppression.

CLINICAL CONSEQUENCES

Sepsis-induced immunosuppression significantly affects survival and infection susceptibility. Early on, it increases acute mortality by impairing the body's defense against the primary infection. In fact, most nonsurviving septic shock patients (78%) die within 48 hours of onset and exhibit clear signs of immunosuppression.[14] During recovery, sepsis survivors are highly vulnerable to secondary and opportunistic infections, including opportunistic bacterial and (invasive) fungal infections.[57] Latent viral reactivation is common, with cytomegalovirus (CMV) and herpes simplex virus reactivating in sepsis survivors, conditions normally controlled by a healthy immune system.[58] Among septic shock patients, 68% show reactivation of herpesviruses, with concurrent CMV and Epstein-Barr virus reactivations linked to increased mortality.[59] Furthermore, a study found that 40% of sepsis patients developed viremia with herpesviruses, polyomaviruses, and anelloviruses, and CMV positivity was associated with a higher risk of fungal infections and death.[60]

Sepsis-induced immunosuppression not only impacts the acute phase but also has long-term consequences. Even patients who appear to recover clinically exhibit heightened susceptibility to recurrent infections and cardiovascular complications.[61,62] Accordingly, sepsis survivors have a substantially increased long-term risk of death compared with age- and sex-matched populations, with excess mortality persisting for years and not fully explained by preexisting comorbidities.[63] Approximately one-third are readmitted within 90 days, more than half due to recurrent sepsis.[64] Other causes of readmission include accelerated progression of preexisting chronic diseases, residual organ injury, and persistent immune dysfunction.[65]

Many sepsis survivors develop sustained functional, cognitive, and physical impairments. These individuals often experience persistent low-grade inflammation, immune suppression, and progressive lean tissue wasting.[66] Emerging evidence suggests that epigenetic changes, including altered chromatin and DNA methylation, contribute to these long-term effects.[67,68] Despite partial recovery at ICU discharge in cellular features like T-cell function and monocyte HLA-DR expression[69] molecular evidence of immune dysregulation persists. One year after discharge, circulating biomarkers of immunosuppression persist, including elevated soluble programmed death ligand 1 (sPD-L1), associated with adverse long-term outcomes.[70] Murine models demonstrate that sepsis induces durable immunoparalysis, with survivors exhibiting impaired control of secondary challenges and accelerated tumor growth up to ~100 days postsepsis despite recovery of lymphocyte counts.[71]

EMERGING THERAPIES

The increasing understanding of the pathophysiology of immunosuppression in sepsis opens the door for the design and testing of novel immunotherapies that may improve the outcome of these patients. **Fig. 3** summarizes these current strategies.

Immune Stimulating Cytokines

Several cytokines have been explored to reverse sepsis-induced immunosuppression. IFN-γ increases monocyte HLA-DR expression in experimental endotoxemia and sepsis patients, improving immune function.[72] Patients with invasive *Candida* and/or *Aspergillus* infections regained partial immune function after IFN -γ treatment.[73] Recombinant IFN-γ has shown effectiveness in treating sepsis-induces immunoparalysis, defined by reduced HLA-DR expression, in the ImmunoSep phase II RCT.[12] Another interferon studied in immunosuppression is IFN-β. IFN-β restored the LPS-induced immunosuppressed state of monocytes in experimental endotoxemia.[74] In murine sepsis, IFN-β significantly improved survival when administered after the onset of sepsis.[75]

IL-7 promotes lymphocyte survival, proliferation, and function and reverses sepsis-induced lymphopenia in animal models.[72] In an RCT, recombinant IL-7 increased CD4+ and CD8+ T cells in septic shock patients with severe lymphopenia, with a favorable safety profile, although it has yet to show an effect on clinical outcomes.[72] IL-15 improves survival in murine sepsis by preventing apoptosis of NK cells, dendritic cells,

Therapies	Mechanism of action	Strongest evidence	Limitations
Interferon-γ (IFN-γ)	Multiple mechanisms activate antigen presenting cells	Improves organ dysfunction in phase II clinical trial (11)	No completed clinical trials on mortality
Interferon-β (IFN-β)	Restores immunosuppressed monocytes	Improves surival in murine sepsis (74)	No human data
Interleukin-7 (IL-7)	Promotes B and T cell development and proliferation	Reverses lymphopenia in phase II clinical trial (71)	No completed clinical trials on clinical outcomes
Interleukin-15 (IL-15)	Prevents apoptosis of lymphocytes and dendritic cells	Improves survival in murine sepsis (75)	No human data, concerns about toxicity (76)
Interleukin-33 (IL-33)	Prevents apoptosis of lymphocytes	Improves survival in murine sepsis (71)	No human data
Granulocyte macrophage colony stimulating factor (GM-CSF)	Accelerates production of innate immune cells	Improves infection clearance in phase II clinical trial (78)	No mortality reduction in clinical trial meta-analysis (78)
Programmed Death 1 (PD-1) inhibitors	Prevents T cell apoptosis	Raises lymphocyte counts in phase I/II clinical trial (34)	No completed clinical trials on clinical outcomes, phase III trial terminated (34)
Cytotoxic T-lymphocyte associated protein 4 (CTLA-4) inhibitor	Prevents T cell apoptosis	Improves survival in murine sepsis (80)	No human data
Thymosin α1 (Tα1)	Restores immunosuppressed monocytes and enhances T cell function	Trend towards lower mortality in clinical trial (81)	Failed to reduce mortality in phase III clinical trial (82)
Toll-like receptor 4 (TLR4) inhibitor	Blocks LPS-induced cytokine responses	Trend towards lower mortality in phase II clinical trial (83)	Failed to reduce mortality in phase III clinical trial (83)
Caspase inhibitors	Prevents lymphocyte apoptosis	Improves survival in murine sepsis (84)	No human data
Intravenous Immunoglobulin (IVIg)	Several immunomodulatory mechanisms	Potential mortality reduction in clinical trial meta-analysis (34)	Guidelines advise against use due to low evidence quality (4)
Mesenchymal Stem Cells (MSCs)	Several immunomodulatory mechanisms	Proved safety in phase I clinical trials (71)	No completed clinical trials on clinical outcomes
Trained Immunity	Reverses tolerance in innate immune cells	Reverses endotoxin tolerance in murine sepsis (85)	Failed to enhance immune responses in human endotoxemia (86)

Fig. 3. Sepsis immunosuppression reversal therapies. (*Created in* BioRender. Research, I. (2026) https://BioRender.com/mqpbbgy.)

and $CD8^+$ T cells and by enhancing IFN-γ production.[76] However, reported toxicities in oncology trials raise concerns regarding its clinical applicability in sepsis.[77] IL-33 has demonstrated protective effects and reduced mortality in murine sepsis.[72] Finally, granulocyte–macrophage colony-stimulating factor (GM-CSF) restores monocyte HLA-DR expression and reduces ICU length of stay in sepsis patients with immune suppression.[78] Although RCTs and meta-analyses report GM-CSF improved leukocyte recovery and infection clearance, these benefits have not translated into reduced mortality.[79]

Immune Checkpoint Inhibition

Immune checkpoint inhibitors, particularly targeting the PD-1/PD-L1 axis, have also been studied in immunosuppression. Monocyte PD-L1 expression predicts 28-day mortality and may serve as a biomarker to identify patients most likely to benefit from checkpoint inhibition.[80] Phase I/II RCTs of anti-PD-L1 therapy in sepsis have been well tolerated, improving lymphocyte counts and monocyte HLA-DR expression.[34] However, effects on major clinical outcomes such as secondary infections and mortality remain unproven, and plans for a phase III RCT were terminated prematurely.[34] Other inhibitory checkpoints like CTLA-4 improve survival in murine models, but human data are lacking.[81]

Other Immune Stimulating Therapies

Thymosin α1 (Tα1) is a thymic peptide proposed to restore immunity in sepsis, showed a trend toward mortality reduction in one RCT[82] but no effect on 28-day mortality in a recent phase III RCT.[83] A Phase II RCT targeting toll-like receptor 4 (TLR4) showed a trend toward lower mortality, while a Phase III RCT failed to reduce 28-day mortality.[84] The use of caspase inhibitors improves survival in murine sepsis by preventing lymphocyte apoptosis, but results in human studies are still lacking.[85] Intravenous immunoglobulin (IVIg) has immunomodulatory properties and may reduce mortality in sepsis, though results are mixed.[34] The Surviving Sepsis Campaign guidelines recommend against intravenous immunoglobulins in patients with sepsis or septic shock due to low quality of evidence.[4] Mesenchymal stem cells (MSCs) have shown potential for immunomodulation and tissue repair in sepsis, with early studies indicating feasibility and tolerance, but further large trials are needed to confirm efficacy.[72]

Innate immunity can develop a form of memory, termed trained immunity, where prior pathogen or vaccine exposure enhances future immune responses.[51] Trained immunity is driven by epigenetic and metabolic reprogramming of monocytes and is epigenetically and functionally the opposite of endotoxin tolerance.[51] β-glucan-induced trained immunity restores monocyte responses, including cytokine production.[51] A fusion protein of apolipoprotein A1 and IL4 reversed endotoxin tolerance in murine models and ex vivo human endotoxemia models by inducing trained immunity.[86] However, induction of trained immunity with gamma-irradiated Bacille Calmette-Guérin (BCG) did not enhance immune responses in human endotoxemia.[87] Future studies are needed to prove clinical effectiveness of trained immunity-based immunotherapies.

FUTURE DEVELOPMENTS

Progress toward effective immunotherapy for sepsis-induced immunosuppression requires moving from prognostic to predictive enrichment, selecting patients based on immune endotypes and biomarkers. Patients with specific endotypes, characterized by defects in particular immune components, are most likely to benefit from immune stimulation. Achieving this requires 2 advances: identifying endotypes responsive to specific immunomodulatory interventions and developing rapid, clinically applicable biomarkers to capture these endotypes at the bedside. Established endotypes such as macrophage activation–like syndrome (MALS) and sepsis-induced immunoparalysis, illustrate the feasibility of this approach with HLA-DR demonstrating therapeutic relevance as a biomarker for immunosuppression.[10]

Advances in multi-omics approaches have led to emerging endotypes, valuable for patient stratification.[88] However, current endotypes almost exclusively reflect the extent of hyperinflammation rather than immune suppression. For future omics-based endotypes, we need those that describe immunosuppression to better select patients and identify new pathways. These should be linked to outcomes like mortality and secondary infections to ensure robustness and associated with a minimal set of functional, rapidly measurable biomarkers suitable for clinical use. Moreover, sepsis is a dynamic syndrome, and endotypes are unlikely to be static. Accordingly, immunomodulatory therapy should be initiated early and reassessed continuously, with treatment adapted as patients transition between endotypes. This need for longitudinal immune monitoring is underscored by evidence that endotypes can change rapidly, often within 48 hours of ICU admission.[89]

Finally, the long-term consequences of sepsis-induced immune dysfunction warrant increased attention. Currently, we cannot identify patients who will develop persistent immune alterations and related late complications, and no targeted therapies exist for this population. A first step is determining whether acute-phase endotypes and biomarkers also predict long-term immune status. If established, further research is needed to explore whether early, personalized immunotherapy can prevent these adverse outcomes, or whether distinct therapies will be required during the recovery phase.

CLINICS CARE POINTS

- Sepsis can lead to immunosuppression, increasing the risk of secondary infections, including opportunistic bacterial, invasive fungal infections, and viral reactivations (eg, cytomegalovirus, herpes simplex virus).
- Effective therapies for sepsis-induced immunosuppression are still lacking, but treatments like IFN-γ, based on decreased monocytic human leukocyte antigen–DR expression, have shown promising results in Phase II randomized clinical trials.

DISCLOSURE

The authors have nothing to disclose.

FUNDING

This research was partially supported through the project Slowing Immune System Aging through Dietary control (ImmunAgeD), PNRR-III-C9-2022-I8, Contract No. 760057/23.05.2023, for the University of Medicine and Pharmacy of Craiova, as part of a grant from the National Recovery and Resilience Plan. Funded by the Dutch Organisation for knowledge and innovation in health, healthcare and well-being (ZonMw) Clinical Fellowship: 09032242410027 This research is part of the project HEAL-SEPSIS with file number OCENW.XL.23.055 of the research programme Open Competition Domain Science XL, which is (partly) financed by the Dutch Research Council (NWO) under the grant https://doi.org/10.61686/CGBGZ00396.

REFERENCES

1. Singer M, Deutschman CS, Seymour CW, et al. The third international consensus definitions for sepsis and septic shock (Sepsis-3). JAMA 2016;315(8):801–10.
2. van der Poll T, Shankar-Hari M, Wiersinga WJ. The immunology of sepsis. Immunity 2021;54(11):2450–64.
3. Boomer JS, To K, Chang KC, et al. Immunosuppression in patients who die of sepsis and multiple organ failure. JAMA 2011;306(23):2594–605.
4. Prescott HC, Antonelli M, Alhazzani W, et al. Surviving sepsis campaign: international guidelines for management of sepsis and septic shock 2026. Crit Care Med 2026;54(4):725–812.
5. Alliance ES. European sepsis report 2021. 2021. Available at: https://static1.squarespace.com/static/5ba4be38a56827832703eb7a/t/613888cb2b988316d6541932/1631094995535/European+Sepsis+Report+FINAL.pdf.
6. Monneret G, Lafon T, Gossez M, et al. Monocyte HLA-DR expression in septic shock patients: insights from a 20-year real-world cohort of 1023 cases. Intensive Care Med 2025;51(10):1820–32.
7. Cavaillon JM, Adib-Conquy M. Bench-to-bedside review: endotoxin tolerance as a model of leukocyte reprogramming in sepsis. Crit Care 2006;10(5):233.
8. Biswas SK, Lopez-Collazo E. Endotoxin tolerance: new mechanisms, molecules and clinical significance. Trends Immunol 2009;30(10):475–87.
9. Gao X, Cai S, Li X, et al. Sepsis-induced immunosuppression: mechanisms, biomarkers and immunotherapy. Front Immunol 2025;16:1577105. https://doi.org/10.3389/fimmu.2025.1577105.
10. Poehlmann H, Schefold JC, Zuckermann-Becker H, et al. Phenotype changes and impaired function of dendritic cell subsets in patients with sepsis: a prospective observational analysis. Crit Care 2009;13(4):R119. https://doi.org/10.1186/cc7969.
11. Monneret G, Venet F, Pachot A, et al. Monitoring immune dysfunctions in the septic patient: a new skin for the old ceremony. Mol Med 2008;14(1–2):64–78.
12. Giamarellos-Bourboulis EJ, Kotsaki A, Kotsamidi I, et al. Precision immunotherapy to improve sepsis outcomes: the immunosep randomized clinical trial. JAMA 2026;335(9):775–86.
13. Landelle C, Lepape A, Voirin N, et al. Low monocyte human leukocyte antigen-DR is independently associated with nosocomial infections after septic shock. Intensive Care Med 2010;36(11):1859–66.
14. Monneret G, Lepape A, Voirin N, et al. Persisting low monocyte human leukocyte antigen-DR expression predicts mortality in septic shock. Intensive Care Med 2006;32(8):1175–83.
15. Schrijver IT, Théroude C, Roger T. Myeloid-derived suppressor cells in sepsis. mini review. Front Immunol 2019;10. https://doi.org/10.3389/fimmu.2019.00327.
16. Gabrilovich DI. Myeloid-derived suppressor cells. Cancer Immunol Res 2017; 5(1):3–8.
17. Mathias B, Delmas AL, Ozrazgat-Baslanti T, et al. Human myeloid-derived suppressor cells are associated with chronic immune suppression after severe sepsis/septic shock. Ann Surg 2017;265(4):827–34.
18. Uhel F, Azzaoui I, Grégoire M, et al. Early expansion of circulating granulocytic myeloid-derived suppressor cells predicts development of nosocomial infections in patients with sepsis. Am J Respir Crit Care Med 2017;196(3):315–27.

19. Hollen MK, Stortz JA, Darden D, et al. Myeloid-derived suppressor cell function and epigenetic expression evolves over time after surgical sepsis. Crit Care 2019;23(1):355.
20. Heidecke CD, Hensler T, Weighardt H, et al. Selective defects of T lymphocyte function in patients with lethal intraabdominal infection. Am J Surg 1999;178(4): 288–92.
21. Manjuck J, Saha DC, Astiz M, et al. Decreased response to recall antigens is associated with depressed costimulatory receptor expression in septic critically ill patients. J Lab Clin Med 2000;135(2):153–60.
22. Venet F, Bohé J, Debard AL, et al. Both percentage of gammadelta T lymphocytes and CD3 expression are reduced during septic shock. Crit Care Med 2005;33(12):2836–40.
23. Drewry AM, Samra N, Skrupky LP, et al. Persistent lymphopenia after diagnosis of sepsis predicts mortality. Shock 2014;42(5):383–91.
24. Hotchkiss RS, Osmon SB, Chang KC, et al. Accelerated lymphocyte death in sepsis occurs by both the death receptor and mitochondrial pathways. J Immunol 2005;174(8):5110–8.
25. Hotchkiss RS, Swanson PE, Freeman BD, et al. Apoptotic cell death in patients with sepsis, shock, and multiple organ dysfunction. Crit Care Med 1999;27(7): 1230–51.
26. Inoue S, Suzuki-Utsunomiya K, Okada Y, et al. Reduction of immunocompetent T cells followed by prolonged lymphopenia in severe sepsis in the elderly. Crit Care Med 2013;41(3):810–9.
27. Heidarian M, Griffith TS, Badovinac VP. Sepsis-induced changes in differentiation, maintenance, and function of memory CD8 T cell subsets. Front Immunol 2023;14:1130009. https://doi.org/10.3389/fimmu.2023.1130009.
28. Shankar-Hari M, Fear D, Lavender P, et al. Activation-associated accelerated apoptosis of memory b cells in critically ill patients with sepsis. Crit Care Med 2017;45(5):875–82.
29. Hotchkiss RS, Karl IE. The pathophysiology and treatment of sepsis. N Engl J Med 2003;348(2):138–50.
30. Spolarics Z, Siddiqi M, Siegel JH, et al. Depressed interleukin-12-producing activity by monocytes correlates with adverse clinical course and a shift toward Th2-type lymphocyte pattern in severely injured male trauma patients. Crit Care Med 2003;31(6):1722–9.
31. O'Sullivan ST, Lederer JA, Horgan AF, et al. Major injury leads to predominance of the T helper-2 lymphocyte phenotype and diminished interleukin-12 production associated with decreased resistance to infection. Ann Surg 1995;222(4):482–90 [discussion: 490–2].
32. Xue M, Xie J, Liu L, et al. Early and dynamic alterations of Th2/Th1 in previously immunocompetent patients with community-acquired severe sepsis: a prospective observational study. J Transl Med 2019;17(1):57.
33. Xu J, Li J, Xiao K, et al. Dynamic changes in human HLA-DRA gene expression and Th cell subsets in sepsis: indications of immunosuppression and associated outcomes. Scand J Immunol 2020;91(1):e12813. https://doi.org/10.1111/sji.12813.
34. Torres LK, Pickkers P, van der Poll T. Sepsis-Induced immunosuppression. Annu Rev Physiol 2022;84:157–81.
35. Monneret G, Debard AL, Venet F, et al. Marked elevation of human circulating CD4+CD25+ regulatory T cells in sepsis-induced immunoparalysis. Crit Care Med 2003;31(7):2068–71.

36. Venet F, Pachot A, Debard AL, et al. Increased percentage of CD4+CD25+ regulatory T cells during septic shock is due to the decrease of CD4+CD25- lymphocytes. Crit Care Med 2004;32(11):2329–31.
37. Hotchkiss RS, Monneret G, Payen D. Sepsis-induced immunosuppression: from cellular dysfunctions to immunotherapy. Nat Rev Immunol 2013;13(12):862–74.
38. Venet F, Pachot A, Debard AL, et al. Human CD4+CD25+ regulatory T lymphocytes inhibit lipopolysaccharide-induced monocyte survival through a Fas/Fas ligand-dependent mechanism. J Immunol 2006;177(9):6540–7.
39. Lin S, Wu H, Wang C, et al. Regulatory T cells and acute lung injury: cytokines, uncontrolled inflammation, and therapeutic implications. review. Front Immunol 2018;9. https://doi.org/10.3389/fimmu.2018.01545.
40. van Vught LA, Wiewel MA, Hoogendijk AJ, et al. The host response in patients with sepsis developing intensive care unit-acquired secondary infections. Am J Respir Crit Care Med 2017;196(4):458–70.
41. Chang K, Svabek C, Vazquez-Guillamet C, et al. Targeting the programmed cell death 1: programmed cell death ligand 1 pathway reverses T cell exhaustion in patients with sepsis. Crit Care 2014;18(1):R3. https://doi.org/10.1186/cc13176.
42. Guignant C, Lepape A, Huang X, et al. Programmed death-1 levels correlate with increased mortality, nosocomial infection and immune dysfunctions in septic shock patients. Crit Care 2011;15(2):R99.
43. Grimaldi D, Louis S, Pène F, et al. Profound and persistent decrease of circulating dendritic cells is associated with ICU-acquired infection in patients with septic shock. Intensive Care Med 2011;37(9):1438–46.
44. Guisset O, Dilhuydy MS, Thiébaut R, et al. Decrease in circulating dendritic cells predicts fatal outcome in septic shock. Intensive Care Med 2007;33(1):148–52.
45. Williams TE, Ayala A, Chaudry IH. Inducible macrophage apoptosis following sepsis is mediated by cysteine protease activation and nitric oxide release. J Surg Res 1997;70(2):113–8.
46. Fu X, Liu Z, Wang Y. Advances in the study of immunosuppressive mechanisms in sepsis. J Inflamm Res 2023;16:3967–81.
47. Hoesel LM, Neff TA, Neff SB, et al. Harmful and protective roles of neutrophils in sepsis. Shock 2005;24(1):40–7.
48. de Kleijn S, Langereis JD, Leentjens J, et al. IFN-γ-stimulated neutrophils suppress lymphocyte proliferation through expression of PD-L1. PLoS One 2013;8(8):e72249. https://doi.org/10.1371/journal.pone.0072249.
49. Oami T, Watanabe E, Hatano M, et al. Suppression of T cell autophagy results in decreased viability and function of t cells through accelerated apoptosis in a murine sepsis model. Crit Care Med 2017;45(1):e77–85.
50. Giza DE, Fuentes-Mattei E, Bullock MD, et al. Cellular and viral microRNAs in sepsis: mechanisms of action and clinical applications. Cell Death Differ 2016;23-(12):1906–18.
51. van der Poll T, van de Veerdonk FL, Scicluna BP, et al. The immunopathology of sepsis and potential therapeutic targets. Nat Rev Immunol 2017;17(7):407–20.
52. Burnham KL, Davenport EE, Radhakrishnan J, et al. Shared and distinct aspects of the sepsis transcriptomic response to fecal peritonitis and pneumonia. Am J Respir Crit Care Med 2017;196(3):328–39.
53. Shalova IN, Lim JY, Chittezhath M, et al. Human monocytes undergo functional re-programming during sepsis mediated by hypoxia-inducible factor-1α. Immunity 2015;42(3):484–98.

54. Bilbault P, Lavaux T, Lahlou A, et al. Transient Bcl-2 gene down-expression in circulating mononuclear cells of severe sepsis patients who died despite appropriate intensive care. Intensive Care Med 2004;30(3):408–15.
55. Cheng SC, Scicluna BP, Arts RJ, et al. Broad defects in the energy metabolism of leukocytes underlie immunoparalysis in sepsis. Nat Immunol 2016;17(4):406–13.
56. Dequin PF, Meziani F, Quenot JP, et al. Hydrocortisone in severe community-acquired pneumonia. N Engl J Med 2023;388(21):1931–41.
57. Otto GP, Sossdorf M, Claus RA, et al. The late phase of sepsis is characterized by an increased microbiological burden and death rate. Crit Care 2011;15(4):R183. https://doi.org/10.1186/cc10332.
58. Venet F, Lukaszewicz AC, Payen D, et al. Monitoring the immune response in sepsis: a rational approach to administration of immunoadjuvant therapies. Curr Opin Immunol 2013;25(4):477–83.
59. Ong DSY, Bonten MJM, Spitoni C, et al. Epidemiology of multiple herpes viremia in previously immunocompetent patients with septic shock. Clin Infect Dis 2017; 64(9):1204–10.
60. Walton AH, Muenzer JT, Rasche D, et al. Reactivation of multiple viruses in patients with sepsis. PLoS One 2014;9(2):e98819. https://doi.org/10.1371/journal.pone.0098819.
61. van der Slikke EC, An AY, Hancock REW, et al. Exploring the pathophysiology of post-sepsis syndrome to identify therapeutic opportunities. EBioMedicine 2020; 61:103044. https://doi.org/10.1016/j.ebiom.2020.103044.
62. Corrales-Medina VF, Musher DM, Wells GA, et al. Cardiac complications in patients with community-acquired pneumonia: incidence, timing, risk factors, and association with short-term mortality. Circulation 2012;125(6):773–81.
63. Prescott HC, Osterholzer JJ, Langa KM, et al. Late mortality after sepsis: propensity matched cohort study. Br Med J 2016;353:i2375. https://doi.org/10.1136/bmj.i2375.
64. Guirgis FW, Brakenridge S, Sutchu S, et al. The long-term burden of severe sepsis and septic shock: sepsis recidivism and organ dysfunction. J Trauma Acute Care Surg 2016;81(3):525–32.
65. Prescott HC, Angus DC. Enhancing recovery from sepsis: a review. JAMA 2018; 319(1):62–75.
66. Fenner BP, Darden DB, Kelly LS, et al. Immunological endotyping of chronic critical illness after severe sepsis. Front Med 2020;7:616694. https://doi.org/10.3389/fmed.2020.616694.
67. Yates KB, Tonnerre P, Martin GE, et al. Epigenetic scars of CD8(+) T cell exhaustion persist after cure of chronic infection in humans. Nat Immunol 2021;22(8): 1020–9.
68. Roquilly A, Jacqueline C, Davieau M, et al. Alveolar macrophages are epigenetically altered after inflammation, leading to long-term lung immunoparalysis. Nat Immunol 2020;21(6):636–48.
69. Zorio V, Venet F, Delwarde B, et al. Assessment of sepsis-induced immunosuppression at ICU discharge and 6 months after ICU discharge. Ann Intensive Care 2017;7(1):80.
70. Yende S, Kellum JA, Talisa VB, et al. Long-term host immune response trajectories among hospitalized patients with sepsis. JAMA Netw Open 2019;2(8): e198686. https://doi.org/10.1001/jamanetworkopen.2019.8686.
71. Danahy DB, Kurup SP, Winborn CS, et al. Sepsis-induced state of immunoparalysis is defined by diminished CD8 T cell-mediated antitumor immunity. J Immunol 2019;203(3):725–35.

72. Cao M, Wang G, Xie J. Immune dysregulation in sepsis: experiences, lessons and perspectives. Cell Death Discov 2023;9(1):465.
73. Delsing CE, Gresnigt MS, Leentjens J, et al. Interferon-gamma as adjunctive immunotherapy for invasive fungal infections: a case series. BMC Infect Dis 2014;14:166.
74. Keramati F, Leijte GP, Bruse N, et al. Systemic inflammation impairs myelopoiesis and interferon type I responses in humans. Nat Immunol 2025;26(5):737–47.
75. Kusakabe Y, Uchida K, Yamamura Y, et al. Early-phase innate immune suppression in murine severe sepsis is restored with systemic interferon-β. Anesthesiology 2018;129(1):131–42.
76. Inoue S, Unsinger J, Davis CG, et al. IL-15 prevents apoptosis, reverses innate and adaptive immune dysfunction, and improves survival in sepsis. J Immunol 2010;184(3):1401–9.
77. Conlon KC, Lugli E, Welles HC, et al. Redistribution, hyperproliferation, activation of natural killer cells and CD8 T cells, and cytokine production during first-in-human clinical trial of recombinant human interleukin-15 in patients with cancer. J Clin Oncol 2015;33(1):74–82.
78. Meisel C, Schefold JC, Pschowski R, et al. Granulocyte-macrophage colony-stimulating factor to reverse sepsis-associated immunosuppression: a double-blind, randomized, placebo-controlled multicenter trial. Am J Respir Crit Care Med 2009;180(7):640–8.
79. Darden DB, Kelly LS, Fenner BP, et al. Dysregulated immunity and immunotherapy after sepsis. J Clin Med 2021;10(8). https://doi.org/10.3390/jcm10081742.
80. Shao R, Fang Y, Yu H, et al. Monocyte programmed death ligand-1 expression after 3-4 days of sepsis is associated with risk stratification and mortality in septic patients: a prospective cohort study. Crit Care 2016;20(1):124.
81. Inoue S, Bo L, Bian J, et al. Dose-dependent effect of anti-CTLA-4 on survival in sepsis. Shock 2011;36(1):38–44.
82. Wu J, Zhou L, Liu J, et al. The efficacy of thymosin alpha 1 for severe sepsis (ETASS): a multicenter, single-blind, randomized and controlled trial. Crit Care 2013;17(1):R8. https://doi.org/10.1186/cc11932.
83. Wu J, Pei F, Zhou L, et al. The efficacy and safety of thymosin α1 for sepsis (TESTS): Multicentre, double blinded, randomised, placebo controlled, phase 3 trial. Br Med J 2025;388:e082583. https://doi.org/10.1136/bmj-2024-082583.
84. Chen F, Zou L, Williams B, et al. Targeting toll-like receptors in sepsis: from bench to clinical trials. Antioxid Redox Signaling 2021;35(15):1324–39.
85. Hotchkiss RS, Chang KC, Swanson PE, et al. Caspase inhibitors improve survival in sepsis: a critical role of the lymphocyte. Nat Immunol 2000;1(6):496–501.
86. Schrijver DP, Röring RJ, Deckers J, et al. Resolving sepsis-induced immunoparalysis via trained immunity by targeting interleukin-4 to myeloid cells. Nat Biomed Eng 2023;7(9):1097–112.
87. Hamers LA, Kox M, Arts RJ, et al. Gamma-irradiated bacille calmette-Guérin vaccination does not modulate the innate immune response during experimental human endotoxemia in adult males. J Immunol Res 2015;2015:261864. https://doi.org/10.1155/2015/261864.
88. Scicluna BP, Cano-Gamez K, Burnham KL, et al. A consensus blood transcriptomic framework for sepsis. Nat Med 2025;31(12):4119–30.
89. Rademaker E, van Amstel RBE, El Bouhaddani S, et al. Temporal robustness of biomarker-based classification algorithms for sepsis. Intensive Care Med 2026; 52(1):22–30.

Sepsis and Systemic Inflammatory Syndromes

Effects of Systemic Inflammation on the Brain

Mayra Romijnders, MSc[1], Bram Snoek, MSc[1], Luc van Oss, MSc[1],
Peter Pickkers, MD, PhD, Wilson F. Käyser-Abdo, MD, PhD*

KEYWORDS

- Sepsis • Sepsis-associated encephalopathy (SAE) • Postsepsis syndrome (PSS)
- Neuroinflammation • Blood-brain-barrier (BBB) • Biomarkers

KEY POINTS

- Sepsis-associated encephalopathy (SAE) is a commonly occurring syndrome and major risk factor for long-term cognitive impairment and mental health problems.
- The underlying biology of SAE is multifactorial, comprising systemic-brain immune cross-talk, blood-brain barrier disruption, glial activation, and synaptic injury.
- Neuroinflammation, a key immunologic process in SAE, involves variable region-specific activation of diverse immune cells, making accurate quantification difficult.

INTRODUCTION

Sepsis is defined as a life-threatening organ dysfunction due to a dysregulated host response to infection and is characterized by immune dysregulation ranging from hyperinflammation to profound immunosuppression.[1] Sepsis affects one in 3 patients in the intensive care unit (ICU)[2] and is one of the leading causes of death worldwide with high mortality rates; 27% in hospitalized patients and up to 42% in ICU patients.[3] Among survivors, the 5-year survival varies between 44% and 62%.[4,5] Sepsis often causes multiorgan failure, including the kidneys, lungs, and liver. The brain is also commonly affected, with dysfunction occurring both in the acute phase as well as in the long-term postsepsis phase. The incidence of clinical characteristics of brain dysfunction and its biological underpinnings related to the immune-brain interplay will be described.

Department of Intensive Care Medicine, Radboud University Medical Center, RadboudumcGeert Grooteplein Zuid 10, Route 707, 6500HB, Nijmegen, The Netherlands
[1] These authors contributed equally.
* Corresponding author.
E-mail address: F.Abdo@radboudumc.nl

Crit Care Clin 42 (2026) 891–907
https://doi.org/10.1016/j.ccc.2026.05.012 criticalcare.theclinics.com

Abbreviations	
ACE	arachnoid cuff exit
BBB	blood-brain barrier
BCSFB	blood–cerebrospinal fluid barrier
CNS	central nervous system
CSF	cerebrospinal fluid
DCE-MRI	Dynamic contrast-enhanced MRI
EEG	electroencephalography
GCS	Glasow Coma Scale
IFNs	Interferons
IL	Interleukin
NFL	neurofilament light chain
PAMP	pathogen-associated molecular patterns
PRR	pattern recognition receptors
PSS	postsepsis syndrome
PTSD	posttraumatic stress disorder
ROS	reactive oxygen species
SAE	sepsis associated encephalopathy
SV2	synaptic vesicle glycoprotein 2
TNF-α	tumor necrosis factor alpha
TSPO	translocator protein

THE CLINICAL SYNDROME IN THE ACUTE AND LONG-TERM PHASE

Sepsis-associated encephalopathy (SAE) is a neurologic syndrome characterized by (diffuse) dysfunction of the brain caused by sepsis (**Fig. 1**). In the acute phase, patients with SAE typically present with an acute onset of encephalopathy ranging from delirium to altered mental states and even coma.[6,7] Other less frequently encountered symptoms are agitation (10%), dysautonomia, convulsive seizures (2%), and focal neurologic signs (1%). Other risk factors such as hyperglycaemia and hypoglycaemia,

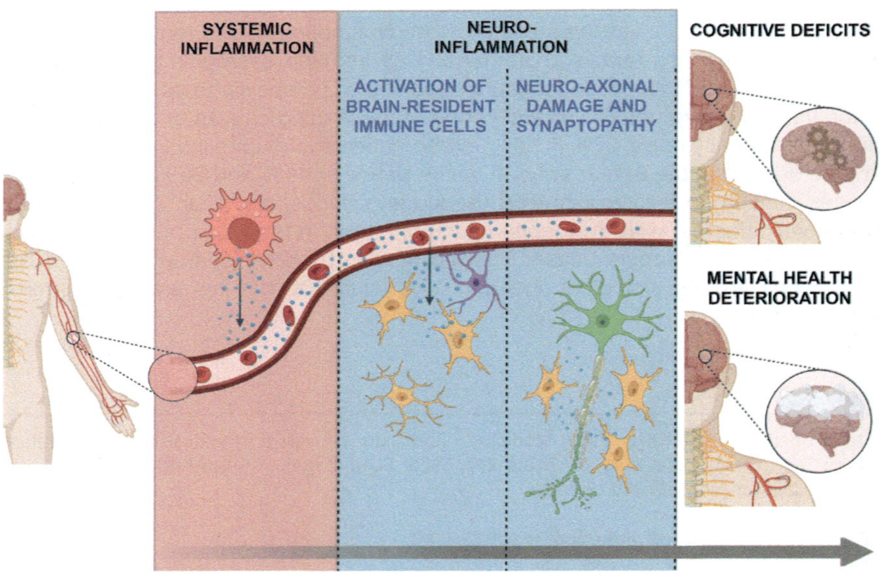

Fig. 1. Left to right. Schematic overview of effects of systemic inflammation on the brain.(-*Created in* BioRender. Research, I. (2026) https://BioRender.com/2feb7lo.)

hypercapnia, hypernatremia, central nervous system (CNS) infection, bacteraemia, may account for these uncommon presentations, rather than being caused by sepsis per se.[7] Without established diagnostic biomarkers or tools, the diagnosis remains purely clinical after excluding other possible causes. This makes the diagnosis of SAE less accurate and at risk to bias, as shown by the wide range of reported SAE incidence, which generally ranges between 30% and 70% of patients with sepsis.[8,9]

Sepsis-Associated Encephalopathy and Survival

In a study with over 2500 patients with sepsis at ICU admission, of whom approximately half had SAE, even mild alterations of mental status, defined by a Glasow Coma Scale (GCS) of 13 or 14, were associated with a 40% higher chance of dying.[8] The degree of SAE severity was also correlated with a more than 3 times increased risk of dying, with patients having a GCS of 3 to 8 showing the worst prognosis. Furthermore, presence of SAE was independently associated with increased need and duration of mechanical ventilation, higher need for sedatives, increased organ supportive therapies such as renal replacement therapy, vasopressor use, and increased ICU length of stay.[10] A recent meta-regression analysis with more than 20.000 patients with sepsis confirmed that patients with SAE at ICU admission had a higher disease severity and longer ICU length of stay.[11]

Postsepsis Syndrome

The long-term sequelae of sepsis are defined as postsepsis syndrome (PSS), which consists of a combination of long-term deterioration of the physical state, mental health disorders, and cognitive decline. Compared to nonseptic patients, patients who survive sepsis develop a higher rate of new functional limitations, in patients who had preexisting limitations as well as patients who did not have any functional limitation beforehand.[12] Importantly, these declines in physical function can persist for many years, impacting independence, mental wellbeing, and quality of life.[13–15] Later, we will focus in more detail on outcomes related to brain dysfunction.

Postsepsis Mental Health

Patients surviving sepsis frequently suffer from subsequent depression, anxiety, posttraumatic stress disorder (PTSD) and sleep disturbances and these sequelae are more likely following SAE.[16] In a cohort of ICU survivors with sepsis or septic shock, anxiety, depression, and PTSD symptoms were present in 67%, 49%, and 46% of patients, respectively, shortly after ICU discharge. After 1 year, 38% of anxiety, 50% of depression, and 31% of PTSD symptoms remained.[17] More severe depression postsepsis was associated with higher levels of PTSD and lower health-related quality of life.[18] PTSD is particularly prevalent in sepsis survivors, with pooled prevalence of 20% within the first year after ICU discharge reported in a meta-analysis of 48 studies.[19] Importantly, PTSD in ICU survivors has been associated with significantly worse functional outcomes, including higher rates of moderate-to-severe disability and more pronounced depressive and anxiety symptoms. In addition to depression and PTSD, survivors frequently report persistent anxiety, fear-related symptoms, and sleep disturbances, reflecting the psychological impact of severe illness and ICU admission.[20] Collectively, these findings demonstrate that mental health disorders are prevalent and persistent after sepsis, and are strongly associated with impaired quality of life.

Postsepsis Cognition

The prevalence of moderate to severe cognitive impairment increased 11% postsepsis[12] and up to a fifth of sepsis survivors shows long-term cognitive deficits.[21] In contrast to patients with sepsis, nonsepsis general hospitalizations did not show a significant change in moderate to severe cognitive impairment.[12] Patients with SAE have an even higher risk of long-term cognitive decline compared to sepsis survivors without SAE.[7,22,23] Within the group of SAE, delirium occurs in up to a third of patients with sepsis and has been shown to be the strongest predictor of long-term cognitive decline.[13]

Pooled data from 8 studies and with follow-up periods up to 11 years, showed that sepsis was associated with a 62% increased risk to develop dementia.[24] This risk was doubled in patients with severe sepsis.[24] In patients with normal neuropsychological assessments, the occurrence of sepsis, compared to patients with no or less severe infectious episodes, was associated an 82% increased risk to develop dementia within the follow-up period.[25] These studies collectively show that sepsis and severity of sepsis are important risk factors for the development of subsequent dementia.

Importantly, the risk of developing dementia postsepsis is strongly linked to higher age.[26] Aging is accompanied by cumulative damage due to repetitive inflammatory hits and due to physiologic age-related decline in cognitive function. This leads to a low-grade, chronic systemically inflamed state, which has been coined as *inflammaging*. Within the brain, this consists of chronically low grade activated (*primed*) (micro)-glial cells, accumulation of aged glial cells and sustained expression of proinflammatory cytokines.[27] Apart from the decline in functional reserves, the inflammaging associated primed neuroimmune state may explain why people of higher age are more likely to develop persistent postsepsis brain dysfunction. Their primed neuroimmune cells mount a more severe and sustained neuroinflammatory response to a sepsis.[28] This is corroborated by animal studies, which showed that primed microglia respond more vigorously to systemic inflammation.[29] In addition, elderly are more likely to already have (undetected) dementia related protein aggregates in the brain, such as amyloid-β, α-synuclein or TAU protein, where additional neuroaxonal loss due to sepsis, accelerates the clinical diagnosis of dementia.

Although sepsis severity and aging are the most important risk factors for developing SAE and subsequent postsepsis cognitive impairments, additional predisposing factors such as (mild) preexisting cognitive deficits, previous acquired severe illnesses, comorbidities, preexistent depression, and metabolic disturbances also strongly add to this risk.[8,26,27]

PATHOPHYSIOLOGY

The pathophysiology of SAE is complex with detailed underlying biological pathways remaining largely unknown. In sepsis, circulating immune cells (neutrophils and monocytes) as well as tissue macrophages are activated through binding of pathogen-associated molecular patterns (PAMPs) to pattern recognition receptors (PRRs), leading to release of proinflammatory cytokines such as tumor necrosis factor alpha (TNF-α), interleukin (IL)-1, IL-6, IL-8, IL-12, IL-18 and type I and II interferons (IFNs), including IFN-γ.[30] These cytokines activate nearby and distal immune cells and this chain reaction may result in a rapid hyperinflammatory immune response.[30] Over recent decades, the brain was shown to be more immunologically active than previously assumed with bidirectional communication between the brain and systemic immune compartments. In patients with sepsis, systemic (hyper) inflammation is hypothesized to dysregulate crosstalk between the systemic and brain compartment. The immune-brain crosstalk occurs at distinct anatomic sites in the brain, which include the blood-brain barrier (BBB), the outer border regions of the brain, and the blood–cerebrospinal fluid barrier (BCSFB).[31,32] Apart from being crosstalk sites, these regions were shown to be important parts of the brain's immune response. Cerebrospinal fluid (CSF) plays an important role in the immune crosstalk at several brain border regions.

The Immune-Brain Crosstalk Regions

Blood–brain barrier

Under normal conditions, the BBB regulates the transfer of molecules between the circulatory system and the CNS and is very selectively permeable in part due to its layer of endothelial cells with tight junctions[33] (**Fig. 2**). During sepsis several processes can disrupt this barrier. First, cytokines damage the endothelium affecting its tight junctions, leading to microvascular leakages and cellular edema.[34] Autopsy studies in patients who died of sepsis showed reduced tight junction proteins in BBB endothelial cells.[35] Second, BBB endothelial cells enhance their expression of intracellular adhesion molecules, increasing leukocyte adhesion to endothelium and promoting leukocyte migration toward the brain.[36] Third, radicals such as reactive nitrogen species and reactive oxygen species (ROS), and matrix metalloproteinases produced during sepsis further amplify the damage to the BBB.[34] This leads to activation of astrocytes and especially microglia within the brain parenchyma, further contributing to BBB breakdown through disruption of the glia limitans and through facilitating transport of immune cells in the neuropil.[37] In the initial stages of systemic inflammation, these processes occur on the luminal side of the BBB, but once the BBB permeability is compromised and inflammatory mediators penetrate into the brain, the BBB may be further disrupted from the abluminal side.

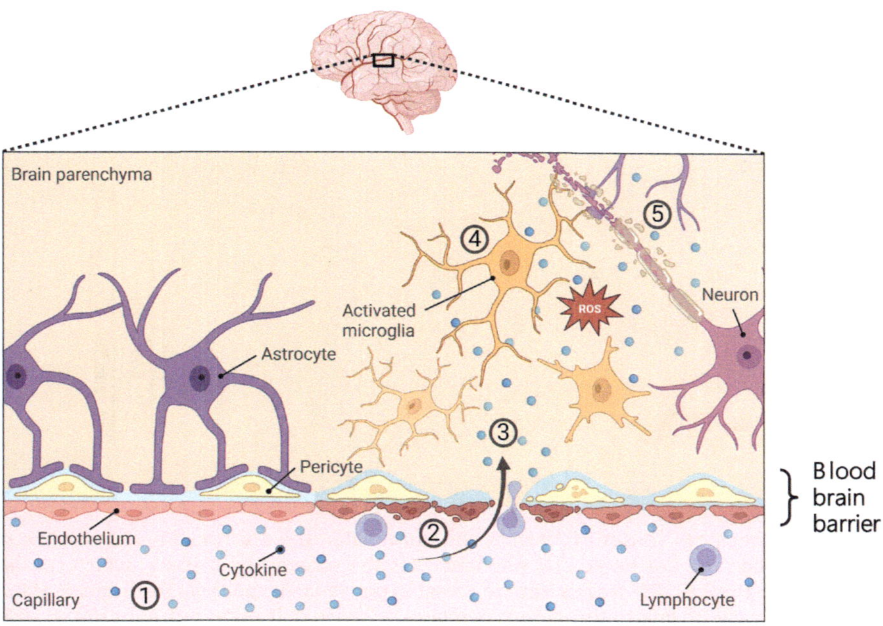

Fig. 2. Systemic inflammation (1) disrupts the BBB and increases its permeability (2), allowing influx of systemically circulating cytokines into the brain (3). Microglia and astrocytes become activated (4) and release proinflammatory cytokines as well as ROS, further enhancing the proinflammatory state in the brain. Prolonged or severe neuroinflammation subsequently results in neuronal dysfunction, synaptic loss and cell death (5).(*Created in* BioRender. Research, I. (2026) https://BioRender.com/u1gdjw6.)

Outer brain border regions

Over the last decade, brain border regions, including the skull bone marrow and meninges, emerged as sites of active crosstalk between the peripheral and brain's immune systems.[38] Beneath the skull bone, there are 3 meningeal layers that separate the skull from the brain parenchyma (**Fig. 3**). These layers allow for bidirectional communication between the peripheral immune system, the brain immune system, and the brain parenchyma. CSF is a key transporter of this communication, as it contains signaling proteins, waste products and cells that originate from the brain parenchyma or were in close contact with it.[38]

Blood vessels of the brain have a perivascular compartment that contains CSF that is in contact with the brain parenchymal interstitium.[39] CSF flow through the interstitium provides nutrients to brain cells, and drains signaling and waste products from the interstitial space of the brain parenchyma (see **Fig. 3**). The mechanism of CSF-interstitial fluid exchange is now regarded as an important part of the glymphatic system of the brain. The CSF flow through the brain parenchyma is regulated by parenchymal border macrophages, also modulating movement of cytokines and antigens.[40] Disruption of this glymphatic flow may increase neuroinflammation. Systemic inflammation was shown to disrupt this glymphatic system.[41,42] Impaired CNS waste removal, indirectly influenced by parenchymal border macrophages, has also been associated with Alzheimer's disease.[40,43] In SAE, increased accumulation of Alzheimer's related protein aggregates (amyloid-β and phosphorylated TAU) was found in both animal and human studies.[44,45]

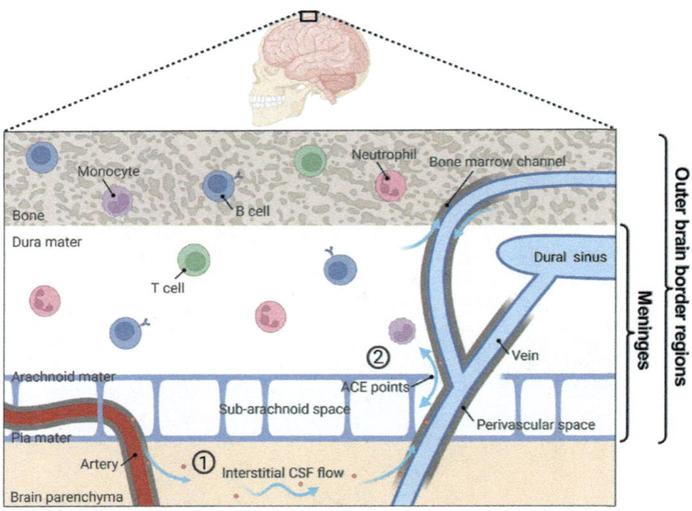

Fig. 3. The meninges consist of 3 layers, the dura mater, the arachnoid mater and the pia mater. Between the arachnoid and pia mater lies the subarachnoid space, which contains CSF and blood vessels. CSF travels from the arterial perivascular space via the interstitial fluid in the brain parenchyma to the venous perivascular space delivering nutrients and clearing waste material. This CSF-interstitial flow is regarded as an intrinsic part of the brain's glymphatic system (1). From the venous perivascular space, CSF flows through the meninges to the dural sinuses or through ACE points via the dura mater to bone marrow (2), allowing exchange of signals from the brain to the bone marrow and flow of immune cells from the bone marrow to the meninges.(*Created in* BioRender. Research, I. (2026) https://BioRender.com/u1gdjw6.)

The brain's blood vessels travel through the brain parenchyma and cross the meninges where some veins end up crossing into the skull (see **Fig. 3**). The bridging veins can relay signals from CSF in their perivascular space via the dura mater to the skull bone marrow through arachnoid cuff exit (ACE) points.[46,47] Additionally, immune cells travel from bone marrow to meninges by channels in the bone marrow and meninges.[48] Thus, bidirectional communication between bone marrow and blood in the skull and the brain is an important component of neuroinflammation, affecting brain immunology and neuronal functioning (see **Fig. 3**). After experimental murine sepsis, skull bone marrow showed decreased amounts of neutrophils, while neutrophil efflux from skull bone marrow into meninges was increased, which enhanced neuroinflammation.[49]

Cerebral veins drain in dural sinuses, which are located in the dura mater of the meninges. In the vicinity of these sinuses, lymphatic vessels of the brain are located. These sites have been shown to be immunologically active hotspots that include various immune cells.[38] Meningeal lymphatics contribute to the drainage of CSF and CNS waste products, and allow immune cells to enter draining lymph nodes.[50] In the meninges, lymphocytes and antigen-presenting cells can present antigens of brain parenchyma encountered in the CSF to T-cells, and can thereby contribute to neuroinflammation.[31] Recently, meninges were found to aid in the removal of CNS-reactive immature B-cells and to be a place for further development of immature B-cells which drifted through channels from the skull bone marrow.[51,52] During neuroinflammation, these immature B-cells were able to mature locally in the meninges, contributing to neuroinflammation.[52]

Blood–cerebrospinal fluid barrier

The choroid plexus, located within the ventricles of the brain, produces CSF and is the site of the BCSFB. The BCSFB consists of vascularized stroma surrounded by CSF producing epithelial cells that are connected by tight junctions (**Fig. 4**).[31] The choroid plexus, including its stromal blood vessels, lacks a tight barrier like the BBB. CSF is separated from the blood compartment by a fenestrated endothelial layer, loosely connective choroid plexus stroma and an epithelial layer of CSF producing cells.[38] This facilitates immune-brain communication between both compartments (see **Fig. 4**). Besides supporting tissue, the choroid plexus stroma is immunologically active as it contains lymphoid and myeloid populations, including T-cells and macrophages. In murine sepsis models, systemically activated antigen presenting cells have been shown to infiltrate the choroid plexus and release IL-1β, triggering stromal cells to produce proinflammatory factors.[53] $CD4^+$ T-helper cells produce IFN-γ and promote transepithelial migration of preactivated T- and B-cells into the CSF.[54] Systemic inflammation has been shown to compromise the tight junctions in the epithelial cells of the choroid plexus.[55] Migration of immune cells and compromised tight junctions could thus promote neuroinflammation at this brain site during sepsis. In addition, oxidative stress was found to be a contributor not only to BBB disruption but also BCSFB disruption during sepsis.[56]

Main Immune Cells in Immune–Brain Crosstalk in Sepsis

The glial cells, microglia and astrocytes, are the main resident tissue immune cells of the brain parenchyma, and maintain cerebral homeostasis and synaptic functioning. Disruption of these glial cells may cause synaptic dysfunction and synaptic apoptosis, leading to function loss.[6,57] The glial cells, and especially microglia, play an important role in neuroinflammatory processes and are presumed to be one of the key drivers of brain dysfunction during sepsis. This is supported by autopsy findings in patients with

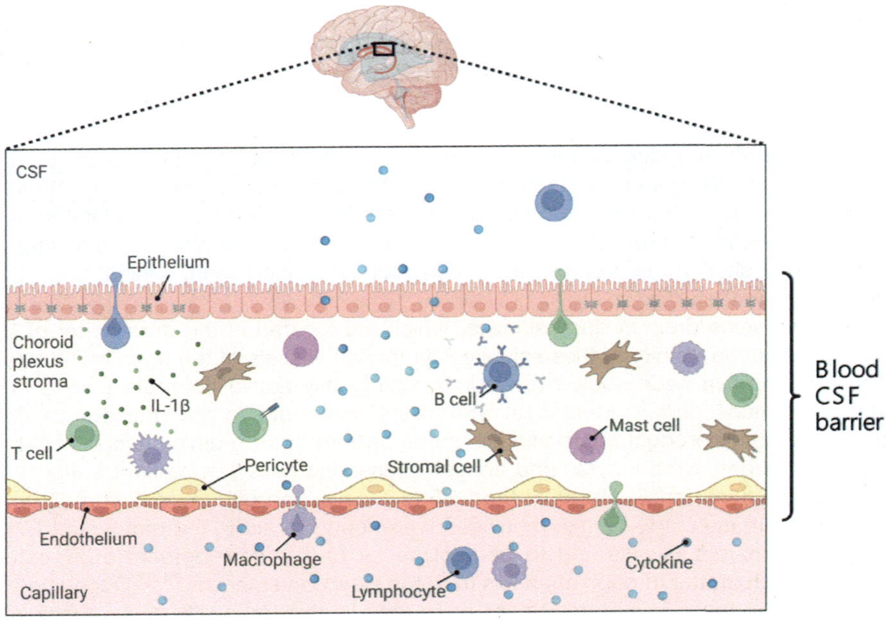

Fig. 4. The BCSFB is a barrier between blood vessels and CSF, located in the choroid plexus, where important bidirectional immune communication occurs between the systemic compartment and the brain through the CSF.(*Created in* BioRender. Research, I. (2026) https://BioRender.com/u1gdjw6.)

sepsis showing microglial activation in absence of bacterial translocation into the brain parenchyma.[58,59] Activated microglia amplify the proinflammatory response, damaging cellular membranes, and contribute to mitochondrial dysfunction. This leads to impaired neuronal functioning and neuronal death.[6,60] The NLR family pyrin domain containing 3 (NLRP3) inflammasome pathway in microglia is gaining much attention in neuroinflammatory research with several drug targets being studied currently in animal and human studies.[61]

Another proposed mechanism by which microglia may cause synaptic dysfunction is through synaptic pruning, which is largely mediated through complement proteins C1q and C3 which give phagocytotic signals to microglia via the C3-C3aR axis.[62] In normal brain development, microglia prune synapses to allow plasticity of the brain and eliminate unnecessary synapses.[63] However, patients with sepsis exhibit extensive phagocytic active $CD68^{+}$ microglia,[58,59,62] and C1q complement activation,[62] suggesting enhanced synaptic pruning. In neurodegenerative diseases, enhanced synaptic pruning is thought to contribute to cognitive decline.[64] It is likely that enhanced synaptic pruning in neuroinflammation could negatively impact cognitive function. This is supported by the finding that synaptic proteins in the CSF were downregulated in patients with infection-associated delirium compared to patients with an infection without delirium.[57] Similar synaptic proteins were also found to be downregulated in the CSF of patients with Alzheimer's disease.[57] To summarize, activated microglia contribute to a proinflammatory milieu, BBB disruption, synaptic dysfunction and apoptosis, leading to transient or permanent brain dysfunction.

While astrocytes are understudied in sepsis, they also promote neuroinflammation by excretion of proinflammatory cytokines and by activating microglia, which both indirectly contribute to neuronal damage.[65] Recently, early astrocyte reactivity was highlighted as a driver of neuroinflammation in sepsis.[66] Activated astrocytes in a murine infection model have also been proposed to promote phagocytosis of synapses through the C3-C3aR axis by releasing C3.[67] Due to this, and importantly, their role as one of the 3 layers that make up the BBB, more research is warranted into their role in neuroinflammation, maintenance of the integrity of the BBB, and neuronal and synaptic homeostasis.

A lot of neuroinflammation related research has focused on the contribution of glial cells, and especially microglia. In part, because much of this research was related to neurodegenerative diseases, where microglia are found near the dementia-related protein aggregates in damaged areas. However, recently it was shown that other immune cells, and especially T-cells, also play a key role via bidirectional communication between the systemic and brain immune compartments in the brain border regions. In addition, single-cell transcriptomics of CSF has shown that approximately 70% of the immune cells in CSF are T-cells, with the remaining being dendritic cells and distinct phenotypes of monocytes.[68]

MEASURES FOR NEUROINFLAMMATION

Measuring neuroinflammation is difficult, as it is not a single measurable entity. It is inferred from proxies reflecting glial activation (microglia, astrocytes), inflammatory mediators, blood-brain barrier dysfunction, immune cell trafficking and proliferation, and downstream neuroaxonal injury. Currently, no measure captures all these proxies simultaneously, but rather most measures correlate with these proxies. This is particularly relevant in postacute infection syndromes, such as in postsepsis patients, where a combination of all these mechanisms can underly the pathogenesis.[69,70]

The most direct way to define and measure neuroinflammation would be through well characterized blood and CSF biomarkers. Proinflammatory and anti-inflammatory cytokines such as IL-1β, IL-6, IL-8, TNF, and IL-10 as well as chemokines such as CCL2 (MCP-1) and CXCL10, reflect (neuro) inflammatory immune signaling.[71,72] Markers of neuroinflammation are elevated in the acute phase but can also be chronically dysregulated in patients with persistent cognitive complaints. CSF concentrations of the proinflammatory cytokines IL-6 and IL-8 are upregulated in patients with SAE.[73] Additionally, IL-6 and IL-8 concentrations, but also IL-1β, IL-10, MCP-1, and TNF have been associated with development of delirium.[74–76] Even at baseline, elevated cytokine concentrations have been shown to hold predictive value for the development of delirium.[77,78] In patients with persistent cognitive complaints (*brain fog*), persistent elevations of IL-6 and CXCL10 have been observed.[79] However, in systemic inflammation higher cytokine levels in the CSF will be seen irrespective of clinical brain involvement, due to influx of systemic inflammatory mediators into the brain compartment.[57,80,81]

Glial proteins, including sTREM2, YKL-40, and to a lesser extent also GFAP and S100b, reflect microglia and astrocyte activation, and thus could be used as more specific biomarkers of neuroinflammation.[72,82–84] Also, neuroaxonal injury markers can be interpreted as downstream consequences and injury due to neuroinflammation. These include neurofilament light chain (NFL), NSE, GFAP, S100 B, UCH-L1, and TAU (total or phosphorylated), all of which are associated with neuronal damage and injury.[72,85–87] They have been shown to be of diagnostic use in discriminating sepsis with and without associated encephalopathy.[72] However, they do not specifically reflect ongoing neuroinflammation as neuroaxonal injury may also occur due to other mechanisms present in sepsis patients, for example, hypoxia or hypotension.[22]

Accurate determination of neuroinflammation using biomarkers remains challenging.[88] CSF sampling is of interest, as it plays a key role in the immune-brain interaction and is in direct anatomic and biochemical contact with CNS immune cells, the different immune brain border niches and brain parenchyma. The main method of obtaining CSF is through invasive lumbar punctures, limiting longitudinal sampling. Due to the relative inaccessibility of the brain, blood-based biomarkers reflecting the degree of neuroinflammation would be an important aid for clinical assessment and research. Unfortunately, blood concentrations correlate poorly to neuroinflammatory profiles.[89] A fundamental limitation of blood-based biomarkers is the fact CSF-blood exchange of biomarkers is restricted and thus highly influenced by blood–brain barrier permeability in addition to peripheral metabolism, renal clearance, extracerebral sources, and anatomic distance to the CNS. As a result, the degree to which circulating biomarker levels reflect CNS inflammation varies substantially.[90,91] For neuroinflammatory processes, blood-based biomarkers have proven unreliable.[89] This is slightly different for neuroaxonal or glial damage related biomarkers such as NFL and GFAP, which show moderate to strong correlations between CSF and plasma, while other biomarkers such as UCHL1 and TAU do not.[87] For example, blood NFL concentrations reflect neuroaxonal damage and predict long-term cognitive dysfunction in patients with severe COVID-19.[85] This highlights the usefulness of blood-based biomarkers related to neuroaxonal damage.[89] In addition, imaging techniques can be used to demonstrate neuroinflammation. The translocator protein (TSPO), which is expressed on microglia, astrocytes, neurons, and peripheral macrophages, is the most frequently used target in imaging neuroinflammation.[92] Expression of TSPO in the healthy brain is low, with expression increasing significantly in neuroinflammatory environments. The expression of TSPO can be imaged in vivo using PET-CT imaging with TSPO radioligand such as [^{11}C]PK11195 (first generation) and [^{18}F]DPA-714, [^{11}C]PBR28 (second generation).[93,94] PET TSPO imaging, however, is limited by a polymorphism in the *TSPO* gene (rs6971), which results in a conformational change that negatively impacts the binding capacity of many (radiolabeled) TSPO antagonists, making imaging a challenge in these patients.[95] An additional important limitation of PET imaging is the lack of detailed spatial resolution and more importantly that it does not provide any insight into (detailed) biological pathways.

Promising new applications of PET-CT imaging include the quantification of synaptic density using radiotracers that bind to synaptic versicles, which are neurotransmitter-containing units located in the axon terminals.[96,97] These radiotracers bind to the synaptic vesicle glycoprotein 2 (SV2), which is highly expressed at presynaptic terminals, with 2 to 5 copies per synaptic vesicle, making it a suitable biomarker for synaptic density.[98,99] While early SV2 ligands showed low labeling yield resulting in a comparatively low resolution,[100,101] the more recent [^{18}F]-SDM-8 ligands showed high resolution synaptic density imaging.[102–104] Synaptic density could prove to be a promising marker for brain dysfunction in patients with sepsis as downregulation of synaptic proteins was previously shown in patients with SAE.[57]

PET-CT imaging is often accompanied by MRI to identify brain and vascular wall lesions, white matter hyperintensities, atrophy patterns, vasogenic edema resulting from neuroinflammation, and BBB dysfunction.[22] In patients with septic shock who developed acute brain dysfunction, MRI imaging has identified leukoencephalopathy and ischemic stroke.[105] Dynamic contrast-enhanced MRI (DCE-MRI) detected BBB leakage associated with inflammatory states but was not able to distinguish between immune activation and vascular injury due to other sources.[106]

Synaptic transmission is one of the first processes to fail during severe metabolic or hypoxic stress.[107] Electroencephalography (EEG) shows cortical synaptic activity of neurons, and in patients with SAE, slowing of the background activity on EEG corresponded with the severity of SAE.[108] As with other measures however, EEG does not measure neuroinflammation and it lacks detailed spatial resolution. It can be used as an additional screening or severity tool of brain dysfunction in combination with other measures.

At present, detailed characterization of neuroinflammation can be inferred from multimodal approaches combining CSF and blood-based and imaging biomarkers. These approaches individually lack specificity because no marker uniquely captures neuroinflammation. Temporal dissociation between systemic and brain immune responses limits blood-based readouts. Finally, even when biomarkers suggest systemic inflammation, CNS inflammation, (neuroaxonal) injury and dysfunction, a causal relationship between these processes cannot be assumed. In the future, multitracer imaging, combining for example, PET tracers for both synaptic density and microglia activation, could enable the assessment of multiple pathologies by in vivo serially capturing the trajectory of these processes in the different disease stages (acute and long-term). Additionally, large scale CSF and blood immune cell profiling using multiomic single-cell sequencing and large-scale proteomics can provide insight into the biological underpinnings of neuroinflammation, and relate these to subsequent injury, impaired mental and cognitive outcomes or even stratifying patients into biological categories at risk for developing long-term brain dysfunction.

CONCLUDING REMARKS

In conclusion, SAE is strongly linked to acute and long-term brain dysfunction, and reduced quality of life, and has a multifactorial pathophysiology. A complex system where the brain and peripheral immune compartments communicate explains the clinical consequences of systemic inflammation on the brain. Neuroinflammation, BBB disruption, and synaptic dysfunction are presumed key contributors. Insight in the mechanistic processes is constrained by phenotypic heterogeneity and limited access to the CNS, resulting in an incomplete understanding of the SAE biology at this moment.

CLINICS CARE POINTS

- Systemic inflammation-induced encephalopathy induces acute (eg, delirium) and long-term brain dysfunction (eg, cognitive decline and neuropsychiatric complaints).
- There is a complex bidirectional crosstalk between the brain and systemic immune compartments involving different brain areas.
- The blood compartment is inadequate for biomarker research or diagnostics of sepsis-associated encephalopathy.
- Large knowledge gaps in the underlying biology currently preclude any biology driven treatment.
- Future research into the underlying biology of systemic inflammation-induced encephalopathy should include biosampling from the brain and use multi-omics techniques.

DISCLOSURE

The authors have nothing to disclose.

FUNDING

Radboudumc and Netherlands Organisation for Health Research and Development (ZonMw) grants to dr. W. Käyser-Abdo (Grant IDs: 10510062320006 and 11080022 430019).

REFERENCES

1. van der Poll T, van de Veerdonk FL, Scicluna BP, et al. The immunopathology of sepsis and potential therapeutic targets. Nat Rev Immunol 2017;17(7):407–20.
2. Wang M, Jiang L, Zhu B, et al. The prevalence, risk factors, and outcomes of sepsis in critically ill patients in China: a multicenter prospective cohort study. Front Med 2020;7:593808.
3. Fleischmann-Struzek C, Mellhammar L, Rose N, et al. Incidence and mortality of hospital- and ICU-treated sepsis: results from an updated and expanded systematic review and meta-analysis. Intensive Care Med 2020;46(8):1552–62.
4. Wang HE, Szychowski JM, Griffin R, et al. Long-term mortality after community-acquired sepsis: a longitudinal population-based cohort study. BMJ Open 2014; 4(1):e004283.
5. Rahmel T, Schmitz S, Nowak H, et al. Long-term mortality and outcome in hospital survivors of septic shock, sepsis, and severe infections: the importance of aftercare. PLoS One 2020;15(2):e0228952.
6. Catarina AV, Branchini G, Bettoni L, et al. Sepsis-associated encephalopathy: from pathophysiology to progress in experimental studies. Mol Neurobiol 2021;58(6):2770–9.
7. Sonneville R, Benghanem S, Jeantin L, et al. The spectrum of sepsis-associated encephalopathy: a clinical perspective. Crit Care 2023;27(1):386.
8. Sonneville R, de Montmollin E, Poujade J, et al. Potentially modifiable factors contributing to sepsis-associated encephalopathy. Intensive Care Med 2017; 43(8):1075–84.
9. Ely EW, Shintani A, Truman B, et al. Delirium as a predictor of mortality in mechanically ventilated patients in the intensive care unit. JAMA 2004;291(14): 1753–62.
10. Sonneville R, Verdonk F, Rauturier C, et al. Understanding brain dysfunction in sepsis. Ann Intensive Care 2013;3(1):15.
11. Fan TH, Premraj L, Roberts J, et al. In-Hospital neurologic complications, neuromonitoring, and long-term neurologic outcomes in patients with sepsis: a systematic review and meta-analysis. Crit Care Med 2024;52(3):452–63.
12. Iwashyna TJ, Ely EW, Smith DM, et al. Long-term cognitive impairment and functional disability among survivors of severe sepsis. JAMA 2010;304(16):1787–94.
13. Pandharipande PP, Girard TD, Jackson JC, et al. Long-term cognitive impairment after critical illness. N Engl J Med 2013;369(14):1306–16.
14. Li Y, Ji M, Yang J. Current understanding of long-term cognitive impairment after sepsis. Front Immunol 2022;13:855006.
15. Torres JSS, Tamayo-Giraldo FJ, Bejarano-Zuleta A, et al. Sepsis and post-sepsis syndrome: a multisystem challenge requiring comprehensive care and management-a review. Front Med 2025;12:1560737.
16. Sherman M, Lim P, Cheema T, et al. From resuscitation to rehabilitation: the post-intensive care syndrome continuum in sepsis care. J Clin Med 2025;14(23). https://doi.org/10.3390/jcm14238374.

17. Calsavara AJ, Costa PA, Nobre V, et al. Prevalence and risk factors for post-traumatic stress, anxiety, and depression in sepsis survivors after ICU discharge. Br J Psychiatry 2021;43(3):269–76.
18. Boede M, Gensichen JS, Jackson JC, et al. Trajectories of depression in sepsis survivors: an observational cohort study. Crit Care 2021;25(1):161.
19. Righy C, Rosa RG, da Silva RTA, et al. Prevalence of post-traumatic stress disorder symptoms in adult critical care survivors: a systematic review and meta-analysis. Crit Care 2019;23(1):213.
20. Dell'Oste V, Martelli M, Fantasia S, et al. Post-traumatic stress disorder in icu survivors: correlations with long-term psychiatric and physical outcomes. Int J Environ Res Public Health 2025;22(3). https://doi.org/10.3390/ijerph22030405.
21. Calsavara AJC, Nobre V, Barichello T, et al. Post-sepsis cognitive impairment and associated risk factors: a systematic review. Aust Crit Care 2018;31(4):242–53.
22. Sekino N, Selim M, Shehadah A. Sepsis-associated brain injury: underlying mechanisms and potential therapeutic strategies for acute and long-term cognitive impairments. J Neuroinflammation 2022;19(1):101.
23. Mazeraud A, Righy C, Bouchereau E, et al. Septic-associated encephalopathy: a comprehensive review. Neurotherapeutics 2020;17(2):392–403.
24. Lei S, Li X, Zhao H, et al. Risk of dementia or cognitive impairment in sepsis survivals: a systematic review and meta-analysis. Front Aging Neurosci 2022;14:839472.
25. Peters van Ton AM, Meijer-van Leijsen EMC, Bergkamp MI, et al. Risk of dementia and structural brain changes following nonneurological infections during 9-year follow-up. Crit Care Med 2022;50(4):554–64.
26. Fritze T, Doblhammer G, Widmann CN, et al. Time course of dementia following sepsis in German health claims data. Neurol Neuroimmunol Neuroinflamm 2021;8(1). https://doi.org/10.1212/nxi.0000000000000911.
27. Manabe T, Heneka MT. Cerebral dysfunctions caused by sepsis during ageing. Nat Rev Immunol 2022;22(7):444–58.
28. Jurcau MC, Jurcau A, Cristian A, et al. Inflammaging and brain aging. Int J Mol Sci 2024;25(19). https://doi.org/10.3390/ijms251910535.
29. O'Neil SM, Hans EE, Jiang S, et al. Astrocyte immunosenescence and deficits in interleukin 10 signaling in the aged brain disrupt the regulation of microglia following innate immune activation. Glia 2022;70(5):913–34.
30. Kox M, Bauer M, Bos LDJ, et al. The immunology of sepsis: translating new insights into clinical practice. Nat Rev Nephrol 2026;22(1):30–49.
31. Castellani G, Croese T, Peralta Ramos JM, et al. Transforming the understanding of brain immunity. Science 2023;380(6640):eabo7649.
32. Meneses G, Cardenas G, Espinosa A, et al. Sepsis: developing new alternatives to reduce neuroinflammation and attenuate brain injury. Ann N Y Acad Sci 2019;1437(1):43–56.
33. Li J, Jia Q, Yang L, et al. Sepsis-associated encephalopathy: mechanisms, diagnosis, and treatments update. Int J Biol Sci 2025;21(7):3214–28.
34. Barichello T, Generoso JS, Collodel A, et al. The blood-brain barrier dysfunction in sepsis. Tissue Barriers 2021;9(1):1840912.
35. Erikson K, Tuominen H, Vakkala M, et al. Brain tight junction protein expression in sepsis in an autopsy series. Crit Care 2020;24(1):385.
36. O'Carroll SJ, Kho DT, Wiltshire R, et al. Pro-inflammatory TNFalpha and IL-1beta differentially regulate the inflammatory phenotype of brain microvascular endothelial cells. J Neuroinflammation 2015;12:131.

37. Konnecke H, Bechmann I. The role of microglia and matrix metalloproteinases involvement in neuroinflammation and gliomas. Clin Dev Immunol 2013;2013: 914104.
38. Rustenhoven J, Kipnis J. Brain borders at the central stage of neuroimmunology. Nature 2022;612(7940):417–29.
39. Hu J, Xie S, Chen T, et al. Glial vascular unit as a bridge between blood-brain barrier and glymphatic system: roles in sepsis-associated encephalopathy. Neuroscience 2025;570:68–71.
40. Drieu A, Du S, Storck SE, et al. Parenchymal border macrophages regulate the flow dynamics of the cerebrospinal fluid. Nature 2022;611(7936):585–93.
41. Chen T, Hu J, Liao Y, et al. The brain washing system in sepsis-associated encephalopathy. J Neuroinflammation 2025;22(1):277.
42. Gu S, Li Y, Jiang Y, et al. Glymphatic dysfunction induced oxidative stress and neuro-inflammation in major depression disorders. Antioxidants 2022;11(11). https://doi.org/10.3390/antiox11112296.
43. Park L, Uekawa K, Garcia-Bonilla L, et al. Brain perivascular macrophages initiate the neurovascular dysfunction of alzheimer abeta peptides. Circ Res 2017;121(3):258–69.
44. Zhao T, Xia Y, Wang D, et al. Association between elevated serum tau protein level and sepsis-associated encephalopathy in patients with severe sepsis. Can J Infect Dis Med Microbiol 2019;2019:1876174.
45. Gasparotto J, Girardi CS, Somensi N, et al. Receptor for advanced glycation end products mediates sepsis-triggered amyloid-beta accumulation, Tau phosphorylation, and cognitive impairment. J Biol Chem 2018;293(1):226–44.
46. Ringstad G, Eide PK. Molecular trans-dural efflux to skull bone marrow in humans with CSF disorders. Brain 2022;145(4):1464–72.
47. Pinho-Correia LM, McCullough SJC, Ghanizada H, et al. CSF transport at the brain-meningeal border: effects on neurological health and disease. Lancet Neurol 2025;24(6):535–47.
48. Cugurra A, Mamuladze T, Rustenhoven J, et al. Skull and vertebral bone marrow are myeloid cell reservoirs for the meninges and CNS parenchyma. Science 2021;373(6553). https://doi.org/10.1126/science.abf7844.
49. Du Y, Li Y, Ye F, et al. Lactate exacerbates neuroinflammation in sepsis-associated encephalopathy via promoting neutrophil migration from skull bone marrow to the meninge. Exp Neurol 2025;391:115318.
50. Louveau A, Herz J, Alme MN, et al. CNS lymphatic drainage and neuroinflammation are regulated by meningeal lymphatic vasculature. Nat Neurosci 2018; 21(10):1380–91.
51. Wang Y, Chen D, Xu D, et al. Early developing B cells undergo negative selection by central nervous system-specific antigens in the meninges. Immunity 2021;54(12):2784–94.e6.
52. Schafflick D, Wolbert J, Heming M, et al. Single-cell profiling of CNS border compartment leukocytes reveals that B cells and their progenitors reside in non-diseased meninges. Nat Neurosci 2021;24(9):1225–34.
53. Shimada A, Hasegawa-Ishii S. Increased cytokine expression in the choroid plexus stroma and epithelium in response to endotoxin-induced systemic inflammation in mice. Toxicol Rep 2021;8:520–8.
54. Kunis G, Baruch K, Rosenzweig N, et al. IFN-gamma-dependent activation of the brain's choroid plexus for CNS immune surveillance and repair. Brain 2013;136(Pt 11):3427–40.

55. Schwerk C, Rybarczyk K, Essmann F, et al. TNFalpha induces choroid plexus epithelial cell barrier alterations by apoptotic and nonapoptotic mechanisms. J Biomed Biotechnol 2010;2010:307231.
56. Goldim MP, Danielski LG, Rodrigues JF, et al. Oxidative stress in the choroid plexus contributes to blood-cerebrospinal fluid barrier disruption during sepsis development. Microvasc Res 2019;123:19–24.
57. Peters van Ton AM, Verbeek MM, Alkema W, et al. Downregulation of synapse-associated protein expression and loss of homeostatic microglial control in cerebrospinal fluid of infectious patients with delirium and patients with Alzheimer's disease. Brain Behav Immun 2020;89:656–67.
58. Zrzavy T, Hoftberger R, Berger T, et al. Pro-inflammatory activation of microglia in the brain of patients with sepsis. Neuropathol Appl Neurobiol 2019;45(3):278–90.
59. Lemstra AW, Groen in't Woud JC, Hoozemans JJ, et al. Microglia activation in sepsis: a case-control study. J Neuroinflammation 2007;4:4.
60. Hu J, Xie S, Zhang H, et al. Microglial activation: key players in sepsis-associated encephalopathy. Brain Sci 2023;13(10). https://doi.org/10.3390/brainsci13101453.
61. Xu W, Huang Y, Zhou R. NLRP3 inflammasome in neuroinflammation and central nervous system diseases. Cell Mol Immunol 2025;22(4):341–55.
62. Chung HY, Wickel J, Hahn N, et al. Microglia mediate neurocognitive deficits by eliminating C1q-tagged synapses in sepsis-associated encephalopathy. Sci Adv 2023;9(21):eabq7806.
63. Paolicelli RC, Bolasco G, Pagani F, et al. Synaptic pruning by microglia is necessary for normal brain development. Science 2011;333(6048):1456–8.
64. Salter MW, Stevens B. Microglia emerge as central players in brain disease. Nat Med 2017;23(9):1018–27.
65. Danielski LG, Giustina AD, Gava FF, et al. The many faces of astrocytes in the septic brain. Mol Neurobiol 2022;59(12):7229–35.
66. Guo Q, Gobbo D, Zhao N, et al. Adenosine triggers early astrocyte reactivity that provokes microglial responses and drives the pathogenesis of sepsis-associated encephalopathy in mice. Nat Commun 2024;15(1):6340.
67. Zhang H, Jin Q, Li J, et al. Astrocyte-derived complement C3 facilitated microglial phagocytosis of synapses in Staphylococcus aureus-associated neurocognitive deficits. PLoS Pathog 2025;21(4):e1013126.
68. Schafflick D, Xu CA, Hartlehnert M, et al. Integrated single cell analysis of blood and cerebrospinal fluid leukocytes in multiple sclerosis. Nat Commun 2020;11(1):247.
69. van der Slikke EC, An AY, Hancock REW, et al. Exploring the pathophysiology of post-sepsis syndrome to identify therapeutic opportunities. EBioMedicine 2020;61:103044.
70. Mostel Z, Perl A, Marck M, et al. Post-sepsis syndrome - an evolving entity that afflicts survivors of sepsis. Mol Med 2019;26(1):6.
71. Kothur K, Wienholt L, Mohammad SS, et al. Utility of CSF cytokine/chemokines as markers of active intrathecal inflammation: comparison of demyelinating, anti-NMDAR and enteroviral encephalitis. PLoS One 2016;11(8):e0161656.
72. Lin X, Zhang J, Ren T, et al. Diagnostic utility of neurogenic biomarkers in differentiating sepsis with and without associated encephalopathy: a systematic review and meta-analytic approach. Front Neurol 2025;16:1640618.
73. Mao Y, Zhang A, Yang H, et al. Identification of IL-8 in CSF as a potential biomarker in sepsis-associated encephalopathy. Cytokine 2023;172:156390.

74. de Rooij SE, van Munster BC, Korevaar JC, et al. Cytokines and acute phase response in delirium. J Psychosom Res 2007;62(5):521–5.
75. Erikson K, Ala-Kokko TI, Koskenkari J, et al. Elevated serum S-100β in patients with septic shock is associated with delirium. Acta Anaesthesiol Scand 2019; 63(1):69–73.
76. Mosharaf MP, Alam K, Gow J, et al. Cytokines and inflammatory biomarkers and their association with post-operative delirium: a meta-analysis and systematic review. Sci Rep 2025;15(1):7830.
77. Lv XC, Lin Y, Wu QS, et al. Plasma interleukin-6 is a potential predictive biomarker for postoperative delirium among acute type a aortic dissection patients treated with open surgical repair. J Cardiothorac Surg 2021;16(1):146.
78. Kaźmierski J, Miler P, Pawlak A, et al. Elevated monocyte chemoattractant protein-1 as the independent risk factor of delirium after cardiac surgery. a prospective cohort study. J Clin Med 2021;10(8). https://doi.org/10.3390/jcm10081587.
79. Greene C, Connolly R, Brennan D, et al. Blood-brain barrier disruption and sustained systemic inflammation in individuals with long COVID-associated cognitive impairment. Nat Neurosci 2024;27(3):421–32.
80. Gryka-Marton M, Grabowska AD, Szukiewicz D. Breaking the barrier: the role of proinflammatory cytokines in BBB dysfunction. Int J Mol Sci 2025;26(8). https://doi.org/10.3390/ijms26083532.
81. Galea I. The blood-brain barrier in systemic infection and inflammation. Cell Mol Immunol 2021;18(11):2489–501.
82. Orhun G, Esen F, Yilmaz V, et al. Elevated sTREM2 and NFL levels in patients with sepsis associated encephalopathy. Int J Neurosci 2023;133(3):327–33.
83. Heneka MT, Gauthier S, Chandekar SA, et al. Neuroinflammatory fluid biomarkers in patients with Alzheimer's disease: a systematic literature review. Mol Psychiatry 2025;30(6):2783–98.
84. Lam AG, Koppal T, Akama KT, et al. Mechanism of glial activation by S100B: involvement of the transcription factor NFkappaB. Neurobiol Aging 2001; 22(5):765–72.
85. Duindam HB, Mengel D, Kox M, et al. Systemic inflammation relates to neuroaxonal damage associated with long-term cognitive dysfunction in COVID-19 patients. Brain Behav Immun 2024;117:510–20.
86. Porchietto E, Morello G, Cicilese G, et al. UCH-L1 in Alzheimer'S disease: a crucial player in dementia-associated mechanisms. Int J Mol Sci 2025;26(18). https://doi.org/10.3390/ijms26189012.
87. Koerbel K, Maiworm M, Schaller-Paule M, et al. Evaluating the utility of serum NfL, GFAP, UCHL1 and tTAU as estimates of CSF levels and diagnostic instrument in neuroinflammation and multiple sclerosis. Mult Scler Relat Disord 2024; 87:105644.
88. Benveniste H, Liu X, Koundal S, et al. The glymphatic system and waste clearance with brain aging: a review. Gerontology 2019;65(2):106–19.
89. Gigase FAJ, Smith E, Collins B, et al. The association between inflammatory markers in blood and cerebrospinal fluid: a systematic review and meta-analysis. Mol Psychiatry 2023;28(4):1502–15.
90. Gaetani L, Paolini Paoletti F, Bellomo G, et al. CSF and blood biomarkers in neuroinflammatory and neurodegenerative diseases: implications for treatment. Trends Pharmacol Sci 2020;41(12):1023–37.
91. Jeppesen R, Orlovska-Waast S, Sørensen NV, et al. Cerebrospinal fluid and blood biomarkers of neuroinflammation and blood-brain barrier in psychotic

disorders and individually matched healthy controls. Schizophr Bull 2022;48(6): 1206–16.

92. Rupprecht R, Wetzel CH, Dorostkar M, et al. Translocator protein (18kDa) TSPO: a new diagnostic or therapeutic target for stress-related disorders? Mol Psychiatry 2022;27(7):2918–26.
93. Peters van Ton AM, Duindam HB, van Tuijl J, et al. Neuroinflammation in cognitive decline post-cardiac surgery (the FOCUS study): an observational study protocol. BMJ Open 2021;11(5):e044062.
94. Peters van Ton AM, Leijte GP, Franssen GM, et al. Human in vivo neuroimaging to detect reprogramming of the cerebral immune response following repeated systemic inflammation. Brain Behav Immun 2021;95:321–9.
95. Mizrahi R, Rusjan PM, Kennedy J, et al. Translocator protein (18 kDa) polymorphism (rs6971) explains in-vivo brain binding affinity of the PET radioligand [(18)F]-FEPPA. J Cereb Blood Flow Metab 2012;32(6):968–72.
96. Lu X, Ji B, Huang G, et al. Advances in synaptic PET imaging and intervention with synapse-targeted small-molecular drugs for dementia diagnosis and therapy. Fundam Res 2025;5(1):63–71.
97. Cai Z, Li S, Matuskey D, et al. PET imaging of synaptic density: a new tool for investigation of neuropsychiatric diseases. Neurosci Lett 2019;691:44–50.
98. Takamori S, Holt M, Stenius K, et al. Molecular anatomy of a trafficking organelle. Cell 2006;127(4):831–46.
99. Mutch SA, Kensel-Hammes P, Gadd JC, et al. Protein quantification at the single vesicle level reveals that a subset of synaptic vesicle proteins are trafficked with high precision. J Neurosci 2011;31(4):1461–70.
100. Cai H, Mangner TJ, Muzik O, et al. Radiosynthesis of (11)C-levetiracetam: a potential marker for PET imaging of SV2A expression. ACS Med Chem Lett 2014; 5(10):1152–5.
101. Rashed HM, Shamma RN, El-Sabagh HA. Preparation of (99m)Tc-levetiracetam intranasal microemulsion as the first radiotracer for SPECT imaging of the synaptic vesicle protein SV2A. Eur J Pharm Sci 2018;121:29–33.
102. Zhang J, Wang J, Xu X, et al. In vivo synaptic density loss correlates with impaired functional and related structural connectivity in Alzheimer's disease. J Cereb Blood Flow Metab 2023;43(6):977–88.
103. Martin SL, Uribe C, Strafella AP. PET imaging of synaptic density in Parkinsonian disorders. J Neurosci Res 2024;102(3):e25253. https://doi.org/10.1002/jnr.25253.
104. Smart K, Uribe C, Desmond KL, et al. Preliminary assessment of reference region quantification and reduced scanning times for [(18)F]SynVesT-1 PET in Parkinson's disease. Mol Imaging 2023;2023:1855985.
105. Polito A, Eischwald F, Maho AL, et al. Pattern of brain injury in the acute setting of human septic shock. Crit Care 2013;17(5):R204.
106. Taheri S, Gasparovic C, Huisa BN, et al. Blood-brain barrier permeability abnormalities in vascular cognitive impairment. Stroke 2011;42(8):2158–63.
107. Putten MjAMv. Basics of the EEG. Dynamics of neural networks. Berlin: Springer-Verlag GmbH Germany; 2020. p. 129–52, chap 6.
108. Young GB, Bolton CF, Archibald YM, et al. The electroencephalogram in sepsis-associated encephalopathy. J Clin Neurophysiol 1992;9(1):145–52.

United States Postal Service

Statement of Ownership, Management and Circulation
(All Periodicals Publications Except Requester Publications)

1. Publication Title	2. Publication Number	3. Filing Date
CRITICAL CARE CLINICS	0 0 0 - 7 0 8	08/21/2026
4. Issue Frequency	**5. Number of Issues Published Annually**	**6. Annual Subscription Price**
JAN, APR, JUL, OCT	4	$297.00

7. Complete Mailing Address of Known Office of Publication (Not printer) (Street, city, county, state, and ZIP+4)
Addr 1: Elsevier INC
Addr 2: 230 Park Ave Ste 800
City, State ZIP: New York NY 10169

Contact Person: Mohana Priya Damodharan
Telephone: 91-44-4299-4077

8. Complete Mailing Address of Headquarters or General Business Office of Publisher (Not Printer)
Addr 1: Elsevier INC
Addr 2: 230 Park Ave Ste 800
City, State ZIP: New York NY 10169

9. Full Names and Complete Mailing Addresses of Publisher, Editor and Managing Editor (do not leave blank)

Publisher (Name and complete mailing address)
Name: Dolores Meloni, ELSEVIER INC.
Addr 1: 1600 JOHN F KENNEDY BLVD. SUITE 1600
Addr 2:
City, State ZIP: PHILADELPHIA, PA 19103-2899

Editor (Name and complete mailing address)
Name: Joanna Gascoine, ELSEVIER INC.
Addr 1: 1600 JOHN F KENNEDY BLVD. SUITE 1600
Addr 2:
City, State ZIP: PHILADELPHIA, PA 19103-2899

Managing Editor (Name and complete mailing address)
Name: PATRICK MANLEY, ELSEVIER INC.
Addr 1: 1600 JOHN F KENNEDY BLVD. SUITE 1600
Addr 2:
City, State ZIP: PHILADELPHIA, PA 19103-2899

10. Owner (Do not leave blank. If the publication is owned by a corporation, give the name and address of the corporation immediately followed by the names and addresses of all stockholders owning or holding 1 Percent or more of the total amount of stock. If not owned by a corporation, give the names and addresses of all the individual owners. If owned by a partnership or other unincorporated firm, give it's name and address as well as those of each individual owner. If the publication is published by a nonprofit organization, give it's name and address.)

Full Name	Complete Mailing Address
WHOLLY OWNED SUBSIDIARY OF REED/ELSEVIER,	1600 JOHN F KENNEDY BLVD. SUITE 1600
US HOLDINGS	PHILADELPHIA, PA 19103-2899

11. Known Bondholders, Mortgagees and Other Security Holders Owning or Holding 1 Percent or more of Total Amount of Bonds, Mortgages, or Other Securities. If none, check box → ☐ None

Full Name	Complete Mailing Address
NA	

12. Tax Status (For completion by nonprofit organizations authorized to mail at nonprofit rates) (Check one)
The purpose, function, and nonprofit status of this organization and the exempt status for federal income tax purposes:
[X] Has Not changed During Preceding 12 Months
[ ] Has Changed During Preceding 12 Months (Publisher must submit explanation of change with this statement below)

PS Form 3526, July 2014

13. Publication Title: CRITICAL CARE CLINICS

14. Issue Date for Circulation Data Below: October 2026

15. Extent and Nature of Circulation			Average No. Copies Each Issue During Preceding 12 Months	No. Copies of Single Issue Published Nearest to filing Date
a. Total Number of Copies (Net press run)			142	130
b. Paid and/or Requested Circulation	(1)	Mailed Outside-County Paid Subscriptions Stated on PS Form 3541 (Include paid distribution above nominal rate, advertiser's proof copies, and exchange copies)	81	74
	(2)	Mailed In-County Paid Subscriptions Stated on PS Form 3541 (Include paid distribution above nominal rate, advertiser's proof copies, and exchange copies)	0	0
	(3)	Paid Distribution Outside the Mails Including Sales Through Dealers and Carriers, Street Vendors, Counter Sales ,and Other Paid Distribution Ouside USPS	42	39
	(4)	Paid Distribution by Other Classes of Mail Through the USPS (e.g. First-Class Mail)	12	10
c. Total Paid Distribution [Sum of 15b. (1), (2), (3), and (4)] ▶			135	123
d. Free or Nominal Rate Distribution (By Mail and Outside the Mail)	(1)	Free or Nominal Rate Outside-County *Copies Included on PS Form 3541*	6	6
	(2)	Free or Nominal In-County Copies Included on PS Form 3541	0	0
	(3)	Free or Nominal Rate Copies Mailed at Other Classes Through the USPS (e.g. First-Class Mail)	0	0
	(4)	Free or Nominal Rate Distribution Outside the Mail *(Carriers or other means)*	1	1
e. Total Free or Nominal Rate Distribution (Sum of 15d. (1), (2), (3) and (4)) ▶			7	7
f. Total Distribution (Sum of 15c. and 15e.) ▶			142	130
g. Copies not Distributed (See Instructions to Publishers #4 (page #3))			0	0
h. Total (Sum of 15f. and g.) ▶			142	130
i. Percent Paid (15c. Divided by 15f. Times 100) ▶			95.07%	94.62%

* If you are claiming electronic copies, go to line 16 on page 3. If you are not claiming electronic copies, skip to line 17 on page 3.

16. Electronic copy Circulation		
If present, check box →		☐
a. Paid Electronic Copies		
b. Total Paid Print Copies (Line 15c) + Paid Electronic Copies (Line 16a) ▶	135	123
c. Total Print Distribution (Line 15F) + Paid Electronic Copies (Line 16a) ▶	142	130
d. Percentage Paid (Both Print & Electronic Copies (16b divided bt 16c x 100) ▶	95.07%	94.62%

[X] I certify that 50% of all my distribution copies (electronic and Print) are paid above a nominal price

17. Publication of Statement of Ownership
[X] Publication required. Will be printed in the **October 2026** issue of this publication. [ ] Publication not required

18. Signature and Title of Editor, Publisher, Business Manager, or Owner

	Title	Date
Mohana Priya Damodharan	**Distribution Controller**	8/21/2026

I certify that all information furnished on this form is true and complete. I understand that anyone who furnishes false or misleading information on this form or who omits material or information requested on the form may be subject to criminal sanctions (including fines and imprisonment) and/or civil sanctions (including civil penalties)

PS Form 3526, July 2014

9780443432804